Nutritional Deficiencies

Guest Editors

PRAVEEN S. GODAY, MBBS, CNSP
TIMOTHY S. SENTONGO, MD

PEDIATRIC CLINICS OF NORTH AMERICA

www.pediatric.theclinics.com

October 2009 • Volume 56 • Number 5

SAUNDERS an imprint of ELSEVIER, Inc.

W.B. SAUNDERS COMPANY
A Division of Elsevier Inc.

1600 John F. Kennedy Boulevard • Suite 1800 • Philadelphia, Pennsylvania 19103-2899

http://www.theclinics.com

THE PEDIATRIC CLINICS OF NORTH AMERICA Volume 56, Number 5
October 2009 ISSN 0031-3955, ISBN-13: 978-1-4377-1257-5, ISBN-10: 1-4377-1257-6

Editor: Carla Holloway
Developmental Editor: Theresa Collier

The Pediatric Clinics of North America (ISSN 0031-3955) is published bimonthly by Elsevier Inc., 360 Park Avenue South, New York, NY 10010-1710. Months of issue are February, April, June, August, October, and December. Periodicals postage paid at New York, NY and additional mailing offices. Subscription prices are $167.00 per year (US individuals), $378.00 per year (US institutions), $227.00 per year (Canadian individuals), $503.00 per year (Canadian institutions), $270.00 per year (international individuals), $503.00 per year (international institutions), $83.00 per year (US students and residents), and $142.00 per year (international and Canadian residents and students). To receive students/resident rare, orders must be accompanied by name of affiliated institution, date of term, and the signature of program/residency coordinator on institution letterhead. Orders will be billed at individual rate until proof of status is received. Foreign air speed delivery is included in all *Clinics* subscription prices. All prices are subject to change without notice. **POSTMASTER:** Send address changes to *The Pediatric Clinics of North America*, Elsevier Health Sciences Division, Subscription Customer Service, 3251 Riverport Lane, Maryland Heights, MO 63043. **Customer Service: 1-800-654-2452 (US and Canada). From outside of the US and Canada: 1-314-447-8871. Fax: 1-314-447-8029. For print support, e-mail: JournalsCustomerService-usa@elsevier.com. For online support, e-mail: JournalsOnlineSupport-usa@elsevier.com.**

Reprints. For copies of 100 or more, of articles in this publication, please contact the Commercial Reprints Department, Elsevier Inc., 360 Park Avenue South, New York, NY 10010-1710. Tel.: 212-633-3812; Fax: 212-462-1935; E-mail: reprints@elsevier.com.

The Pediatric Clinics of North America is also published in Spanish by McGraw-Hill Inter-americana Editores S.A., Mexico City, Mexico; in Portuguese by Riechmann and Affonso Editores, Rua Comandante Coelho 1085, CEP 21250, Rio de Janeiro, Brazil; and in Greek by Althayia SA, Athens, Greece.

The Pediatric Clinics of North America is covered in *MEDLINE/PubMed (Index Medicus), Excerpta Medica, Current Contents, Current Contents/Clinical Medicine, Science Citation Index, ASCA, ISI/BIOMED,* and *BIOSIS*.

Printed and bound by CPI Group (UK) Ltd, Croydon, CR0 4YY

Transferred to Digital Print 2011

GOAL STATEMENT

The goal of the *Pediatric Clinics of North America* is to keep practicing physicians and residents up to date with current clinical practice in pediatrics by providing timely articles reviewing the state-of-the-art in patient care.

ACCREDITATION

The *Pediatric Clinics of North America* is planned and implemented in accordance with the Essential Areas and Policies of the Accreditation Council for Continuing Medical Education (ACCME) through the joint sponsorship of the University Of Virginia School Of Medicine and Elsevier. The University Of Virginia School of Medicine is accredited by the ACCME to provide continuing medical education for physicians.

The University of Virginia School of Medicine designates this educational activity for a maximum of 15 *AMA PRA Category 1 Credits*™ for each issue, 90 credits per year. Physicians should only claim credit commensurate with the extent of their participation in the activity.

The American Medical Association has determined that physicians not licensed in the US who participate in this CME activity are eligible for a maximum of 15 *AMA PRA Category 1 Credits*™ for each issue, 90 credits per year.

Credit can be earned by reading the text material, taking the CME examination online at http://www.theclinics.com/home/cme, and completing the evaluation. After taking the test, you will be required to review any and all incorrect answers. Following completion of the test and evaluation, your credit will be awarded and you may print your certificate.

FACULTY DISCLOSURE/CONFLICT OF INTEREST

The University of Virginia School of Medicine, as an ACCME accredited provider, endorses and strives to comply with the Accreditation Council for Continuing Medical Education (ACCME) Standards of Commercial Support, Commonwealth of Virginia statutes, University of Virginia policies and procedures, and associated federal and private regulations and guidelines on the need for disclosure and monitoring of proprietary and financial interests that may affect the scientific integrity and balance of content delivered in continuing medical education activities under our auspices.

The University of Virginia School of Medicine requires that all CME activities accredited through this institution be developed independently and be scientifically rigorous, balanced and objective in the presentation/discussion of its content, theories and practices.

All authors/editors participating in an accredited CME activity are expected to disclose to the readers relevant financial relationships with commercial entities occurring within the past 12 months (such as grants or research support, employee, consultant, stock holder, member of speakers bureau, etc.). The University of Virginia School of Medicine will employ appropriate mechanisms to resolve potential conflicts of interest to maintain the standards of fair and balanced education to the reader. Questions about specific strategies can be directed to the Office of Continuing Medical Education, University of Virginia School of Medicine, Charlottesville, Virginia.

The faculty and staff of the University of Virginia Office of Continuing Medical Education have no financial affiliations to disclose.

The authors/editors listed below have identified no financial or professional relationships for themselves or their spouse/partner:

Elaine Danner, RD, CD, CNSD; Christopher P. Duggan, MD, MPH; Looi C. Ee, MBBS, FRACP; Lina M. Felípez, MD; Judy Fuentebella, MD; Praveen S. Goday, MBBS, CNSP (Guest Editor); Zubin Grover, MBBS, MD; Maria D. Hanna, MS, RD, LDN; Carla Holloway (Acquisitions Editor); John A. Kerner, MD; Midge Kirby, MS, RD, CD, CSP; Asim Maqbool, MD; Maria Mascarenhas, MBBS; Nilesh M. Mehta, MD; Suzanne H. Michel, MPH, RD, LDN; Charmaine H. Mziray-Andrew, MD; Vicky Loo Ng, MD, FRCP; Scott Nightingale, BMed (Hons), FRACP; Karen Rheuban, MD (Test Author); Timothy S. Sentongo, MD (Guest Editor); Malika D. Shah, MD, FAAP; Shilpa R. Shah, MBBS, MD, MRCPCH; David L. Suskind, MD; and, Stavra A. Xanthakos, MD, MS.

Disclosure of Discussion of Non-FDA Approved Uses for Pharmaceutical Products and/or Medical Devices

The University of Virginia School of Medicine, as an ACCME provider, requires that all faculty presenters identify and disclose any off-label uses for pharmaceutical and medical device products. The University of Virginia School of Medicine recommends that each physician fully review all the available data on new products or procedures prior to clinical use.

TO ENROLL

To enroll in the Pediatric Clinics of North America Continuing Medical Education program, call customer service at 1-800-654-2452 or visit us online at www.theclinics.com/home/cme. The CME program is available to subscribers for an additional fee of $195.00

Contributors

GUEST EDITORS

PRAVEEN S. GODAY, MBBS, CNSP
Associate Professor, Pediatric Gastroenterlogy and Nutrition, Medical College
of Wisconsin, Milwaukee, Wisconsin

TIMOTHY S. SENTONGO, MD
Assistant Professor of Pediatrics, Director, Pediatric Nutrition Support,
Pediatric Gastroenterology, Hepatology and Nutrition, The University of Chicago Medical
Center, Chicago, Illinois

AUTHORS

ELAINE DANNER, RD, CD, CNSD
Pediatric Dietitian, Clinical Nutrition Lead, Children's Hospital of Wisconsin, Milwaukee,
Wisconsin

CHRISTOPHER P. DUGGAN, MD, MPH
Director, Clinical Nutrition Service; Associate Professor of Pediatrics, Division of
Gastroenterology/Nutrition, Children's Hospital, Harvard Medical School, Boston,
Massachusetts

LOOI C. EE, MBBS, FRACP
Senior Staff Specialist, Queensland Paediatric Gastroenterology, Hepatology & Nutrition
Services, Department of Gastroenterology, Royal Children's Hospital, Brisbane,
Queensland, Australia

LINA FELÍPEZ, MD
Department of Pediatrics, Section of Pediatric Gastroenterology and Nutrition, University
of Chicago, Chicago, Illinois

JUDY FUENTEBELLA, MD
Fellow, Division of Pediatric Gastroenterology, Hepatology, and Nutrition, Lucile Packard
Children's Hospital, Stanford University Medical Center, Palo Alto, California

ZUBIN GROVER, MBBS, MD
Fellow, Queensland Paediatric Gastroenterology, Hepatology & Nutrition Services,
Department of Gastroenterology, Royal Children's Hospital, Brisbane, Queensland,
Australia

MARIA D. HANNA, MS, RD, LDN
Department of Clinical Nutrition, The Children's Hospital of Philadelphia, Philadelphia,
Pennsylvania

JOHN A. KERNER, MD
Professor of Pediatrics, Medical Director of the Nutrition Support Team and the Children's
Home Pharmacy, Division of Pediatric Gastroenterology, Hepatology, and Nutrition, Lucile
Packard Children's Hospital, Stanford University Medical Center, Palo Alto, California

MIDGE KIRBY, MS, RD, CD, CSP
Pediatric Dietitian, Clinical Nutrition Lead, Children's Hospital of Wisconsin, Milwaukee, Wisconsin

MARIA MASCARENHAS, MBBS
Associate Professor of Pediatrics, Division of Gastroenterology, Hepatology, and Nutrition, The Children's Hospital of Philadelphia, University of Pennsylvania School of Medicine, Philadelphia, Pennsylvania

ASIM MAQBOOL, MD
Assistant Professor of Pediatrics, Division of Gastroenterology, Hepatology, and Nutrition, The Children's Hospital of Philadelphia, University of Pennsylvania School of Medicine, Philadelphia, Pennsylvania

NILESH M. MEHTA, MD
Faculty in Division of Critical Care Medicine, Instructor in Anesthesia/Critical Care, Children's Hospital, Harvard Medical School, Boston, Massachusetts

SUZANNE H. MICHEL, MPH, RD, LDN
Department of Clinical Nutrition, The Children's Hospital of Philadelphia, Philadelphia, Pennsylvania

CHARMAINE H. MZIRAY-ANDREW, MD
Fellow, Pediatric Gastroenterology, Hepatology and Nutrition, University of Chicago, Chicago, Illinois

VICKY LEE NG, MD, FRCP
SickKids Transplant Center and Division of Gastroenterology, Hepatology, and Nutrition, The Hospital for Sick Children, Toronto, Ontario, Canada; Department of Pediatrics, University of Toronto, Ontario, Canada

SCOTT NIGHTINGALE, BMed (Hons), FRACP
SickKids Transplant Center and Division of Gastroenterology, Hepatology, and Nutrition, The Hospital for Sick Children, Toronto, Ontario, Canada

TIMOTHY A. SENTONGO, MD
Assistant Professor of Pediatrics, Director of Pediatric Nutrition Support, Pediatric Gastroenterology, Hepatology and Nutrition, University of Chicago, Chicago, Illinois

MALIKA D. SHAH, MD, FAAP
Assistant Professor of Pediatrics and Attending Physician, Northwestern University Feinberg School of Medicine, Chicago, Illinois

SHILPA R. SHAH, MBBS, MD, MRCPCH
Pediatric Registrar, Royal Belfast Hospital for Sick Children, Belfast, Northern Ireland, United Kingdom

DAVID L. SUSKIND, MD
Associate Professor, Department of Pediatrics, Division of Pediatric Gastroenterology Hepatology and Nutrition, Seattle Children's Hospital, University of Washington, Seattle, Washington

STAVRA A. XANTHAKOS, MD, MS
Assistant Professor, Division of Gastroenterology, Hepatology and Nutrition; Medical Director, Surgical Weight Loss Program for Teens, Cincinnati Children's Hospital Medical Center, Cincinnati, Ohio

Contents

Nutritional deficiencies have always been a major consideration in pediatrics. Although the classic forms of many of the well-documented nutritional deficiencies are memorized during training as a physician, nutritional deficiencies that can occur in otherwise asymptomatic normally growing children are often overlooked. The two most common deficiencies seen in children who are growing normally are iron and vitamin D deficiencies. These deficiencies are surprisingly common and can have a significant impact on the overall health of a child. This article reviews these nutritional deficiencies and other less commonly seen deficiencies in children who are otherwise growing normally.

Protein energy malnutrition (PEM) is a common problem worldwide and occurs in both developing and industrialized nations. In the developing world, it is frequently a result of socioeconomic, political, or environmental factors. In contrast, protein energy malnutrition in the developed world usually occurs in the context of chronic disease. There remains much variation in the criteria used to define malnutrition, with each method having its own limitations. Early recognition, prompt management, and robust follow up are critical for best outcomes in preventing and treating PEM.

Premature infants are a population prone to nutrient deficiencies. Because the early diet of these infants is entirely amenable to intervention, understanding the pathophysiology behind these deficiencies is important for both the neonatologists who care for them acutely and for pediatricians who are responsible for their care through childhood. This article reviews the normal accretion of nutrients in the fetus, discusses specific nutrient deficiencies that are exacerbated in the postnatal period, and identifies key areas for future research.

Pediatric nutritional deficiencies are associated not only with poverty and developing countries, but also in children in the developed world who adhere to restricted diets. At times, these diets are medically necessary, such as the gluten-free diet for management of celiac disease or exclusion diets in children with food allergies. At other times, the diets are self-selected by children with behavioral disorders, or parent-selected because of nutrition misinformation, cultural preferences, alternative nutrition therapies, or misconceptions regarding food tolerance. Health care providers must be vigilant in monitoring both growth and feeding patterns to identify inappropriate dietary changes that may result in nutritional deficiencies.

Stavra A. Xanthakos

The presence of nutritional deficiencies in overweight and obesity may seem paradoxical in light of excess caloric intake, but several micronutrient deficiencies appear to be higher in prevalence in overweight and obese adults and children. Causes are multifactorial and include decreased consumption of fruits and vegetables, increased intake of high-calorie, but nutritionally poor-quality foods, and increased adiposity, which may influence the storage and availability of some nutrients. As the obesity epidemic continues unabated and the popularity of bariatric surgery rises for severely obese adults and adolescents, medical practitioners must be aware of pre-existing nutritional deficiencies in overweight and obese patients and appropriately recognize and treat common and rare nutritional deficiencies that may arise or worsen following bariatric surgery. This article reviews current knowledge of nutritional deficits in obese and overweight individuals and those that commonly present after bariatric surgery and summarizes current recommendations for screening and supplementation.

Suzanne H. Michel, Asim Maqbool, Maria D. Hanna,
and Maria Mascarenhas

Since the identification of cystic fibrosis (CF) in the 1940s, nutrition care of patients who have CF has been a challenge. Through optimal caloric intake and careful management of malabsorption, patients are expected to meet genetic potential for growth. Yet factors beyond malabsorption, including nutrient activity at the cellular level, may influence growth and health. This article reviews nutrition topics frequently discussed in relationship to CF and presents intriguing new information describing nutrients currently being studied for their impact on overall health of patients who have CF.

Nilesh M. Mehta and Christopher P. Duggan

A significant proportion of critically ill children admitted to the pediatric intensive care unit (PICU) present with nutritional deficiencies. Malnourished hospitalized patients have a higher rate of complications, increased mortality, longer length of hospital stay, and increased hospital costs. Critical illness may further contribute to nutritional deteriorate with poor outcomes. Younger age, longer duration of PICU stay, congenital heart disease, burn injury, and need for mechanical ventilation support are some of the factors that are associated with worse nutritional deficiencies. Failure to estimate energy requirements accurately, barriers to bedside delivery of nutrients, and reluctance to perform regular nutritional assessments are responsible for the persistence and delayed detection of malnutrition in this cohort.

Malnutrition is common in infants and children with chronic liver disease (CLD) and may easily be underestimated by clinical appearance alone. The cause of malnutrition in CLD is multifactorial, although insufficient dietary intake is probably the most important factor and is correctable. Fat malabsorption occurs in cholestatic disorders, and one must also consider any accompanying fat-soluble vitamin and essential fatty acid deficiencies. The clinician should proactively evaluate, treat, and re-evaluate response to treatment of nutritional deficiencies. Because a better nutritional state is associated with better survival before and after liver transplantation, aggressive nutritional management is an important part of the care of these children.

Intestinal failure (IF) is the ultimate malabsorption state, with multiple causes, requiring long-term therapy with enteral or intravenous fluids and nutrient supplements. The primary goal during management of children with potentially reversible IF is to promote intestinal autonomy while supporting normal growth, nutrient status, and preventing complications from parenteral nutrition therapy. This article presents how an improved understanding of digestive pathophysiology is essential for diagnosis, successful management, and prevention of nutrient deficiencies in children with IF.

Refeeding syndrome (RFS) is the result of aggressive enteral or parenteral feeding in a malnourished patient, with hypophosphatemia being the hallmark of this phenomenon. Other metabolic abnormalities, such as hypokalemia and hypomagnesemia, may also occur, along with sodium and fluid retention. The metabolic changes that occur in RFS can be severe enough to cause cardiorespiratory failure and death. This article reviews the pathophysiology, the clinical manifestations, and the management of RFS. The key to prevention is identifying patients at risk and being aware of the potential complications involved in rapidly reintroducing feeds to a malnourished patient.

> Good clinical care extends beyond mere diagnosis and treatment of disease to appreciation that nutrient deficiencies can be the price of effective drug therapy. The major risk factors for developing drug-induced nutrient deficiencies are lack of awareness by the prescribing physician and long duration of drug therapy. The field of pharmacogenomics has potential to improve clinical care by detecting patients at risk for complications from drug therapy. Further improvements in patient safety rely on physicians voluntarily reporting serious suspected adverse drug reactions.

Preface

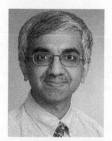 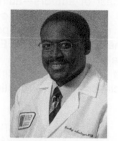

Praveen S. Goday, MBBS, CNSP   Timothy S. Sentongo, MD
Guest Editors

We are honored to edit this issue on "Nutritional Deficiencies" in the *Pediatric Clinics of North America*. The last issue of *Pediatric Clinics of North America* addressing nutritional problems was published 7 years ago. We have highlighted a spectrum of nutritional deficiencies ranging from those occurring despite normal health to those associated with a variety of disease states. Our aim is to provide pediatric practitioners and trainees across the globe with a comprehensive and practical clinical review that links pathophysiology with clinical manifestations and management strategies.

The first part of this issue discusses nutrient deficiencies associated with growth in normal children, premature infants, children with protein-energy malnutrition, children on restricted diets, and adolescents who have undergone bariatric surgery. Despite increased knowledge about growth and nutrient requirements, protein-energy malnutrition and nutrient deficiencies remain globally pervasive problems. Preventable childhood illness and decreased access to food due to geopolitical factors are the main causes of malnutrition in less-developed countries. In contrast, chronic disease and excess calories are major risk factors for malnutrition in more-developed countries. The forced maldigestion and malabsorption of nutrients induced by bariatric surgery have been responsible for the re-emergence of nutrient deficiencies previously consigned to textbooks. Restricted diets used during therapy for food allergies and intolerances, and, sometimes, empirically in children with autism are also associated with increased risk for nutrient deficiencies.

Nutrient deficiencies may manifest differently based on disease and medical therapy; therefore, the second part of this issue discusses pathophysiology, diagnosis, and management of nutrient deficiencies encountered in critically ill children and chronic disease states, including cystic fibrosis, chronic liver disease, and intestinal failure. These are representative conditions that have a unique impact on nutrient intake, digestion, absorption, and use. We have also included a sobering reminder that regardless of the cause of malnutrition, nutritional intervention should proceed cautiously because of risk of precipitating refeeding syndrome. Finally, this issue is rounded off by a discussion about the nutritional implications of drug therapy and an

Pediatr Clin N Am 56 (2009) xiii–xiv
doi:10.1016/j.pcl.2009.09.001
0031-3955/09/$ – see front matter © 2009 Elsevier Inc. All rights reserved.

introduction to the role of pharmacogenomics in avoidance of adverse drug-nutrient interactions.

We are proud of a global cast of authors—authors from the United Kingdom, Canada, and Australia joined authors from all over the United States in this venture—whose contributions made this issue possible. We also thank Carla Holloway, Peggy Ennis, and the editorial team at Elsevier for their invaluable help in assembling this issue. Finally, we would like to dedicate this issue to our families—Thangam, Arvind, and Tara Goday and Mirika, David, Samuel, and Joanna Sentongo—and extend appreciation for their continued love, understanding, and support.

Praveen S. Goday, MBBS, CNSP
Pediatric Gastroenterology and Nutrition
Medical College of Wisconsin
8701 Watertown Plank Road
Milwaukee, WI 53226

Timothy S. Sentongo, MD
Hepatology & Nutrition
The University of Chicago Medical Center
5839 South Maryland Avenue, MC 4065 WP C-474
Chicago, IL 60637

E-mail addresses:
pgoday@mcw.edu (P.S. Goday)
tsentong@peds.bsd.uchicago.edu (T.S. Sentongo)

Nutritional Deficiencies During Normal Growth

David L. Suskind, MD

KEYWORDS

- Growth • Pediatric mineral • Vitamin deficiency
- Micronutrient deficiency development • Pediatric
- Iron deficiency • Vitamin D deficiency

Nutritional deficiencies have always been a major consideration in pediatrics. Although the classic forms of many of the well-documented nutritional deficiencies are memorized during training as a physician, nutritional deficiencies that can occur in otherwise asymptomatic normally growing children are often overlooked. The two most common deficiencies seen in children who are growing normally are iron and vitamin D deficiencies. These deficiencies are surprisingly common and can have a significant impact on the overall health of a child. This article reviews these nutritional deficiencies and other less commonly seen deficiencies in children who are otherwise growing normally.

IRON DEFICIENCY

Iron deficiency (ID) is the most common nutritional deficiency in children. The usual presentation of ID anemia is an otherwise asymptomatic, well-nourished infant with a mild-to-moderate microcytic, hypochromic anemia. In some developing countries, up to 50% of preschool children and pregnant mothers have ID anemia (IDA).[1]

Although the prevalence of ID among 1-year-old infants in the United States has declined as a result of improved iron supplementation during the first year of life,[2,3] the rate of ID in older children and toddlers has remained relatively unchanged over the last 4 decades. National Health and Nutrition Examination Surveys (NHANES) II and IV revealed that 8% of children aged 12 to 36 months between 1999 and 2002 were iron deficient.[4] ID is higher among children living at or below the poverty level, among premature and low-birth-weight infants, among black and Hispanic toddlers, and among infants fed only non-iron fortified formulas.[4–6] Other risk factors for

Department of Pediatrics, Division of Pediatric Gastroenterology Hepatology and Nutrition, Seattle Children's Hospital, University of Washington, 4800 Sand Point Way NE, Seattle, WA 98105, USA
E-mail address: david.suskind@seattlechildrens.org

Pediatr Clin N Am 56 (2009) 1035–1053
doi:10.1016/j.pcl.2009.07.004
0031-3955/09/$ – see front matter © 2009 Elsevier Inc. All rights reserved.

developing IDA in children 1 to 3 years of age include obesity, being of Hispanic origin, and not attending day care.[4] Immigrant populations are also at higher risk for IDA.[7]

Infants born to mothers with ID or who are breast-fed by iron-deficient mothers are also at risk. A decreased hemoglobin concentration at birth directly affects nonstorage iron and increases the risk of IDA during the first 3 to 6 months of life. Prematurity, fetal-maternal hemorrhage, twin-twin transfusion syndrome and insufficient dietary intake can all lead to the early development of IDA.

Dietary issues contribute significantly to the evolution of ID anemia in infancy and early childhood. Common factors leading to IDA include insufficient iron intake or poor dietary sources of iron (eg, vegetarian/vegan diet), early introduction of whole cow's milk,[8–10] occult blood loss secondary to cow's milk intolerance, medications (eg, nonsteroidal antiinflammatory drugs), and malabsorptive states.[11]

The early introduction of whole cow's milk in infants increases intestinal blood loss. In one study, infants 5 to 6 months of age consuming cow's milk had a higher rate of heme-positive stools (up to 30%) during the first 28 days, whereas only 5% of infants maintained on formula had heme-positive stools.[12] There is also an increased risk of ID with continued bottle-feeding compared with cup feeding in the second and third year of life, most likely also because of greater consumption of cow's milk.[13]

ID in industrialized countries presents most commonly as a mild-to-moderate microcytic, hypochromic anemia in an asymptomatic, well-nourished infant. Uncommon but also reported are infants with severe anemia who present with pallor, lethargy, irritability, poor feeding, and cardiomegaly. Although typically presenting as a nutritional anemia, IDA may present secondary to other diseases including celiac disease,[14] *Helicobacter pylori* infections,[15] and the anemia of chronic disease.

Pica (the craving for substances largely non-nutritive such as clay or paper products) and pagophagia (craving for ice) are common features associated with ID. It may be present in children who are not anemic and will respond rapidly to treatment with iron, often before any increase is noted in the hemoglobin concentration.[16]

Despite several well-documented studies, there is still debate about the effect of ID on the neurodevelopment of infants and children. Impaired psychomotor or mental development has been described in iron-deficient infants and cognitive impairment has been noted in iron-deficient adolescents.[17,18] ID may also negatively affect the infant's social-emotional behavior.[19,20] It may be a risk factor for children with attention-deficit/hyperactivity disorder.[21,22] Decreased iron, even in the absence of anemia, is associated with decreased exercise performance in laboratory animals and children, particularly in adolescent athletes. ID has been associated with altered immunity and with cerebral vein thrombosis in children.[23]

Diagnosing ID in a healthy-appearing infant/child can be challenging. Analysis of the NHANES III database demonstrated that anemia (hemoglobin level <11 g/dL) is neither a sensitive nor a specific screen for ID.[24] Only one-third of iron-deficient children have evidence of IDA. A careful dietary history is an important screening tool in determining whether a child is iron deficient.[25] Dietary ID can be suspected from one or more of the following: less than five servings each of meat, grains, vegetables, and fruit per week; more than 480 mL of milk per day; or daily intake of fatty snacks, sweets, or more than 480 mL of soft drinks. Other studies have not shown dietary history to be useful.[26]

For infants/children presenting with a mild microcytic, hypochromic anemia with a presumptive diagnosis of ID anemia, the most cost-effective strategy is a therapeutic trial of iron.[27] Several laboratory tests can be helpful in confirming the diagnosis of ID anemia. Although an elevated red cell distribution width is the earliest hematologic manifestation of ID,[27] ID in infants and young children is usually identified by a serum ferritin concentration of less than 12 ng/mL. IDA is diagnosed by a low hemoglobin concentration in conjunction with a low serum ferritin. The major drawback with using serum ferritin as an indicator of ID is that ferritin is an acute phase reactant, with serum levels increasing with inflammatory and infectious processes.[28] A more complete evaluation for IDA would also include a serum iron, total iron-binding capacity, and transferrin saturation. Other laboratory tests, although not routinely used, such as erythrocyte protoporphyrin, serum transferrin receptor, and reticulocyte hemoglobin content, may prove useful tools for measuring ID.[29,30]

Once the diagnosis of ID anemia is established, every child should have a careful dietary history, be screened for lead poisoning and have three separate stools screened for occult blood. Among older children and adolescents with moderate-to-severe IDA, more detailed investigations for gastrointestinal blood loss should be considered unless the menstrual history in an adolescent girl is thought to be the cause of the deficiency.

For infants with confirmed IDA, ferrous sulfate (3–4 mg/kg of elemental iron, in divided doses, between meals with a citrus juice) is the standard of care.[27] Ferrous sulfate at 3 mg/kg should produce an increase of greater than 1 g/dL per week in patients with ID. Iron absorption is increased if the ferrous sulfate is given with juice rather than milk. Iron should be continued in responders for 2 to 3 months after normalization of hemoglobin values to replace iron stores. If the patient fails to respond after 4 weeks of therapy, a review of the patient's history should take place for medication dosing and administration errors, appropriate dietary modifications, or history of a recent illness. Other laboratory studies, including a serum ferritin level, should be obtained to evaluate the anemia further and to rule out conditions simulating (ie, thalassemias and the anemia of chronic disease) or complicating (eg, concomitant vitamin B_{12} or folic acid deficiency) ID anemia. Close follow-up should occur after appropriate treatment to ensure the patient's response to iron therapy.

VITAMIN D DEFICIENCY

Vitamin D is a prohormone that is essential for the normal absorption of calcium in the gastrointestinal tract. Deficiency in vitamin D leads to hypocalcemia and hypophosphatemia with resultant rickets in children and osteomalacia in adults. In adults, vitamin D deficiency has been linked to cardiovascular disease, insulin resistance, and hypertension.

In addition to a number of large case studies, NHANES III has emphasized the high prevalence of vitamin D deficiency in industrialized nations, with up to 14% in the United States.[31,32] In NHANES III, children aged 1 to 5 years had the highest mean serum vitamin D concentrations followed by children aged 6 to 11 years, with adolescents having the lowest mean vitamin D levels. The resurgence of vitamin D deficiency is likely a result of several dietary and environmental factors, including body mass index, milk ingestion, and sun exposure.[33] In nonindustrialized nations vitamin D deficiency remains a major public health problem.

Vitamin D deficiency causes nutritional rickets. The primary abnormality may be dietary deficiency or decreased vitamin D activity, which leads to a decrease in intestinal absorption of calcium. Although the majority of pediatric patients with low vitamin D level are asymptomatic, some may develop secondary hyperparathyroidism and characteristic changes in the growth plates and metaphyseal bones.

Rickets due to vitamin D deficiency has three stages of increasing severity.[34] Stage one arises from impaired intestinal calcium absorption, resulting in hypocalcemia.

Hyperaminoaciduria and hyperphosphaturia are absent and serum inorganic phosphorus is normal. Hypophosphatemia develops in stages two and three. Serum calcium is normal in stage two, but low in stage three, when the clinical and radiological findings of rickets are most striking. Serum parathyroid hormone concentrations are elevated in all three stages.

The vitamin D status of an infant depends upon the amount of vitamin D transferred from the mother prenatally and on the amount of vitamin D ingested or produced by the skin during exposure to ultraviolet light postnatally.[35] Maternal-fetal transfer of vitamin D is mostly in the form of calcidiol (25-OH vitamin D), which readily crosses the placenta.[35] The half-life of calcidiol is approximately 3 to 4 weeks.[36] Thus, the serum concentration of vitamin D falls rapidly after birth unless additional sources are available.

In North America, infant formula, cow's milk, and cereals are fortified with vitamin D. All infant formulas in the United States contain at least 400 IU/L of vitamin D. Nonetheless, the diet of most breast-fed infants and many formula-fed infants does not provide the recommended intake of vitamin D. Vitamin D deficiency rickets commonly presents between 3 months and 3 years of age, when growth rates (and calcium needs) are high, and exposure to sunlight may be limited.[37–39] The main reasons for inadequate vitamin D supply in infants from Western countries are prolonged breast-feeding without vitamin D supplementation, and concomitant avoidance of sun exposure.[39,40] The recommended intake of vitamin D to prevent deficiency in normal infants and young children is 200 to 400 IU/day.[41] Human milk typically contains less than 25 IU of vitamin D per liter.[42] Dark skin is an additional risk factor for developing rickets in breast-fed infants as dark-skinned individuals produce less vitamin D in response to sunlight.[39] The vitamin D concentration of the breast milk of dark-skinned mothers is less than that of lighter-skinned individuals.[43] In high-risk populations, most mothers of breast-fed infants with rickets are deficient in vitamin D. Consequently, all at-risk mothers should be evaluated for vitamin D deficiency.[38]

Other causes of vitamin D deficiency caused by diminished absorption are gastrectomy, celiac disease, malabsorption, extensive bowel surgery, inflammatory bowel disease, and advanced cystic fibrosis.

Although vitamin D deficiency is often asymptomatic, skeletal findings can occur with advanced disease. The classic findings of advanced rickets include delay in the closure of the fontanels, frontal bossing, craniotabes (soft skull bones), enlargement of the costochondral junction visible as beading along the anterolateral aspects of the chest (the "rachitic rosary"), Harrison groove caused by the muscular pull of the diaphragm on the "softened" lower ribs, enlargement of the wrist, bowing of the distal radius and ulna, and progressive lateral bowing of the femur and tibia.

The most widely used treatment for vitamin D deficiency is vitamin D_2 (ergocalciferol). Infants younger than 1 month with vitamin D deficient rickets should receive 1000 IU daily, infants aged 1 to 12 months should receive between 1000 and 5000 IU daily, and children older than 1 year should receive 5000 IU daily. Treatment is continued at these doses until radiographic evidence of healing is observed. The dose of vitamin D is then reduced to 400 IU daily. Radiographic evidence of healing usually occurs after 3 months of treatment.[41] Calcium intake should be maintained at approximately 1000 mg per day to avoid the so-called hungry bone syndrome (worsening hypocalcemia after the start of vitamin D therapy). This is usually accomplished by administering supplements of 30 to 75 mg/kg of elemental calcium per day in three divided doses.[41]

Nutritional management should lead to resolution of biochemical and radiological abnormalities within 3 months. A key signal that this is occurring is the increase in urinary calcium excretion. If after appropriate nutritional treatment for 3 months the patient still has no detectable urinary calcium, continuation of the same treatment regimen for an additional 3 months is recommended. Serum calcium, phosphorus, alkaline phosphatase, and urinary calcium/creatinine ratio should be measured 4 weeks after the initiation of therapy in children who are being treated for vitamin D deficiency. These studies should be repeated after 3 months of therapy, at which point radiographs should be obtained to document healing of rachitic lesions.

An alternative treatment protocol is the so-called stosstherapy, which consists of a high dose of oral vitamin D (600,000 IU) given on a single day.[44] This amount of vitamin D approximately corresponds to a 3-month course of 5000 IU per day and should be sufficient to induce healing within 3 months. Stosstherapy may be advantageous when compliance with therapy or follow-up is a problem.[45] However, such high doses of vitamin D can lead to hypercalcemia. Doses of 150,000 or 300,000 IU appear to be equally effective, but with less risk of hypercalcemia.[46]

CALCIUM DEFICIENCY

Nutritional rickets remains prevalent in many parts of the world. Because ample sunlight exists in many of the countries where the incidence of rickets is high, researchers have suggested that insufficient calcium intake rather than primary vitamin D deficiency may be the main causative factor.[47] Most of the children in these studies had normal serum 25-OH vitamin D concentrations and high serum 1,25-OH_2 vitamin D concentrations, indicating adequate intake of vitamin D. A randomized, double-blind, controlled trial of 123 Nigerian children with rickets showed that baseline intake of calcium was very low (about 200 mg/d).[48] These children responded better to treatment with calcium alone or in combination with vitamin D than to treatment with vitamin D alone. However, other factors in addition to calcium intake may play a role because control children without rickets had similarly low calcium intake. Although most of the studies on calcium deficiency rickets have been performed in Africa, similar dietary deficiencies occur in North America.[49]

Although vitamin D and iron are the most common nutritional deficiencies in normally growing infants and children, an array of other nutritional deficiencies can occur in specific clinical scenarios. These occur in certain diseases and in special diets, such as vegetarian/vegan diets. Less common causes of nutritional deficiencies in normal-growing infants and children are reviewed in the following sections.

WATER-SOLUBLE VITAMIN DEFICIENCIES
Vitamin B₁ (Thiamine)

Thiamine deficiency has been associated with three disorders: beriberi (infantile and adult), Wernicke-Korsakoff syndrome, and Leigh syndrome. Although these patients usually present with severe malnutrition, there have been case reports of thiamine deficiency in well-nourished patients.[50] Thiamine is found in larger quantities in food products such as yeast, legumes, pork, rice, and cereals, whereas milk products, fruits, and vegetables are poor sources of thiamine. The thiamine molecule is denatured at high pH and high temperatures. Hence, cooking, baking, and canning of some foods and pasteurization can destroy thiamine.

Beriberi in infants becomes clinically apparent between the ages of 2 and 3 months. The clinical features are variable and may include a fulminant cardiac syndrome with cardiomegaly, tachycardia, a loud piercing cry, cyanosis, dyspnea, and vomiting.[51] A form of aseptic meningitis has also been described, in which the affected infants show vomiting, nystagmus, purposeless movements, and seizures, despite a "normal" cerebrospinal fluid.[52] Wernicke disease is a triad of nystagmus, ophthalmoplegia, and ataxia, along with confusion. Korsakoff psychosis is impaired short-term memory and confabulation with otherwise grossly normal cognition.

Beriberi has been reported as a complication of weight loss surgery, presenting as a polyneuropathy with a burning sensation in the extremities, weakness, and falls.[53,54] Thiamine deficiency can occur as a complication of total parenteral nutrition if adequate thiamine supplements are not provided.[55] Although a number of adult studies have suggested that patients on chronic loop diuretics can develop thiamine deficiency, pediatric data on cardiac patients suggest the cause of the thiamine deficiency is multifactorial.[56]

Vitamin B₂ (Riboflavin)

Vitamin B_2, or riboflavin, is one of a group of naturally occurring compounds known as flavins. Flavoproteins are catalysts in several mitochondrial oxidative and reductive reactions, and function as electron transporters. Although riboflavin is supplied in many foods, including meats, fish, eggs, milk, green vegetables, yeast, and enriched foods, riboflavin deficiency may be more common than generally appreciated. One study of adolescents of low socioeconomic status in New York City found a prevalence of riboflavin deficiency of 26.6% among those not on vitamin supplements. Deficiency was determined from estimation of erythrocyte glutathione reductase activity, an accurate reflector of riboflavin nutritional status. The prevalence was neither sex nor age dependent. Prevalence was highest among those consuming less than 1 cup of milk/week and least among those taking 3 or more cups of milk a day.[57] The same group found riboflavin deficiency in 11% of children from the same socioeconomic background.[58] In the United Kingdom, the National Diet and Nutrition Survey reported a high prevalence of poor riboflavin status in adolescent girls (15–18 years) and young women (19–24 years). It has been reported that 95% of adolescent girls (15–18 years) and 75% of young women (19–24 years) in the United Kingdom have poor riboflavin status as measured by the erythrocyte glutathione reductase activation coefficient assay.[59]

Most cases of riboflavin deficiency go undetected because of the mild nature and nonspecific signs and symptoms of the deficiency. Significant deficiency is characterized by sore throat, hyperemia of pharyngeal mucous membranes, edema of mucous membranes, cheilitis, stomatitis, glossitis, normocytic-normochromic anemia, and seborrheic dermatitis.

Vitamin B₃ (Niacin)

Pellagra (meaning "raw skin") is characterized by a photosensitive-pigmented dermatitis (typically located in sun-exposed areas), diarrhea, dementia, and death. Pellagra was epidemic in the southeastern part of the United States during the early 20th century secondary to malnutrition and the consumption of tryptophan-deficient corn, because tryptophan is a precursor of niacin. Currently, pellagra is uncommon in the industrialized world except as a complication of alcoholism, anorexia nervosa, and malabsorptive diseases. Primary nutritional deficiencies secondary to inadequate niacin intake are uncommon, because niacin is widely distributed in plant and animal foods, with the exception of cereal, corn, or sorghum.

The most characteristic finding is the presence of a symmetrical hyperpigmented rash in sun-exposed areas. Other clinical findings are a red tongue and several nonspecific symptoms, such as diarrhea and vomiting. Neurologic symptoms include insomnia, anxiety, disorientation, delusions, dementia, encephalopathy, and death.

Subclinical niacin deficiency has been reported in an adult patient with carcinoid syndrome in which the conversion of tryptophan is to 5-OH tryptophan and serotonin rather than to nicotinic acid.[60] These patients can also develop full-blown pellagra. Niacin deficiency has not been identified in normal-growing children.

Pyridoxine (B_6)

Pyridoxine deficiency is seen classically in one of six pyridoxine-dependent syndromes: pyridoxine-dependent seizures, B_6 responsive anemia, xanthurenic acidemia, cystathionemia, homocystinuria, and type 2 hyperprolinemia.[61] Unusual as an isolated nutritional deficiency, pyridoxine deficiency has been associated with isoniazid treatment and in exclusively breast-fed infants older than 6 months.[62–64] Pyridoxine deficiency has also been associated with low-income pregnant adolescents. Although low vitamin B_6 in pregnancy has been associated with low Apgar scores, the true benefit of supplementation is unclear.[65] In adults, vitamin B_6 deficiency has been associated with increased risk of venous thromboembolism.[66]

VITAMIN B_{12} DEFICIENCY/FOLATE-ASSOCIATED MEGALOBLASTIC ANEMIA

Nutritional megaloblastic anemia features macrocytic red cells and mean corpuscular volumes greater than 100 fL. The megaloblast, the morphologic hallmark of the syndrome, is a result of impaired DNA formation secondary to deficiencies of vitamin B_{12} (cobalamin, Cbl) or folic acid.[67]

Cobalamin

Animal products (meat and dairy products) provide the only dietary source of vitamin B_{12} for humans. Although the true prevalence of vitamin B_{12} deficiency is unknown in the United States, the NHANES III (1991–1994) estimated a frequency of 1 in 200 children aged 4 to 19 years with decreased vitamin B_{12} levels (<200 pg/mL).[68]

Clinically evident vitamin B_{12} deficiency is uncommon in infants and children without predisposing factors. In infancy, cobalamin deficiency is usually secondary to maternal deficiency in breast-feeding mothers who follow strict vegan diets or are moderate vegetarians.[69] In addition, reported cases of cobalamin deficiency during infancy include breast-feeding mothers with a history of gastric bypass, malabsorptive syndromes, and pernicious anemia.[69,70] Depending on the age of presentation, these infants often present with poor growth, movement disorders, developmental delays, and hematologic abnormalities. If identified early, however, the infants may have no physical stigmata of cobalamin deficiency, emphasizing the importance of pre- and postnatal care.

In older children and adolescents, cobalamin deficiency is often associated with autoimmune diseases. There are case reports of pediatric patients with polyglandular autoimmune disease, Hashimoto thyroiditis, and pernicious anemia.[70–72] Cobalamin deficiency in pernicious anemia is thought to occur as a result of an autoimmune attack on gastric intrinsic factor.[73] Other reported causes include H pylori infection, intestinal bacterial overgrowth, ileal disease including Crohn disease, long-term use of biguanides, antacids, H_2 receptor antagonists/proton pump inhibitors,[74] bariatric surgery,[75] pancreatic insufficiency, and Sjögren syndrome.

Vitamin B_{12} can cause not only megaloblastic anemia but also neurologic changes. Because vitamin B_{12} stores are so large in relation to daily requirements, years of inadequate intake or absorption are required before the onset of symptoms. The classic picture of a patient with vitamin B_{12} deficiency (ie, an elderly Caucasian woman with anemia, icterus, and atrophic glossitis, who has a shuffling gait and is mentally sluggish) is less common and has been replaced by more subtle presentations, especially in pediatrics. Children may present with hard-to-characterize neuropsychiatric problems consisting of paresthesias, numbness, weakness, loss of dexterity, impaired memory, and personality changes.[76] It is clinically important to note that not all patients with neurologic abnormalities secondary to vitamin B_{12} deficiency are either anemic or have macrocytic red cell indices.[77]

Folic Acid

Folate occurs in animal products and in leafy vegetables.[78] Normal daily requirements are from 200 to 400 μg/d; this increases to 500 to 800 μg/d in pregnancy and lactation. Folate at physiologic levels enters cells by binding to a folate receptor. Once inside the cell, Folic acid is polyglutamated, a form that is biologically active and cannot rediffuse into the plasma.[78] Folic acid deficiency in pediatrics is generally secondary to an inadequate dietary intake or to drug interference. Since 1998, the US Food and Drug Administration has required the fortification of enriched cereal-grain products with folic acid. As a result there has been an increase in serum folate levels in the United States across all ages, sexes, and ethnicities. Adolescents have experienced the biggest relative increase, with children aged 5 years or younger having the smallest increase.[79]

The most common cause of folate deficiency is a lack of dietary intake. Although folate is plentiful in liver, greens, and yeast, it is easily destroyed by heat during cooking. Body stores are small (5–10 mg) and individuals on a folate-deficient diet can develop a megaloblastic anemia within 4 to 5 months. Individuals with increased requirements (ie, patients with hemolytic anemias, exfoliative skin diseases, and drug-induced interference with folate metabolism) are at higher risk for developing folate deficiency. Medications that interfere with folic acid metabolism include pyrimethamine (an antimalarial agent) and methotrexate, both of which cause a megaloblastic anemia by inhibiting dihydrofolate reductase. Phenytoin blocks folic acid absorption and increases use of folic acid by an unknown mechanism.[80]

The classic presentation of folate deficiency differs from vitamin B_{12} deficiency in two important ways. Although the hematologic manifestations of folate deficiency are similar, neurologic abnormalities do not occur with folate deficiency. In addition, symptoms of folate deficiency can occur within a few months of a decreased intake, in contrast with vitamin B_{12}.

Diagnosis of vitamin B_{12} or folate deficiency requires an examination of red blood cell histology. Macrocytosis (mean cell volume >100) is not specific for vitamin B_{12} or folate deficiency, and hypersegmented neutrophils can also occur in renal failure, ID, or as a familial trait. However, the combination of macrocytosis and hypersegmented neutrophils is pathognomonic of a megaloblastic anemia.

Other hematologic abnormalities that occur in vitamin B_{12} and folate deficiencies include decreased reticulocyte count, increased serum iron, evidence of mild hemolysis, decreased serum haptoglobin, elevated lactate dehydrogenase , and slightly elevated unconjugated bilirubin. The marrow is typically hypercellular and megaloblastic.

When the anemia is severe, there may also be thrombocytopenia and neutropenia (ie, pancytopenia), suggesting diagnoses such as myelodysplastic syndrome/acute myeloid leukemia, or aplastic anemia, all of which may present with macrocytosis, a reduced reticulocyte count, and pancytopenia. Assays of serum or red cell folate, serum B_{12}, methylmalonate, and homocysteine will confirm the diagnosis of folic acid or vitamin B_{12} deficiency.

Vitamin C (Ascorbic Acid)

Ascorbic acid deficiency presents with the clinical manifestations of scurvy. In all primates, ascorbic acid is an essential nutrient derived from the diet. In industrialized countries vitamin C deficiency has often been thought of as a disease of the past or to occur primarily in malnourished individuals living below the poverty line. In fact vitamin C deficiency, based on data from NHANES III, is not uncommon: 14% of males and 10% of females were vitamin C deficient as determined by serum vitamin C levels; the percentage of 12- to 17-year-old males and females was 5% to 6%. Smoking, not taking vitamin supplements, and being male were all associated with an increased risk of vitamin C deficiency.[81]

Although ascorbic acid has a number of biologic actions, the clinical symptoms of ascorbic acid deficiency are largely due to impaired collagen synthesis. Symptoms, which occur as early as 3 months after the initiation of a deficient intake, include bleeding gums, ecchymoses, petechiae, coiled hairs, hyperkeratosis, arthralgias, and impaired wound healing. Two cases of well-nourished children with vitamin C deficiency presented solely with painful limp secondary to a periosteal hematoma.[82,83] As deficiency progresses, patients may develop generalized systemic symptoms, including weakness, malaise, joint swelling, edema, depression, and vasomotor instability.

The incidence of vitamin C deficiency in normal-growing infants is unknown, but likely low since breast milk and infant formulas provide an adequate source of ascorbic acid. Although vitamin C deficiency is not uncommon in industrialized countries, overt scurvy has only been noted in case reports. It occurs in children with restricted or low dietary vitamin C. These children are usually growing normally without evidence of protein energy malnutrition.[84] Vitamin C deficiency has been described in normal-growing infants fed exclusively cow's milk formula and in children with neurodevelopmental disabilities.[85] Resolution of symptoms occurs with pharmacologic dosing of vitamin C.

Biotin Deficiency

Biotin is an essential component of several enzyme complexes in mammals, all of which are involved in carbohydrate and lipid metabolism. Because of its role in lipid metabolism, biotin deficiency can lead to defects in the metabolism of long-chain fatty acids. The resulting deficiency of essential fatty acids is often manifested by dermatologic changes, including seborrheic dermatitis and alopecia.

The clinical significance of biotin deficiency was first demonstrated in humans by Sydenstricker in 1942 in an experiment in which he gave human volunteers a diet deficient solely in biotin. He ensured biotin deficiency by feeding participants raw eggs, which contain avidin, which binds to biotin. Volunteers developed nonpruritic, scaly dermatitis, atrophic glossitis, anorexia and nausea, pallor, muscle pains and localized paresthesia, lassitude, somnolence, depression, anemia, and electrocardiographic abnormalities. With administration of biotin all symptoms reversed within 5 days.[86] In pediatrics, biotin deficiency is best characterized by biotinidase deficiency, a genetic disorder characterized by a patient's inability to reutilize biotin. Clinical features include hypotonia, ataxia, hearing loss, optic atrophy, skin rash, and alopecia.

Although primary nutritional biotin deficiency is unusual, case reports have been described. In Japan, where biotin was not a required supplement in infant formulas, cases of biotin deficiency presented primarily with an exfoliative rash and lethargy.[87] Cases of biotin deficiency have also been associated with parenteral nutrition without biotin supplementation.[88] Although presenting with associated protein calorie malnutrition, reports of patients consuming diets high in raw eggs, in which avidin binds to biotin and affects absorption, have also produced biotin deficiency.[89] As in the Sydenstricker study, dietary biotin supplementation reversed the primary clinical symptoms associated with biotin deficiency.

OTHER FAT-SOLUBLE VITAMIN DEFICIENCIES
Vitamin A

Vitamin A deficiency, a common nutrient deficiency in developing countries, causes primarily ophthalmologic disease.[90] Vitamin A is essential for maintaining the integrity of epithelial tissues, particularly the surface linings of the eye, respiratory, urinary, and intestinal tracts. The first clinical signs of vitamin A deficiency are drying of the conjunctiva, the development of Bitot spots and drying of the cornea (xerophthalmia); the patient also complains of an inability to see in dim light (night blindness).[91] As the disease progresses, vitamin A deficiency leads to a breakdown of the cornea (keratomalacia) and permanent blindness. Vitamin A deficient children often have evidence of protein energy malnutrition and other complicating nutritional deficiencies.[92,93] The World Health Organization (WHO) estimates that 70 to 80 million children worldwide suffer from subclinical vitamin A deficiency without overt clinical signs or symptoms.[94] Subclinical vitamin A deficiency has also been identified in the pediatric age group within the United States.[95]

Subclinical vitamin A deficiency increases the child's susceptibility to infection, reduces physical growth, and decreases the possibility of survival from serious illness.[96] Recent epidemiologic studies in developing countries have identified a relationship between subclinical vitamin A deficiency and higher rates of morbidity and mortality from common infectious diseases such as respiratory and diarrheal infections.[97] In nonindustrialized nations, vitamin A deficiency has been associated with measles. This association, and increasing morbidity associated with measles, has also been identified in the United States.[98] As a result, WHO, the United Nations Children's Fund (UNICEF), and the American Academy of Pediatrics have all issued recommendations regarding supplementation of vitamin A in children with measles.[95]

Tocopherol (Vitamin E) Deficiency

Vitamin E is a generic term for a group of fat-soluble compounds, of which α-tocopherol is most important. These compounds function as free radical scavengers at the cellular level. Vitamin E provides protective effects against free radical damage, which fosters chronic disease. Data suggest it may help prevent ischemic heart disease, atherosclerosis, diabetes, cataracts, Parkinson disease and Alzheimer disease. It may also have a protective effect against cancer.[99] Clinically evident vitamin E deficiency is uncommon in humans except in unusual circumstances secondary to the abundance of tocopherols in our diet. Vitamin E deficiency can occur in patients with fat malabsorption and in certain genetic disorders, including abetalipoproteinemia and Friedreich ataxia.

The major features of vitamin E deficiency are myopathy, ataxia, and pigmented retinopathy with loss of vision.[100] Sensory-motor neuropathy occurs late in the course of vitamin E deficiency and is manifested by loss of vibration and position sense, loss of reflexes, and generalized weakness. The progressive course of the neurologic disorder in vitamin E deficiency was described in a series of children with chronic forms of intrahepatic neonatal cholestasis or extrahepatic biliary atresia.

Data on the adequacy of vitamin E levels in healthy normal-growing children are primarily based upon serum α-tocopherol levels. Reports of less than adequate vitamin E levels have been reported in preschool children and adolescents within the United States, but the clinical significance of these lower levels based upon serum α-tocopheral levels have not been validated.[101,102]

Vitamin K

Vitamin K deficiency causes a coagulation disorder as shown by an elevated prothrombin time and international normalization ratio (INR) in the presence of normal platelets and fibrinogen. Vitamin K deficiency in the neonate, previously named hemorrhagic disease of the newborn, manifests itself in three ways.

Early vitamin K deficiency at birth (VKDB) presents within 24 hours of birth. Infants affected by early VKDB are usually born to mothers taking medications that inhibit vitamin K, including vitamin K antagonists such as warfarin, anticonvulsants such as carbamazepine, phenytoin, and barbiturates, and antibiotics such as cephalosporins, isoniazid, and rifampicin. At-risk infants have a 6% to 12% chance of developing VKDB if vitamin K is not administered at birth.

Classic VKDB occurs between the second and seventh day of life and is usually associated with a delay in feeding or insufficient feeding. Clinical presentation is usually mild, with bruising or minimal bleeding from the gastrointestinal tract/umbilicus. Rarely has significant blood loss or intracranial bleeding been described. Without vitamin K supplementation the incidence of classic VKDB is 0.01% to 0.44%.[103]

Late VKDB is associated with exclusive breast-feeding and occurs between 8 days and 6 months. Clinical presentation is usually severe, with mortality as high as 20% and intracranial hemorrhage occurring in 50% of infants. Infants with cholestasis or malabsorptive syndrome are at greatest risk, although the disease has been described in normal-growing infants. The cholestasis associated with late VKDB may be mild and self-limiting.[104] In fully breast-fed infants who did not receive vitamin K at birth, the incidence is 1 per 15,000 to 20,000 live births.[105]

Vitamin K given after birth prevents development of VKDB. There have been a number of epidemiologic studies and reviews examining the efficacy of different administration rates and dosing.[106] Both intramuscular and oral administration of 1 mg protects against classic VKDB. A single dose of intramuscular vitamin K at birth in exclusively breast-fed infants appears to be effective in preventing late VKDB, but oral administration should be repeated to prevent late VKDB.[107]

OTHER MINERAL DEFICIENCIES
Zinc

Zinc is an essential micronutrient for human growth, development, and immune function. Zinc intake is closely related to protein intake. Moderate-to-severe symptoms attributable to zinc deficiency include growth failure, primary hypogonadism, skin lesions including alopecia, impaired taste/smell, impaired immunity, and resistance to infection. Primary dietary sources of zinc include animal products such as meat, seafood, and milk. Sufficient dietary zinc sources are available in a typical mixed diet, but lacto-ovovegetarians require additional milk, eggs, grains, legumes, nuts, and seeds to achieve an adequate intake. Zinc absorption is inhibited by the presence of dietary phytates and fiber, which bind zinc and inhibit its absorption.[108]

Although nutritional zinc deficiency has often been associated with protein energy malnutrition, Crohn disease,[109] sickle cell anemia,[110] and nephrotic syndrome, mild zinc deficiencies can occur in vegan/vegetarian diets high in phytates,[111] and in healthy adolescent gymnasts.[112] The true prevalence of mild zinc deficiency is unknown because of the nonspecific nature of deficiency symptoms and imprecise diagnostic methods. Experimental zinc deficiency has been produced in normal volunteers and leads to a decreased immune response, as shown by a decrease in lymphocyte and natural killer cell activity, and endocrine changes, including primary hypogonadism with a decrease in serum androgens, an increase in serum gonadotropins, and oligospermia.[113,114]

Iodine

Iodine is an essential component of thyroxin (T4) and triiodothyronine (T3). It is acquired solely from the diet. Although mention of iodine deficiency suggests cretinism and severe developmental delay, it presents as a spectrum of diseases dependent on the degree of iodine deficiency. Since 1985, the International Council for the Control of Iodine Deficiency Disorders (http://www.iccidd.org), supported by WHO and UNICEF, has focused on the elimination of iodine deficiency disorders.[115] Despite significant progress with the introduction of iodinated salt, iodine deficiency is still a significant public health problem in many developing and industrialized countries.[116] Based on urinary iodine data collected from 1993 to 2003, WHO estimates the prevalence of iodine deficiency in school-aged children to be 36.4% worldwide. The lowest prevalence of iodine deficiency is found in the Americas (10.1%), where the proportion of households consuming iodized salt is the highest in the world (90%). The prevalence of iodine deficiency in Europe is much higher (59.9%), where the proportion of households consuming iodized salt is the lowest (27%).[117]

Iodine deficiency disorders include goiter, hypothyroidism, mental retardation, cretinism, and increased neonatal and infant mortality. Iodine deficiency goiter is often only a cosmetic problem for many individuals, who have no other clinical features of the disease. Decreased iodine intake leads to decreased T4 and T3 production. This in turn causes an increase in thyrotropin (TSH) secretion, which is an attempt by the body to restore T4 and T3 levels. TSH also stimulates thyroid growth; thus, goiter occurs as part of the compensatory response to iodine deficiency.[118,119] Mild-to-moderate iodine deficiency during pregnancy can lead to minor neuropsychological defects in offspring.[120] Smoking reduces iodine in breast milk. Mothers who smoke have reduced iodine levels in their breast milk (26 µg /L vs 54 µg /L in nonsmokers despite identical urine iodine concentrations), and their infants have reduced urinary iodine concentrations (33 µg /L vs 40 µg /L in nonsmokers).[121,122] Iodine supplementation should be considered in smokers. In infants and children, the effects of iodine deficiency on growth and development are well documented, but children may present with subclinical manifestations of mild iodine deficiency with only mild-to-moderate neurologic and neuropsychological deficits [123]

Selenium

Selenium is an essential nutrient that acts as a cofactor in several enzymatic reactions important in redox function, production of active thyroid hormone, and immune function. Selenium is a component of selenoproteins, including glutathione peroxidase, selenoprotein-P, and thioredoxin reductase. Nutritional selenium deficiency occurs in areas with low selenium content in the soil. In industrialized nations, which have soils rich in selenium, deficiencies are seen in infants and children with dietary restrictions and prolonged parenteral nutrition. Severe endemic selenium deficiency can result in Keshan disease (an endemic cardiomyopathy) and Kashin-Bek disease (a deforming arthritis). The effects of selenium deficiency can also be less overt. Selenium deficiency has been shown to negatively affect immunocompetency, spermatogenesis, mood, thyroid function, and cardiovascular disease.[124,125]

Copper

Copper deficiency is best characterized by Menkes syndrome, an X-linked recessive disorder characterized by generalized copper deficiency leading to early growth retardation, peculiar hair, and focal cerebral and cerebellar degeneration. Nutritional copper deficiency in children can occur in burn patients,[126] patients with short bowel syndrome, and patients dependent on total parenteral nutrition,[127] and has been identified in normally growing individuals.[128] In a cohort of children from low-income families in the United States, despite identification of other nutritional deficiencies, copper deficiency was not identified, making the true prevalence of nutritional copper deficiency most likely very low in normal-growing children.[129]

SUMMARY

Health care providers often focus their attention on overt disease processes and fail to recognize deficiencies. This is especially true for nutritional deficiencies. It is evident from the medical literature that children, even when growing normally, are at risk for nutritional deficiencies. These deficiencies are common and can have significant negative short-term and long-term effects on their lives. Health care providers should continue to stress the importance of proper diet and nutrition to their patients, colleagues, and the wider community.

REFERENCES

1. Galloway R, McGuire J. Determinants of compliance with iron supplementation: supplies, side effects, or psychology? Soc Sci Med 1994;39(3):381–90.
2. Yip R, Binkin NJ, Fleshood L, et al. Declining prevalence of anemia among low-income children in the United States. JAMA 1987;258(12):1619–23.
3. Sherry B, Bister D, Yip R. Continuation of decline in prevalence of anemia in low-income children: the Vermont experience. Arch Pediatr Adolesc Med 1997; 151(9):928–30.
4. Brotanek JM, Gosz J, Weitzman M, et al. Iron deficiency in early childhood in the United States: risk factors and racial/ethnic disparities. Pediatrics 2007;120(3): 568–75.
5. Brotanek JM, Gosz J, Weitzman M, et al. Secular trends in the prevalence of iron deficiency among US toddlers, 1976–2002. Arch Pediatr Adolesc Med 2008; 162(4):374–81.
6. Cusick SE, Mei Z, Cogswell ME. Continuing anemia prevention strategies are needed throughout early childhood in low-income preschool children. J Pediatr 2007;150(4):422–8, 8, e1–2.
7. Stellinga-Boelen AA, Storm H, Wiegersma PA, et al. Iron deficiency among children of asylum seekers in the Netherlands. J Pediatr Gastroenterol Nutr 2007; 45(5):591–5.
8. Tunnessen WW Jr, Oski FA. Consequences of starting whole cow milk at 6 months of age. J Pediatr 1987;111(6 Pt 1):813–6.
9. Pizarro F, Yip R, Dallman PR, et al. Iron status with different infant feeding regimens: relevance to screening and prevention of iron deficiency. J Pediatr 1991; 118(5):687–92.
10. Hopkins D, Emmett P, Steer C, et al. Infant feeding in the second 6 months of life related to iron status: an observational study. Arch Dis Child 2007;92(10):850–4.

11. de Vizia B, Poggi V, Conenna R, et al. Iron absorption and iron deficiency in infants and children with gastrointestinal diseases. J Pediatr Gastroenterol Nutr 1992;14(1):21–6.

12. Ziegler EE, Fomon SJ, Nelson SE, et al. Cow milk feeding in infancy: further observations on blood loss from the gastrointestinal tract. J Pediatr 1990; 116(1):11–8.

13. Sutcliffe TL, Khambalia A, Westergard S, et al. Iron depletion is associated with daytime bottle-feeding in the second and third years of life. Arch Pediatr Adolesc Med 2006;160(11):1114–20.

14. De Caterina M, Grimaldi E, Di Pascale G, et al. The soluble transferrin receptor (sTfR)-ferritin index is a potential predictor of celiac disease in children with refractory iron deficiency anemia. Clin Chem Lab Med 2005;43(1):38–42.

15. Kurekci AE, Atay AA, Sarici SU, et al. Is there a relationship between childhood *Helicobacter pylori* infection and iron deficiency anemia? J Trop Pediatr 2005; 51(3):166–9.

16. Brown WD, Dyment PG. Pagophagia and iron deficiency anemia in adolescent girls. Pediatrics 1972;49(5):766–7.

17. Sherriff A, Emond A, Bell JC, et al. Should infants be screened for anaemia? A prospective study investigating the relation between haemoglobin at 8, 12, and 18 months and development at 18 months. Arch Dis Child 2001;84(6):480–5.

18. Halterman JS, Kaczorowski JM, Aligne CA, et al. Iron deficiency and cognitive achievement among school-aged children and adolescents in the United States. Pediatrics 2001;107(6):1381–6.

19. Williams J, Wolff A, Daly A, et al. Iron supplemented formula milk related to reduction in psychomotor decline in infants from inner city areas: randomised study. BMJ 1999;318(7185):693–7.

20. Lozoff B, Clark KM, Jing Y, et al. Dose-response relationships between iron deficiency with or without anemia and infant social-emotional behavior. J Pediatr 2008;152(5):696–702, 31–3.

21. Konofal E, Lecendreux M, Deron J, et al. Effects of iron supplementation on attention deficit hyperactivity disorder in children. Pediatr Neurol 2008;38(1):20–6.

22. Lozoff B, Jimenez E, Smith JB. Double burden of iron deficiency in infancy and low socioeconomic status: a longitudinal analysis of cognitive test scores to age 19 years. Arch Pediatr Adolesc Med 2006;160(11):1108–13.

23. Maguire JL, deVeber G, Parkin PC. Association between iron-deficiency anemia and stroke in young children. Pediatrics 2007;120(5):1053–7.

24. White KC. Anemia is a poor predictor of iron deficiency among toddlers in the United States: for heme the bell tolls. Pediatrics 2005;115(2):315–20.

25. Boutry M, Needlman R. Use of diet history in the screening of iron deficiency. Pediatrics 1996;98(6 Pt 1):1138–42.

26. Bogen DL, Duggan AK, Dover GJ, et al. Screening for iron deficiency anemia by dietary history in a high-risk population. Pediatrics 2000;105(6):1254–9.

27. Oski FA. Iron deficiency in infancy and childhood. N Engl J Med 1993;329(3): 190–3.

28. Wright RO, Shannon MW, Wright RJ, et al. Association between iron deficiency and low-level lead poisoning in an urban primary care clinic. Am J Public Health 1999;89(7):1049–53.

29. Brugnara C, Zurakowski D, DiCanzio J, et al. Reticulocyte hemoglobin content to diagnose iron deficiency in children. JAMA 1999;281(23):2225–30.

30. Ullrich C, Wu A, Armsby C, et al. Screening healthy infants for iron deficiency using reticulocyte hemoglobin content. JAMA 2005;294(8):924–30.

31. Robinson PD, Hogler W, Craig ME, et al. The re-emerging burden of rickets: a decade of experience from Sydney. Arch Dis Child 2006;91(7):564–8.
32. Ward LM. Vitamin D deficiency in the 21st century: a persistent problem among Canadian infants and mothers. CMAJ 2005;172(6):769–70.
33. Looker AC, Pfeiffer CM, Lacher DA, et al. Serum 25-hydroxyvitamin D status of the US population: 1988–1994 compared with 2000–2004. Am J Clin Nutr 2008; 88(6):1519–27.
34. Kruse K. Pathophysiology of calcium metabolism in children with vitamin D-deficiency rickets. J Pediatr 1995;126(5 Pt 1):736–41.
35. Kovacs CS, Kronenberg HM. Maternal-fetal calcium and bone metabolism during pregnancy, puerperium, and lactation. Endocr Rev 1997;18(6):832–72.
36. Rothberg AD, Pettifor JM, Cohen DF, et al. Maternal-infant vitamin D relationships during breast-feeding. J Pediatr 1982;101(4):500–3.
37. Weisberg P, Scanlon KS, Li R, et al. Nutritional rickets among children in the United States: review of cases reported between 1986 and 2003. Am J Clin Nutr 2004;80(6 Suppl):1697S–705S.
38. Nozza JM, Rodda CP. Vitamin D deficiency in mothers of infants with rickets. Med J Aust 2001;175(5):253–5.
39. Kreiter SR, Schwartz RP, Kirkman HN Jr, et al. Nutritional rickets in African American breast-fed infants. J Pediatr 2000;137(2):153–7.
40. Welch TR, Bergstrom WH, Tsang RC. Vitamin D-deficient rickets: the reemergence of a once-conquered disease. J Pediatr 2000;137(2):143–5.
41. Misra M, Pacaud D, Petryk A, et al. Vitamin D deficiency in children and its management: review of current knowledge and recommendations. Pediatrics 2008;122(2):398–417.
42. Hollis BW, Roos BA, Draper HH, et al. Vitamin D and its metabolites in human and bovine milk. J Nutr 1981;111(7):1240–8.
43. Specker BL, Tsang RC, Hollis BW. Effect of race and diet on human-milk vitamin D and 25-hydroxyvitamin D. Am J Dis Child 1985;139(11):1134–7.
44. Shah BR, Finberg L. Single-day therapy for nutritional vitamin D-deficiency rickets: a preferred method. J Pediatr 1994;125(3):487–90.
45. Mimouni F. Single-day therapy for rickets. J Pediatr 1995;126(6):1019–20.
46. Cesur Y, Caksen H, Gundem A, et al. Comparison of low and high dose of vitamin D treatment in nutritional vitamin D deficiency rickets. J Pediatr Endocrinol Metab 2003;16(8):1105–9.
47. Marie PJ, Pettifor JM, Ross FP, et al. Histological osteomalacia due to dietary calcium deficiency in children. N Engl J Med 1982;307(10):584–8.
48. Thacher TD, Fischer PR, Pettifor JM, et al. A comparison of calcium, vitamin D, or both for nutritional rickets in Nigerian children. N Engl J Med 1999;341(8): 563–8.
49. DeLucia MC, Mitnick ME, Carpenter TO. Nutritional rickets with normal circulating 25-hydroxyvitamin D: a call for reexamining the role of dietary calcium intake in North American infants. J Clin Endocrinol Metab 2003;88(8): 3539–45.
50. San Sebastian M, Jativa R. Beriberi in a well-nourished Amazonian population. Acta Trop 1998;70(2):193–6.
51. Reid DH. Acute infantile beriberi. J Pediatr 1961;58:858–63.
52. Abad MB, Pecache L. The pseudomeningitic form of infantile beriberi. Acta Med Philipp 1949;5(4):21–7.
53. Towbin A, Inge TH, Garcia VF, et al. Beriberi after gastric bypass surgery in adolescence. J Pediatr 2004;145(2):263–7.

54. Lawson ML, Kirk S, Mitchell T, et al. One-year outcomes of Roux-en-Y gastric bypass for morbidly obese adolescents: a multicenter study from the Pediatric Bariatric Study Group. J Pediatr Surg 2006;41(1):137–43 [discussion: 43].

55. Hahn JS, Berquist W, Alcorn DM, et al. Wernicke encephalopathy and beriberi during total parenteral nutrition attributable to multivitamin infusion shortage. Pediatrics 1998;101(1):E10.

56. Suter PM, Vetter W. Diuretics and vitamin B1: are diuretics a risk factor for thiamin malnutrition? Nutr Rev 2000;58(10):319–23.

57. Lopez R, Schwartz JV, Cooperman JM. Riboflavin deficiency in an adolescent population in New York City. Am J Clin Nutr 1980;33(6):1283–6.

58. Lopez F, Cole HS, Montoya MF, et al. Riboflavin deficiency in a pediatric population of low socioeconomic status in New York City. J Pediatr 1975;87(3):420–2.

59. Hill MH, Mushtaq S, Williams EA, et al. Study Protocol: Randomised controlled trial to investigate the functional significance of marginal riboflavin status in young women in the UK (RIBOFEM). BMC Public Health 2009;9(1):90.

60. Shah GM, Shah RG, Veillette H, et al. Biochemical assessment of niacin deficiency among carcinoid cancer patients. Am J Gastroenterol 2005;100(10):2307–14.

61. Rajesh R, Girija AS. Pyridoxine-dependent seizures: a review. Indian Pediatr 2003;40(7):633–8.

62. Snider DE Jr. Pyridoxine supplementation during isoniazid therapy. Tubercle 1980;61(4):191–6.

63. Heiskanen K, Siimes MA, Perheentupa J, et al. Risk of low vitamin B6 status in infants breast-fed exclusively beyond six months. J Pediatr Gastroenterol Nutr 1996;23(1):38–44.

64. Schuster K, Bailey LB, Mahan CS. Vitamin B6 status of low-income adolescent and adult pregnant women and the condition of their infants at birth. Am J Clin Nutr 1981;34(9):1731–5.

65. Thaver D, Saeed MA, Bhutta ZA. Pyridoxine (vitamin B6) supplementation in pregnancy. Cochrane Database Syst Rev 2006;(2):CD000179.

66. Hron G, Lombardi R, Eichinger S, et al. Low vitamin B6 levels and the risk of recurrent venous thromboembolism. Haematologica 2007;92(9):1250–3.

67. Allen RH, Stabler SP, Savage DG, et al. Metabolic abnormalities in cobalamin (vitamin B12) and folate deficiency. FASEB J 1993;7(14):1344–53.

68. Wright JD, Bialostosky K, Gunter EW, et al. Blood folate and vitamin B12: United States, 1988–94. Vital Health Stat 20. 1998;11(243):1–78.

69. Marble M, Copeland S, Khanfar N, et al. Neonatal vitamin B12 deficiency secondary to maternal subclinical pernicious anemia: identification by expanded newborn screening. J Pediatr 2008;152(5):731–3.

70. Rosenblatt DS, Whitehead VM. Cobalamin and folate deficiency: acquired and hereditary disorders in children. Semin Hematol 1999;36(1):19–34.

71. Greenwood DL, Crock P, Braye S, et al. Autoimmune gastritis and parietal cell reactivity in two children with abnormal intestinal permeability. Eur J Pediatr 2008;167(8):917–25.

72. Katz S, Berernheim J, Kaufman Z, et al. Pernicious anemia and adenocarcinoma of the stomach in an adolescent: clinical presentation and histopathology. J Pediatr Surg 1997;32(9):1384–5.

73. Toh BH, van Driel IR, Gleeson PA. Pernicious anemia. N Engl J Med 1997;337(20):1441–8.

74. Hirschowitz BI, Worthington J, Mohnen J. Vitamin B12 deficiency in hypersecretors during long-term acid suppression with proton pump inhibitors. Aliment Pharmacol Ther 2008;27(11):1110–21.

75. Shah M, Simha V, Garg A. Review: long-term impact of bariatric surgery on body weight, comorbidities, and nutritional status. J Clin Endocrinol Metab 2006; 91(11):4223–31.
76. Green R, Kinsella LJ. Current concepts in the diagnosis of cobalamin deficiency. Neurology 1995;45(8):1435–40.
77. Lindenbaum J, Healton EB, Savage DG, et al. Neuropsychiatric disorders caused by cobalamin deficiency in the absence of anemia or macrocytosis. N Engl J Med 1988;318(26):1720–8.
78. Pruthi RK, Tefferi A. Pernicious anemia revisited. Mayo Clin Proc 1994;69(2): 144–50.
79. Pfeiffer CM, Caudill SP, Gunter EW, et al. Biochemical indicators of B vitamin status in the US population after folic acid fortification: results from the National Health and Nutrition Examination Survey, 1999–2000. Am J Clin Nutr 2005;82(2):442–50.
80. Lambie DG, Johnson RH. Drugs and folate metabolism. Drugs 1985;30(2): 145–55.
81. Hampl JS, Taylor CA, Johnston CS. Vitamin C deficiency and depletion in the United States: the Third National Health and Nutrition Examination Survey, 1988 to 1994. Am J Public Health 2004;94(5):870–5.
82. Shetty AK, Steele RW, Silas V, et al. A boy with a limp. Lancet 1998;351(9097): 182.
83. Tamura Y, Welch DC, Zic JA, et al. Scurvy presenting as painful gait with bruising in a young boy. Arch Pediatr Adolesc Med 2000;154(7):732–5.
84. Gomez-Carrasco JA, Lopez-Herce Cid J, Bernabe de Frutos C, et al. Scurvy in adolescence. J Pediatr Gastroenterol Nutr 1994;19(1):118–20.
85. Baumbach J. Scurvy by any other name: a case report. R I Med 1994;77(1):24–5.
86. Sydenstricker VP, Singal SA, Briggs AP, et al. Preliminary observations on "egg white injury" in man and its cure with a biotin concentrate. Science 1942; 95(2459):176–7.
87. Higuchi R, Noda E, Koyama Y, et al. Biotin deficiency in an infant fed with amino acid formula and hypoallergenic rice. Acta Paediatr 1996;85(7):872–4.
88. Mock DM, Baswell DL, Baker H, et al. Biotin deficiency complicating parenteral alimentation: diagnosis, metabolic repercussions, and treatment. J Pediatr 1985; 106(5):762–9.
89. Sweetman L, Surh L, Baker H, et al. Clinical and metabolic abnormalities in a boy with dietary deficiency of biotin. Pediatrics 1981;68(4):553–8.
90. Underwood BA, Arthur P. The contribution of vitamin A to public health. Faseb J 1996;10(9):1040–8.
91. Sommer A. Vitamin A: its effect on childhood sight and life. Nutr Rev 1994;52(2 Pt 2):S60–6.
92. Brown KH, Gaffar A, Alamgir SM. Xerophthalmia, protein-calorie malnutrition, and infections in children. J Pediatr 1979;95(4):651–6.
93. West KP Jr, Djunaedi E, Pandji A, et al. Vitamin A supplementation and growth: a randomized community trial. Am J Clin Nutr 1988;48(5):1257–64.
94. Underwood BA. Hypovitaminosis A: international programmatic issues. J Nutr 1994;124(Suppl 8):1467S–72S.
95. Stephens D, Jackson PL, Gutierrez Y. Subclinical vitamin A deficiency: a potentially unrecognized problem in the United States. Pediatr Nurs 1996;22(5): 377–89, 456.
96. Underwood BA. Maternal vitamin A status and its importance in infancy and early childhood. Am J Clin Nutr 1994;59(Suppl 2):517S–22S [discussion: 22S–24S].

97. Semba RD. Vitamin A, immunity, and infection. Clin Infect Dis 1994;19(3): 489–99.
98. Butler JC, Havens PL, Sowell AL, et al. Measles severity and serum retinol (vitamin A) concentration among children in the United States. Pediatrics 1993;91(6):1176–81.
99. Brigelius-Flohe R, Traber MG. Vitamin E: function and metabolism. Faseb J 1999;13(10):1145–55.
100. Aparicio JM, Belanger-Quintana A, Suarez L, et al. Ataxia with isolated vitamin E deficiency: case report and review of the literature. J Pediatr Gastroenterol Nutr 2001;33(2):206–10.
101. Looker AC, Underwood BA, Wiley J, et al. Serum alpha-tocopherol levels of Mexican Americans, Cubans, and Puerto Ricans aged 4–74 y. Am J Clin Nutr 1989;50(3):491–6.
102. Drewel BT, Giraud DW, Davy SR, et al. Less than adequate vitamin E status observed in a group of preschool boys and girls living in the United States. J Nutr Biochem 2006;17(2):132–8.
103. Sutor AH, von Kries R, Cornelissen EA, et al. Vitamin K deficiency bleeding (VKDB) in infancy. ISTH Pediatric/Perinatal Subcommittee. International Society on Thrombosis and Haemostasis. Thromb Haemost 1999;81(3):456–61.
104. von Kries R, Shearer MJ, Gobel U. Vitamin K in infancy. Eur J Pediatr 1988; 147(2):106–12.
105. Autret-Leca E, Jonville-Bera AP. Vitamin K in neonates: how to administer, when and to whom. Paediatr Drugs 2001;3(1):1–8.
106. Puckett RM, Offringa M. Prophylactic vitamin K for vitamin K deficiency bleeding in neonates. Cochrane Database Syst Rev 2000;(4):CD002776.
107. Van Winckel M, De Bruyne R, Van De Velde S, et al. An update for the paediatrician. Eur J Pediatr 2009;168(2):127–34.
108. Lonnerdal B. Dietary factors influencing zinc absorption. J Nutr 2000; 130(Suppl 5S):1378S–83S.
109. Naber TH, van den Hamer CJ, Baadenhuysen H, et al. The value of methods to determine zinc deficiency in patients with Crohn's disease. Scand J Gastroenterol 1998;33(5):514–23.
110. Phebus CK, Maciak BJ, Gloninger MF, et al. Zinc status of children with sickle cell disease: relationship to poor growth. Am J Hematol 1988;29(2):67–73.
111. Donovan UM, Gibson RS. Iron and zinc status of young women aged 14 to 19 years consuming vegetarian and omnivorous diets. J Am Coll Nutr 1995;14(5): 463–72.
112. Brun JF, Dieu-Cambrezy C, Charpiat A, et al. Serum zinc in highly trained adolescent gymnasts. Biol Trace Elem Res 1995;47(1-3):273–8.
113. Prasad AS, Meftah S, Abdallah J, et al. Serum thymulin in human zinc deficiency. J Clin Invest 1988;82(4):1202–10.
114. Abbasi AA, Prasad AS, Rabbani P, et al. Experimental zinc deficiency in man. Effect on testicular function. J Lab Clin Med 1980;96(3):544–50.
115. Hetzel BS. Towards the global elimination of brain damage due to iodine deficiency: the role of the International Council for Control of Iodine Deficiency Disorders. Int J Epidemiol 2005;34(4):762–4.
116. Manz F, van't Hof MA, Haschke F. Iodine supply in children from different European areas: the Euro-growth study. Committee for the Study of Iodine Supply in European Children. J Pediatr Gastroenterol Nutr 2000;31(Suppl 1):S72–5.
117. Zimmermann MB. Assessing iodine status and monitoring progress of iodized salt programs. J Nutr 2004;134(7):1673–7.

118. Wilders-Truschnig MM, Warnkross H, Leb G, et al. The effect of treatment with levothyroxine or iodine on thyroid size and thyroid growth stimulating immuno-globulins in endemic goitre patients. Clin Endocrinol (Oxf) 1993;39(3):281–6.
119. Rasmussen LB, Ovesen L, Bulow I, et al. Relations between various measures of iodine intake and thyroid volume, thyroid nodularity, and serum thyroglobulin. Am J Clin Nutr 2002;76(5):1069–76.
120. Aghini Lombardi FA, Pinchera A, Antonangeli L, et al. Mild iodine deficiency during fetal/neonatal life and neuropsychological impairment in Tuscany. J Endocrinol Invest 1995;18(1):57–62.
121. Laurberg P, Nohr SB, Pedersen KM, et al. Iodine nutrition in breast-fed infants is impaired by maternal smoking. J Clin Endocrinol Metab 2004;89(1):181–7.
122. Pearce EN, Leung AM, Blount BC, et al. Breast milk iodine and perchlorate concentrations in lactating Boston-area women. J Clin Endocrinol Metab 2007;92(5):1673–7.
123. Bleichrodt N, Escobar del Rey F, Morreale de Escobar G, et al. Iodine deficiency. Implications for mental and psychomotor development in children. New York: Plenum Press; 1989.
124. Rayman MP. The importance of selenium to human health. Lancet 2000; 356(9225):233–41.
125. Chanoine JP. Selenium and thyroid function in infants, children and adolescents. Biofactors 2003;19(3-4):137–43.
126. Liusuwan RA, Palmieri T, Warden N, et al. Impaired healing because of copper deficiency in a pediatric burn patient: a case report. J Trauma 2008;65(2): 464–6.
127. Angotti LB, Post GR, Robinson NS, et al. Pancytopenia with myelodysplasia due to copper deficiency. Pediatr Blood Cancer 2008;51(5):693–5.
128. Harless W, Crowell E, Abraham J. Anemia and neutropenia associated with copper deficiency of unclear etiology. Am J Hematol 2006;81(7):546–9.
129. Schneider JM, Fujii ML, Lamp CL, et al. The prevalence of low serum zinc and copper levels and dietary habits associated with serum zinc and copper in 12- to 36-month-old children from low-income families at risk for iron deficiency. J Am Diet Assoc 2007;107(11):1924–9.

Protein Energy Malnutrition

Zubin Grover, MBBS, MD*, Looi C. Ee, MBBS, FRACP

KEYWORDS

• Protein energy malnutrition • Pediatrics

The World Health Organization (WHO) defines malnutrition as "the cellular imbalance between the supply of nutrients and energy and the body's demand for them to ensure growth, maintenance, and specific functions."[1] Although malnutrition is a state of deficiency or excess of energy, protein, and other nutrients, this article deals with undernutrition and specifically protein energy malnutrition (PEM). Children with primary PEM generally are found in developing countries as a result of inadequate food supply caused by socioeconomic, political, and occasionally environmental factors such as natural disasters. Among the four principal causes of mortality in young children worldwide, undernutrition has been ascribed to be the cause of death in 60.7% of children with diarrheal diseases, 52.3% of those with pneumonia, 44.8% of measles cases, and 57.3% of children with malaria.[2] More than 50% of all the childhood deaths are attributable to undernutrition, with relative risks of mortality being 8.4 for severe malnutrition, 4.6 for moderate malnutrition, and 2.5 for mild malnutrition as estimated by analyses of 28 epidemiologic studies done across 53 countries.[3–5] Most of the deaths (> 80%) occur among those with mild or moderate malnutrition (weight for age 60% to 80%). This is explained by the fact that although the risk of death is greatest for those with severe malnutrition, these extreme cases only make up a small fraction of total number of children with malnutrition.[3,5]

Malnutrition in the developed world is not rare, but its prevalence and importance often are underappreciated. Several studies using various measures of malnutrition have reported a prevalence of between 6% and 51% of hospitalized children in developed nations.[6–9] The genesis of secondary malnutrition in the developed world may be attributed to abnormal nutrient loss, increased energy expenditure, or decreased food intake, frequently in the context of associated chronic diseases like cystic fibrosis, chronic renal failure, childhood malignancies, congenital heart disease, and neuromuscular diseases.

Department of Gastroenterology, Royal Children's Hospital, Herston Road, Brisbane, Queensland 4029, Australia
* Corresponding author.
E-mail address: zubin_grover@health.qld.gov.au (Z. Grover).

Pediatr Clin N Am 56 (2009) 1055–1068
doi:10.1016/j.pcl.2009.07.001
0031-3955/09/$ – see front matter © 2009 Elsevier Inc. All rights reserved.

pediatric.theclinics.com

EPIDEMIOLOGY

According to the United Nations Children's Fund (UNICEF), PEM is an invisible emergency much like the tip of an iceberg, where its deadly consequences are hidden from view. In 2005, 20% of children younger than 5 years in low-to-middle income countries were estimated to be underweight (weight for age z-score <-2), while 32% (178 million) children younger than 5 years in developing countries were estimated to be stunted (height for age z score <-2).[10] The highest prevalence of stunting was in central Africa and south-central Asia, although the largest numbers of children, 74 million, live in southern Asia.[10] Worldwide, only 36 countries account for 90% of all stunted children when countries with stunting prevalence of at least 20% were considered.[10] India alone has 34% of the world's stunted children because of its large population, although there is significant variation between its states. The global estimate of wasting (weight for height z score <-2) is 10%, with south-central Asia estimated to have the highest prevalence and total number affected, 16% and 29 million respectively. Sub-Saharan Africa has about 25% of the world's underweight children younger than 5 years of age, with Congo, Ethiopia, and Nigeria being the nations affected worst.

In 1990, the World Summit for Children announced key requirements for improving child health and nutrition. Subsequently, the United Nations incorporated this into its first Millennium Goal in September 2000. A key target for MDG1 (Millennium Development Goal 1) is to halve the proportion of people who suffer from hunger between 1990 and 2015. Unfortunately, despite progress in reducing the prevalence of undernutrition, the current rate of decline is not fast enough to reach this target for most of the world except for Latin America and the Caribbean, Pacific, and eastern Asia. In Africa, the number of underweight children was forecasted to increase because of political and social instability and the acquired immunodeficiency syndrome (AIDS) epidemic.[11,12]

MALNUTRITION IN THE DEVELOPED WORLD

Several reports from Germany, the United Kingdom, the United States, and France as recently as the last decade reported the prevalence of acute malnutrition in hospitalized pediatric patients to be between 6.1% and 24%.[6,7,9] In 2008, Pawellek and colleagues,[7] using Waterlow's criteria, reported 24.1% of patients in a tertiary pediatric hospital in Germany to be malnourished (<90th percentile weight for height), of which 17.9% were mild, 4.4% moderate, and 1.7% severely malnourished. The prevalence of malnutrition varied depending on their underlying medical conditions and ranged from 40% in patients with neurologic diseases, to 34.5% in those with infectious disease, 33.3% in those with cystic fibrosis, 28.6% in those with cardiovascular disease, 27.3% in oncology patients, and 23.6% in those with gastrointestinal diseases.[7] Patients with multiple diagnoses were most likely to be malnourished (43.8%). The prevalence and degree of acute PEM in hospitalized pediatric patients are similar to those observed by Hendricks and colleagues[9] almost a decade ago using the same criteria.

Secker and colleagues[8] used subjective global nutritional assessment in children admitted for elective surgery in a tertiary referral pediatric hospital in Toronto and found that 51% of children were malnourished (36% had moderate malnutrition, and 15% had severe malnutrition). Despite differences in methods of assessing malnutrition, these studies clearly document a significant prevalence of malnutrition even in the developed world, particularly in hospitalized pediatric patients. These results may be skewed, because most of the reports have been from tertiary centers with relatively larger proportions of patients with chronic and severe disorders. A cross-sectional study on patients attending outpatient clinics in Brazil, however, reported an overall prevalence of underweight, stunting, and wasting as 14.3%, 17.3%, and 4.4%, respectively, with reference to National Center for Health Statistics (NCHS) growth curves.[13]

One of the difficulties in being able to compare prevalence between studies and centers is the lack of consensus on a uniform definition of malnutrition and its grades of severity. A recent review highlighted the issues of lack of uniform screening tools, poor nutritional data collection, and early identification of those at risk of developing PEM.[6]

DEFINITION

There remains much variation and controversy as to the best and most useful method of assessing and defining malnutrition. In 1956, Gomez introduced a classification based on weight below a specified percentage of median weight for age.[14] Seoane and Latham then proposed calculating weight for height and height for age as a means to distinguish between wasting and stunting.[15] Wasting, where weight for height is reduced, is indicative of acute growth disturbance from malnutrition, whereas stunting, where height for age is reduced is more suggestive of chronic malnutrition with faltering of long-term growth.[16] In 1977, Waterlow recommended the use of z-scores and SDs below the median to define underweight, wasting, and stunting.[17,18] These definitions continue to be used widely with subsequent WHO modifications. WHO adopted the US National Center for Health Statistics (NCHS) classification in 1983 as the international reference for weight and height in children. It has since been used to classify children as underweight, wasted, or stunted based on z-scores.[19-21] The major issues with using NCHS criteria as the population standard are the extrapolation from an ethnically homogenous population, which likely does not represent developing world countries, inclusion of bottle-fed infants, and the assumption that all children of a given height will have the same average weight regardless of age. In 2006, a new population standard was adopted by WHO based on an international multicenter study using exclusively breast-fed children of diverse ethnic backgrounds.[22] Subsequent studies have highlighted that these new WHO growth reference curves will result in a higher measured prevalence of malnutrition when compared with NCHS standards.[23,24]

An alternative proposed approach to assessing malnutrition is to measure mid-upper arm circumference (MUAC) as a proxy for weight, and head circumference as a proxy for height.[25] This may be useful when accurate measures of height and weight are unavailable, particularly in children younger than 3 years and also in small regional centers. The degree of malnutrition is calculated by dividing the MUAC by occipito-frontal head circumference. The use of MUAC and presence of edema have been reported to be better indicators than weight for height (either NCHS or WHO) for case definition of severe acute malnutrition.[26] There is significant evidence indicating that using MUAC less than 110 mm as a definition for severe malnutrition may be the best method to assess nutrition in terms of age independence, simplicity, accuracy, specificity, and sensitivity. Additionally, it is a good anthropometric predictor of mortality related to malnutrition.[26-31] Although the evidence favors use of MUAC for estimating malnutrition and for admission to therapeutic feeding programs, more information is needed on the use of MUAC as a discharge and follow-up tool.

More recently, a new definition of thinness has been proposed by Cole,[32] who performed meta-analyses on population studies from six high- and middle-income countries, with a total of 192,727 subjects, whose ages ranged from 0 to 25 years.

He proposed using body mass index for age to grade thinness according to age as a method of assessing malnutrition. This methodology, however, has not been tested in population studies, and its validity in predicting morbidity is unknown.

A summary of the several different methods of assessing malnutrition is shown in **Table 1**.

CLINICAL SYNDROMES

The two main clinical syndromes of the extreme forms of PEM are marasmus and kwashiorkor, although a mixed picture also is seen frequently. These are differentiated on the basis of clinical findings, with the primary distinction between kwashiorkor and marasmus being the presence edema in kwashiorkor.

Marasmus

Marasmus, the more common syndrome, is characterized clinically by depletion of subcutaneous fat stores, muscle wasting, and absence of edema. It results from the body's physiologic adaptation to starvation in response to severe deprivation of calories and all nutrients. It most commonly occurs in children younger than 5 years because of their increased caloric requirements and increased susceptibility to infections. These children often appear emaciated, are weak and lethargic, and have associated bradycardia, hypotension, and hypothermia. Their skin is xerotic, wrinkled, and loose because of the loss of subcutaneous fat but is not characterized by any specific dermatosis. Muscle wasting often starts in the axilla and groin, then thigh and buttocks, followed by chest and abdomen, and finally the facial muscles, which are metabolically less active. The loss of buccal fat pads commonly gives the child an appearance of monkey-like or aged facies in severe cases (**Fig. 1**). Severely affected

Table 1
Definitions of malnutrition

Classification	Definition	Grading	
Gomez	Weight below % median WFA	Mild (grade 1)	75%–90% WFA
		Moderate (grade 2)	60%–74% WFA
		Severe (grade 3)	<60% WFA
Waterlow	z-scores (SD) below median WFH	Mild	80%–90% WFH
		Moderate	70%–80% WFH
		Severe	<70% WFH
WHO (wasting)	z-scores (SD) below median WFH	Moderate	$-3 \leq$ z-score <-2
		Severe	z-score <-3
WHO (stunting)	z-scores (SD) below median HFA	Moderate	$-3 \leq$ z-score <-2
		Severe	z-score <-3
Kanawati	MUAC divided by occipitofrontal head circumference	Mild	<0.31
		Moderate	<0.28
		Severe	<0.25
Cole	z-scores of BMI for age	Grade 1	BMI for age z-score <-1
		Grade 2	BMI for age z-score <-2
		Grade 3	BMI for age z-score <-3

Abbreviations: BMI, body mass index; HFA, height for age; MUAC, mid-upper arm circumference; NCHS, US National Center for Health Statistics; SD, standard deviation; WFA, weight for age; WFH, weight for height; WHO, World Health Organization.

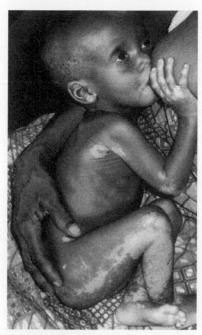

Fig. 1. Marasmus with wasting, loss of subcutaneous tissue, and old man's facies. *Courtesy of* Tom D. Thacher, MD, Rochester, MN.

children are often apathetic but become irritable and difficult to console when handled.

Kwashiorkor

The term kwashiorkor, which first was introduced by Cicely D. Williams in 1935,[33] is taken from the Ga language of Ghana and means the sickness of the weaning. Kwashiorkor tends to occur mainly in older infants and young children, and results from a diet with inadequate protein but reasonably normal caloric intake, often exacerbated by superimposed infection. A common scenario is when the older infant or toddler is displaced from breastfeeding by the birth of a younger sibling and has to wean rapidly but is unable to increase protein intake adequately. The clinical picture is characterized by almost normal weight for age, marked generalized edema, dermatoses, hypopigmented hair, distended abdomen, and hepatomegaly (see **Fig. 2**). The term sugar baby also has been used to describe these children, as their typical diet is low in protein but high in carbohydrate. Edema usually results from a combination of low serum albumin, increased cortisol, and inability to activate antidiuretic hormone. Hair is usually dry, sparse, brittle, and depigmented, appearing reddish yellow. With adequate protein intake, hair color is restored and may result in alternating bands of pale and normal-colored hair, also known as the flag sign, reflecting periods of poor and good nutrition. Cutaneous manifestations are characteristic and progress over days from dry atrophic skin with confluent areas of hyperkeratosis and hyperpigmentation, which then splits when stretched, resulting in erosions and underlying paler, erythematous skin. These patchy areas of dark and pale skin give the impression of crazy paving or flaky paint, particularly over limbs and buttocks. Various skin changes in children with kwashiorkor include: shiny, varnished-looking skin (64%), dark

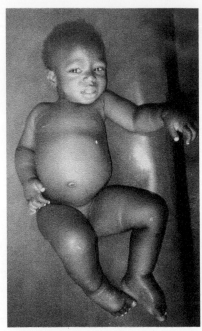

Fig. 2. Kwashiorkor with edema and abdominal distension. *Courtesy of* Tom D. Thacher, MD, Rochester, MN.

erythematous pigmented macules (48%), xerotic crazy paving skin (28%), residual hypopigmentation (18%), and hyperpigmentation and erythema (11%).[34]

Marasmic Kwashiorkor

A child with marasmic kwashiorkor presents with a mixed picture with features of both marasmus and kwashiorkor. Characteristically, these children have concurrent gross wasting and edema and frequently are stunted. They usually have mild hair and skin changes and an enlarged palpable fatty liver.

PATHOPHYSIOLOGY AND ADAPTATION

Inadequate energy intake leads to various physiologic adaptations, including growth restriction; loss of fat, muscle, and visceral mass; reduced basal metabolic rate, and reduced total energy expenditure. The biochemical changes in prolonged starvation involve complex metabolic, hormonal, and glucoregulatory mechanisms. Metabolic changes progress from the early phase, where there is rapid gluconeogenesis with resultant loss of skeletal muscle caused by use of amino acids, pyruvate and lactate, to the later protein conservation phase, with fat mobilization leading to lipolysis and ketogenesis. Major electrolyte changes including sodium retention and intracellular potassium depletion can be explained by decreased activity of glycoside-sensitive energy-dependent sodium pump to increased permeability of cell membranes in kwashiorkor.[35]

Some studies suggest that marasmus represents an adaptive response to starvation, while kwashiorkor is a maladaptive response. Aflatoxins have been proposed to have a role in the pathogenesis of kwashiorkor.[36] Reactive oxygen species also have been postulated to have a role in its pathogenesis.[37] This is supported by the observation that supplementation with N-acetylcysteine, a free radical scavenger, leads to more rapid resolution of signs and symptoms and improved erythrocyte glutathione levels.[38]

ALTERATIONS IN ORGAN SYSTEMS
Endocrine System

The main hormones affected are the thyroid hormones, insulin, and growth hormone. Changes include reduced levels of tri-iodothyroxine (T_3), insulin, insulin-like growth factor-1 (IGF-1), and raised levels of growth hormone and cortisol. Glucose levels are often initially low, with depletion of glycogen stores. Patients frequently also develop some degree of glucose intolerance of unclear etiology and are at risk of profound hypoglycemia during the renourishment phase.

Immune System

Cellular immunity is affected most because of atrophy of the thymus, lymph nodes, and tonsils. Changes include reduced CD4 but relatively preserved CD8-T lymphocytes, loss of delayed hypersensitivity, impaired phagocytosis, and reduced secretory immunoglobulin A (IgA). These changes increase the susceptibility of malnourished children to invasive infections.

Gastrointestinal System

Villous atrophy with resultant loss of disaccharidases, crypt hypoplasia, and altered intestinal permeability results in malabsorption, but losses often rapidly recover once nutrition is improved. Bacterial overgrowth is common with reduced gastric acid secretion. Pancreatic atrophy is also common and results in fat malabsorption. Although fatty infiltration of the liver is common, synthetic function usually is preserved. Protein synthesis, gluconeogenesis, and drug metabolism are decreased.

Cardiovascular System

Cardiac myofibrils are thinned with impaired contractility. Cardiac output is reduced proportionate to weight loss. Bradycardia and hypotension are also common in the severely affected. Intravascular volume frequently is decreased. The combination of bradycardia, impaired cardiac contractility, and electrolyte imbalances predispose these children to arrhythmias.

Respiratory

Reduced thoracic muscle mass, decreased metabolic rate, and electrolyte imbalances (hypokalemia and hypophosphatemia) may result in decreased minute ventilation, leading to impaired ventilatory response to hypoxia.

Neurologic

Specific neurodevelopmental sequelae attributable to just PEM are difficult to ascertain, as PEM frequently coexists with other nutritional deficiencies. Malnutrition has been recognized to cause reductions in the numbers of neurons, synapses, dendritic arborizations, and myelinations, all of which result in decreased brain size.[39] The cerebral cortex is thinned and brain growth slowed. Delays in global function, motor function, and memory have been associated with PEM, with neonates and infants being most susceptible despite the plasticity of the infant's brain.[39]

Hematological

Normochromic anemia is often present but can be exacerbated by other nutrient (iron and folate) deficiencies and infections such as malaria or other parasitic infections. Blood clotting usually is preserved.

CLINICAL FINDINGS

Malnutrition has the potential to affect all organ systems in the body. Initially, clinical findings include lack of adiposity and subcutaneous tissue, poor muscle bulk, irritability, and edema. As malnutrition progresses, growth is delayed, leading to stunting, and other systems become involved, with changes in hair, skin, nails, mucous membranes, and other organs. Micronutrient deficiencies, particularly deficiencies of vitamins and minerals, are common in malnourished patients, so many patients also will exhibit signs of these deficiencies. The most commonly reported micronutrient deficiencies are of iron, zinc, iodine, and vitamin A.[40] Deficiencies of other micronutrients, however, including calcium, vitamin D, vitamin C, folic acid, thiamine, and riboflavin are increasingly being recognized. A summary of the clinical findings in PEM is shown in **Table 2**.

LABORATORY INVESTIGATIONS

Laboratory investigations can be useful to identify deficiencies before clinical symptoms develop, confirm deficiencies associated with specific disease states, and monitor recovery from malnutrition. The most useful tests in assessing nutritional state are hemoglobin and red cell indices, and serum albumin. Electrolytes, specifically potassium, magnesium, and phosphate, should be monitored closely in the early treatment phase to avoid refeeding syndrome. WHO recommends performing the following tests in malnourished children: blood glucose, hemoglobin and blood smear, electrolytes, serum albumin, urine microscopy and culture, stool microscopy and culture including for parasites, and human immunodeficiency virus testing.[41] Specific testing should be directed by the history and physical examination.

Complete blood cell count measuring hemoglobin, red cell indices, and blood film is helpful to demonstrate anemia, which is usually normochromic but can be microcytic from iron deficiency. Blood film can identify malarial parasites, if appropriate. Additional testing including iron studies, vitamin B_{12}, and folic acid measurements are also useful when assessing for deficiencies.

Biochemical testing is useful in determining hypoglycemia; electrolyte imbalances, particularly of sodium, potassium, phosphate, magnesium, and protein stores with serum albumin and prealbumin levels. Fat-soluble vitamin measurement may be indicated if there is evidence of malabsorption.

Culture and microscopy of urine and stool are important, as concurrent infections are common in malnourished children. If clinically indicated, blood cultures and lumbar puncture also may be necessary. Other additional tests such as QuantiFERON testing for tuberculosis, celiac serology, sweat test, and thyroid function testing also may be warranted depending on history and physical examination.

Radiology and other imaging studies are often unnecessary but may be performed if clinically indicated. Skeletal radiographs maybe useful in assessing bone age and detecting early evidence of scurvy or rickets. Body composition testing, including air displacement plethysmography, bioimpedance analysis, dual energy x-ray absorptiometry (DEXA), and total body potassium are potentially helpful in identifying lean

Table 2
Clinical signs of malnutrition

Site	Signs
Face	Moon face (kwashiorkor), simian facies (marasmus)
Eye	Dry eyes, pale conjunctiva, Bitot's spots (vitamin A), periorbital edema
Mouth	Angular stomatitis, cheilitis, glossitis, spongy bleeding gums (vitamin C), parotid enlargement
Teeth	Enamel mottling, delayed eruption
Hair	Dull, sparse, brittle hair, hypopigmentation, flag sign (alternating bands of light and normal color), broomstick eyelashes, alopecia.
Skin	Loose and wrinkled (marasmus), shiny and edematous (kwashiorkor), dry, follicular hyperkeratosis, patchy hyper- and hypopigmentation (crazy paving or flaky paint dermatoses), erosions, poor wound healing
Nail	Koilonychia, thin and soft nail plates, fissures or ridges
Musculature	Muscle wasting particularly buttocks and thighs. Chvostek or Trousseau signs (hypocalcemia)
Skeletal	Deformities usually a result of calcium, vitamin D or vitamin C deficiencies
Abdomen	Distended—hepatomegaly with fatty liver; ascites may be present
Cardiovascular	Bradycardia, hypotension, reduced cardiac output, small vessel vasculopathy
Neurologic	Global developmental delay, loss of knee and ankle reflexes, impaired memory
Hematological	Pallor, petechiae, bleeding diathesis
Behavior	Lethargic, apathetic, irritable on handling

mass or lack of it in malnourished patients. These investigations, however, are expensive, require highly specialized equipment, and are done in the research setting.

MANAGEMENT

WHO has developed guidelines for managing severe malnutrition.[41] These guidelines, with some adaptation to local conditions, have been demonstrated to reduce case fatality rates when administered in Bangladesh, Africa, and South America.[42–48] Infection and sepsis continue to be the main causes of death in severe acute malnutrition, although other causes include dehydration, electrolyte imbalances, and heart failure.[42,47,49] Death also can occur once treatment is instituted because of refeeding syndrome with its associated electrolyte and metabolic changes. The decision as to whether to treat in the hospital or community depends on the patient's clinical condition and availability of resources. Controlled trials show that community- or home-based management for children with uncomplicated acute severe malnutrition results in equivalent or superior outcomes to hospital care.[50,51] The authors have adopted algorithm suggested by Collins and colleagues to help clinicians decide whether the malnourished child can be managed at home or in the hospital (**Fig. 3**).[52]

WHO has formulated a three-phase management approach, where the patient initially is resuscitated and stabilized (phase 1), before starting nutritional rehabilitation (phase 2), and eventual follow-up and recurrence prevention (phase 3).

Phase 1: Resuscitate and Stabilize

The main aim during this phase is to resuscitate, rehydrate, treat infections, prevent sepsis, and monitor closely to avoid developing complications of treatment. Patients

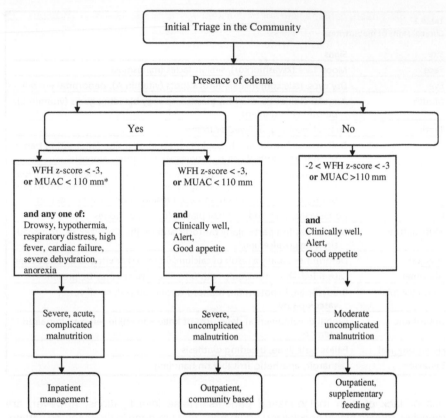

Fig. 3. Algorithm to help clinicians decide whether the malnourished child needs hospitalization. *Abbreviations:* MUAC, mid-upper arm circumference; WFH, weight-for-height. WFH z-score based on WHO criteria. *For children between 6 and 59 months or length/height 65 to 110 cm as a proxy for age.

are most vulnerable during this period, which usually lasts about 1 week. Feeding should be instituted carefully and slowly, with restriction of caloric intake to 60% to 80% of caloric requirement for age. This is to avoid refeeding syndrome, but many severely malnourished children also have some degree of malabsorption because of disaccharidase deficiencies, villous atrophy, and relative pancreatic insufficiency. Continuous nasogastric feeding or small frequent meals including at night may be necessary to avoid hypoglycemia. Vitamins, especially thiamine and oral phosphate, also are administered, in addition to supplemental feeds to prevent the potentially fatal hypophosphatemia with refeeding.

Refeeding syndrome is thought to be explained by the sudden availability of glucose, leading to inhibition of gluconeogenesis and an insulin surge. This causes rapid influx of potassium, magnesium, and phosphate intracellularly and thus low serum levels and poor myocardial contractility. This clinical syndrome, which can manifest with excessive sweatiness, muscle weakness, tachycardia, and heart failure, may be prevented by avoiding rapid carbohydrate feeding, supplementing phosphate and thiamine during the initial increase in nutritional intake, and monitoring the patient carefully for alterations in serum phosphate, potassium, and magnesium.[53–55]

During this phase, patients also should be kept warm, as they are often hypothermic and may need restriction of physical activities because of decreased cardiac output. Antibiotics additionally may be necessary even in the absence of fever if infection is suspected.

Phase 2: Nutritional Rehabilitation

The rehabilitation phase starts once acute complications have been addressed adequately with gradual return of appetite, resolution of diarrhea and sepsis, and correction of electrolyte imbalances. The main goals of this phase are to increase dietary caloric intake, treat occult infections, complete vaccination, improve family involvement, and stimulate psychomotor activity. Weight loss is common initially in children with kwashiorkor as their edema resolves. Most children will need 120% to 140% of their estimated caloric requirements to achieve desired weight gain and maintain catch-up growth. This phase usually lasts between 2 to 6 weeks. WHO recommends delaying iron therapy until rehabilitation occurs because of concerns about increased infection risk, although a recent review does not support this practice.[56,57] Elemental iron 2 to 6 mg/kg should be prescribed for 3 months.

Phase 3: Follow-up and Recurrence Prevention

Discharge planning and follow-up are recommended, as these patients have tendency to relapse. Interventions that have been reported to be helpful in preventing undernutrition in children include promoting breast-feeding, complementary and supplemental feeding, zinc and vitamin A supplementation, universal salt iodization, and hand-washing and other hygiene measures.[58] Universal provision of iodized salt could reduce stunting by 36% and mortality for children younger than 3 years by 25%.[58-60]

REFERENCES

1. de Onis M, Monteiro C, Clugston G. The worldwide magnitude of protein energy malnutrition: an overview from the WHO global database on child growth. Bull World Health Organ 1993;71(6):703–12.
2. Caulfield LE, de Onis M, Blössner M, et al. Undernutrition as an underlying cause of child deaths associated with diarrhea, pneumonia, malaria, and measles. Am J Clin Nutr 2004;80:193–8.
3. Pelletier DL, Frongillo EA Jr, Habicht JP. Epidemiologic evidence for a potentiating effect of malnutrition on child mortality. Am J Public Health 1993;83(8):1130–3.
4. Pelletier DL, Frongilllo EA Jr. Changes in child survival are strongly associated with changes in malnutrition in developing countries. J Nutr 2003;133:107–19.
5. Pelletier DL, Frongillo EA Jr, Habicht JP. The effects of malnutrition on child mortality in developing countries. Bull World Health Organ 1995;73:443–8.
6. Joosten KFM, Hulst JM. Prevalence of malnutrition in paediatric hospital patients. Curr Opin Pediatr 2008;20:590–6.
7. Pawellek I, Dokoupil K, Koletzko B. Prevalence of malnutrition in paediatric hospital patients. Clin Nutr 2008;27:72–6.
8. Secker DJ, Jeejeebhoy KN. Subjective global nutritional assessment for children. Am J Clin Nutr 2007;85:1083–9.
9. Hendricks KM, Duggan C, Gallagher L, et al. Malnutrition in hospitalized pediatric patients. Current prevalence. Arch Pediatr Adolesc Med 1995;149:1118–22.
10. Black RE, Allen LH, Bhutta ZA, et al. Maternal and child undernutrition: global and regional exposures and health consequences. Lancet 2008;371:243–60.

11. Department of Economic and Social Affairs. UN Population Division. World population prospects: the sex and age distribution of the world population, the 2000 revision. New York: United Nations; 2001.
12. de Onis M, Blössner M, Borghi E, et al. Estimates of global prevalence of childhood underweight in 1990 and 2015. JAMA 2004;291:2600–6.
13. Maia MM, Fausto MA, Vieira EL, et al. The prevalence of malnutrition and its risk factors in children attending outpatient clinics in the city of Manaus, Amazonas, Brazil. Arch Latinoam Nutr 2008;58:234–40.
14. Gomez F, Ramos-Galvan R, Frenk S, et al. Mortality in second- and third-degree malnutrition. J Trop Pediatr 1956;2:77–83.
15. Seoane N, Latham MC. Nutritional anthropometry in the identification of malnutrition in childhood. J Trop Pediatr Environ Child Health 1971;17:1271–4.
16. Bear MT, Harris AB. Pediatric nutrition assessment: identifying children at risk. J Am Diet Assoc 1997;97(10S2):107–15.
17. Waterlow JC. Classification and definition of protein calorie malnutrition. BMJ 1972;3:566–9.
18. Waterlow JC, Buzina R, Keller W, et al. The presentation and use of height and weight data for comparing the nutritional status of groups of children under the age of 10years. Bull World Health Organ 1977;55:489–98.
19. Hamill PW, Drizd TA, Johnson CL, et al. NCHS growth curves for children birth–18years. Washington, DC: National Center for Health Statistics; 1977.
20. Lavoi-Pierre GJ, Keller W, Dixon H, et al. Measuring change in nutritional status. Guidelines for assessing the nutritional impact of supplementary feeding programmes for vulnerable groups. Geneva (Switzerland): World Health Organization; 1983.
21. World Health Organization. Physical status: the use and interpretation of anthropometry. Geneva (Switzerland): World Health Organization; 1995.
22. WHO Multicentre Growth Reference Study Group. WHO child growth standards based on length/height, weight, and age. Acta Paediatr 2006;450:76–85.
23. Seal A, Kerac M. Operational implications of using 2006 World Health Organization growth standards in nutrition programmes: secondary data analysis. BMJ 2007;334:733.
24. Prost MA, Jahn A, Floyd S, et al. Implication of new WHO growth standards on identification of risk factors and estimated prevalence of malnutrition in rural Malawian infants. PLoS One 2008;3(7):e2684.
25. Kanawati AA, McLaren DS. Assessment of marginal malnutrition. Nature 1970;228:573–5.
26. Myatt M, Khara T, Collins S. A review of methods to detect cases of severely malnourished children in the community for their admission into community-based therapeutic care programs. Food Nutr Bull 2006;27:S7–23.
27. Briend A, Zimicki S. Validation of arm circumference as an indicator of risk of death in one to four year old children. Nutr Res 1986;6:249–61.
28. Briend A, Dykewicz C, Graven K, et al. Usefulness of nutritional indices and classifications in predicting death of malnourished children. Br Med J (Clin Res Ed) 1986;293:373–5.
29. Briend A, Wojtyniak B, Rowland MGM. Arm circumference and other factors in children at heightened risk of death in rural Bangladesh. Lancet 1987;26:725–7.
30. Chen LC, Chowdhury MK, Huffman SL. Anthropometric assessment of energy protein malnutrition and subsequent risk of mortality among preschool children. Am J Clin Nutr 1980;33:1836–45.

31. Alam N, Wojtyniak B, Rahaman MM. Anthropometric indicators and risk of death. Am J Clin Nutr 1989;49:884–8.
32. Cole TJ, Flegal KM, Nicholls D, et al. Body mass index cutoff to define thinness in children and adolescents: international survey. BMJ 2007;335:194–202.
33. Williams CD. Kwashiorkor: a nutritional disease of children associated with a maize diet. Lancet 1935;229:1151–2.
34. Lowy G, Meilman I. Kwashiorkor. Dermatological and clinical aspects. Analysis of 100 cases. Med Cutan Ibero Lat Am 1975;3(3):181–9.
35. Patrick J, Golden M. Leukocyte electrolytes and sodium transport in protein energy malnutrition. Am J Clin Nutr 1977;30:1478–81.
36. Lamplugh SM, Hendrickse RG. Aflatoxins in the livers of children with kwashiorkor. Ann Trop Paediatr 1982;2:101–4.
37. Golden MH, Ramdath D. Free radicals in the pathogenesis of kwashiorkor. Proc Nutr Soc 1987;46:53–68.
38. Badaloo A, Reid M, Forrester T, et al. Cysteine supplementation improves the erythrocyte glutathione synthesis rate in children with severe edematous malnutrition. Am J Clin Nutr 2002;76:646–52.
39. Georgieff MK. Nutrition and the developing brain: nutrient priorities and measurement. Am J Clin Nutr 2007;85:614S–20S.
40. Bhutta ZA. Micronutrient needs of malnourished children. Curr Opin Clin Nutr Metab Care 2008;11:309–14.
41. World Health Organization. Management of severe malnutrition: a manual for physicians and other senior health workers. Geneva (Switzerland): World Health Organization; 1999.
42. Ashworth A, Chopra M, McCoy D, et al. WHO guidelines for management of severe malnutrition in rural South African hospitals: effect on case fatality and the influence of operational factors. Lancet 2004;363(9415):1110–5.
43. Ahmed T, Ali M, Ullah MM, et al. Mortality in severely malnourished children with diarrhea and use of standard management protocol. Lancet 1999;353(9168):1919–22.
44. Deen JL, Funk M, Guevera VC, et al. Implementation of WHO guidelines on management of severe malnutrition in hospitals in Africa. Bull World Health Organ 2003;81:237–43.
45. Briend A. Management of severe malnutrition: efficacious or effective? J Pediatr Gastroenterol Nutr 2001;32:521–2.
46. Cavalcante AA, Pinheiro LM, Monte C, et al. Treatment of malnutrition in Brazil: simple solutions to a common problem. Trop Doct 1998;28:95–7.
47. Bernal C, Velasquez C, Alcaraz G, et al. Treatment of severe malnutrition in children: experience in implementing the World Health Organisation guidelines in Turbo, Columbia. J Pediatr Gastroenterol Nutr 2008;46:322–8.
48. Falbo AR, Alves JG, Filho MB, et al. Decline in hospital mortality rate after the use of the World Health Organization protocol for management of severe malnutrition. Trop Doct 2009;39:71–2.
49. Bachou H, Tumwine JK, Mwadime R, et al. Risk factors in hospital deaths in severely malnourished children in Kampala, Uganda. BMC Pediatr 2006;6:7–16.
50. Ciliberto MA, Sandige H, Ndekha MJ, et al. A comparison of home-based therapy with ready-to-use therapeutic food with standard therapy in the treatment of malnourished Malawian children: a controlled clinical effectiveness trial. Am J Clin Nutr 2005;81:864–70.
51. Linneman Z, Matilsky D, Ndekha M, et al. A large-scale operation study of home-based therapy with ready-to-use therapeutic food in childhood malnutrition in Malawi. Matern Child Nutr 2007;3:206–15.

52. Collins S, Yates R. The need to update the classification of acute malnutrition. Lancet 2003;362(9379):249.

53. Crook MA, Hally V, Panteli JV. The importance of the refeeding syndrome. Nutrition 2001;17:632–7.

54. Stanga Z, Brunner A, Leuenberger M, et al. Nutrition in clinical practice—the refeeding syndrome: illustrative cases and guidelines for prevention and treatment. Eur J Clin Nutr 2008;62:687–94.

55. Manary MJ, Hart CA, Whyte MP. Severe hypophosphatemia in children with kwashiorkor is associated with increased mortality. J Pediatr 1998;133:789–91.

56. Smith IF, Taiwo O, Golden MH. Plant protein rehabilitation diets and iron supplementation of protein energy malnourished child. Eur J Clin Nutr 1989;43:763–8.

57. Gera T, Sachdev HP. Effect of iron supplementation on incidence of infectious illness in children: systemic review. BMJ 2002;325:1142–7.

58. Bhutta ZA, Ahmed T, Black RE, et al. What works? Interventions for maternal and child undernutrition and survival. Lancet 2008;371:417–40.

59. Manary MJ, Sandige H. Management of acute moderate and severe childhood malnutrition. BMJ 2008;337:2180.

60. Collins S. Treating severe acute malnutrition seriously. Arch Dis Child 2007;92: 453–61.

Nutrient Deficiencies in the Premature Infant

Malika D. Shah, MD, FAAP[a],*, Shilpa R. Shah, MBBS, MD, MRCPCH[b]

KEYWORDS

- Premature • Nutrition • Fetus • Accretion
- Postdischarge • Deficiency

Premature infants are a population prone to nutrient deficiencies. Because the early diet of these infants is entirely amenable to intervention, understanding the pathophysiology behind these deficiencies is important for both the neonatologists who care for them acutely and for pediatricians who are responsible for their care through childhood. This article reviews the normal accretion of nutrients in the fetus, discusses specific nutrient deficiencies that are exacerbated in the postnatal period, and identifies key areas for future research.

IN UTERO ACCRETION OF NUTRIENTS

The potential for adverse effects of inadequate or excess intake of any nutrient on any organ system is based on the timing, dose, and duration of exposure.[1] The lungs, gastrointestinal system, immune system, and brain undergo rapid growth and maturation during the last two trimesters and throughout the first year of life. Growth rates mirroring intrauterine growth are presumed to result in optimal postnatal development. Although this strategy has come under scrutiny because premature infants who show greater catch-up growth seem to be at increased risk for metabolic disease in later years,[2–7] the known positive effects of catch-up growth on neurodevelopment seem to outweigh these concerns and most published studies on premature infant growth patterns continue to use the intrauterine growth standard.[8–10]

The fetus is ideally adapted for survival, taking most nutrients it needs irrespective of the nutritional status of the mother. Except in extreme situations of nutrient deprivation, most vital nutrients are transported in a fashion that ensures proper substrate delivery to the fetus for growth. Placental transfer of several macronutrients and important micronutrients has been well studied (**Table 1**).

[a] Department of Pediatrics, Division of Neonatology, Northwestern University's Feinberg School of Medicine, 250 East Superior Street, Suite 05-2146, Chicago, IL 60611
[b] Department of Paediatric, Royal Belfast Hospital for Sick Children, 180 Falls Road, Belfast BT 12 6BE, Northern Ireland, UK
* Corresponding author.
E-mail address: m-shah@northwestern.edu (M.D. Shah).

Pediatr Clin N Am 56 (2009) 1069–1083
doi:10.1016/j.pcl.2009.08.001
0031-3955/09/$ – see front matter © 2009 Elsevier Inc. All rights reserved.

Table 1
Placental transfer of key nutrients

Nutrient	Mode of Transport	Fetal Accretion During Third Trimester
Glucose	Facilitated diffusion[108]	1% throughout gestation[11]
Fatty acids	Simple and receptor-mediated diffusion (ARA and DHA preferentially transported)[109]	3 g adipose tissue/kg[11] 552 mg/d N-6[100] 67 mg/d N-3[100]
Protein	Active transport[101]	1.8–2.2 g/d[11]
Iron	Active transport[102]	60%[48]
Calcium	Active transport[103]	80%[103]
Phosphorus	Active transport[103]	80%[103]

Abbreviations: ARA, arachidonic acid; DHA, docohexanoic acid.

In 1976, in a landmark paper published in *Growth*, Ziegler and colleagues[11] described the body of the reference fetus using reports of whole-body chemical analysis of infants born prematurely who were stillborn or passed away within 48 hours. He found fetal body composition to be dynamic: although percentages of body water, extracellular water, sodium, and chloride decrease during gestation, percentages of intracellular water, protein, fat, calcium, iron, and magnesium increase. Between 24 and 40 weeks gestation, water content declines from approximately 87% to 71%, protein rises from 8.8% to 12%, and fat from 1% to 13.1%. Early gestation is characterized by accumulation of lean tissue, whereas late gestation is characterized by accumulation of fat.[11] Current recommended intake levels for premature infants are based on fetal accretion rates of specific nutrients during the third trimester and do not compensate for additional needs for sick infants.

As a result, the more premature an infant, the more nutrient deficient he or she is at birth. Umbilical cord blood samples confirm that premature infants have lower plasma levels of certain nutrients. These results likely underestimate the deficiencies, because plasma levels can be in a normal range at the expense of tissue deficits (**Table 2**).

Table 2
Umbilical cord blood levels of nutrients in preterm infants

Nutrient	Age if Preterm (wk)	Premature Infant Cord Blood (SD)	Term Infant Cord Blood (37–41 wk)	Reference
Ferritin (μg/dL)	23	63	171	Siddappa et al, 2007[104]
TIBC (μmol/L) Iron (μmol/L)	24–29	31 (27–35) 17.4 (10.7)	42 (36–49.5) 20.8 (8.8)	Sweet et al, 2001[105]
Selenium (μg/dL)	23	45.85 (15.4)	68.4 (26.6)	Makhoul et al, 2004[106]
Total protein (g/dL) Albumin (g/dL) Calcium (mg/dL) Triglycerides (mg/dL) Total cholesterol (mg/dL) Magnesium (mg/dL) Zinc (μg/dL)	<37	4.24 (0.5) 1.84 (0.264) 5.67 (0.89) 52.10 (18.87) 51.46 (19.39) 1.62 (0.31) 70.25 (24.25)	5.50 (0.735) 2.494 (0.391) 8.08 (0.96) 66.66 (20.3) 69.79 (19.81) 1.96 (0.19) 92.24 (19.40)	Elizabeth et al, 2001[107]

Hospital Course Predisposes to Nutrient Deficiencies

At birth, clamping of the cord immediately disrupts all nutrient delivery from the placenta. Premature infants are then abruptly exposed to an environment that exacerbates virtually every existing nutrient deficiency. Although incubators and mechanical ventilators are used to minimize energy expenditure in preterm infants, other factors including enteral feeding, respiratory distress, chronic lung disease, and therapy with methylxanthines result in higher energy needs than in utero.[12] Management of respiratory distress syndrome, chronic lung disease, patent ductus arteriosus, intraventricular hemorrhage, and feeding intolerance frequently involves restriction of fluids and delayed advancement of enteral feeds. To support optimal growth, energy delivery must surpass energy requirements and this can be difficult to achieve with such restrictions in place.

Parenteral and enteral nutrition do not achieve the same nutrient delivery as the placenta. As a result, premature infants accrue protein and energy deficits rather quickly. Embleton and colleagues[13] studied preterm infants less than 34 weeks and found that nutrient intakes meeting current recommended dietary intakes were rarely achieved during early life. Despite initiation of parenteral nutrition by day of life 2, enteral feeds by day of life 4, and over 80% of participants receiving full enteral feeds by 12 days of life, cumulative energy and protein deficits were 400 kcal/kg in infants less than 30 weeks gestation in the first week of life. By the end of the fifth week, cumulative energy and protein deficits were over 813 kcal/kg for such infants. Variation in dietary intake accounted for 45% of the variation in changes in z score suggesting that the growth restriction may be partially amenable to intervention.[13]

Breast milk is always preferred for its immune properties, tolerance, and protective effect against necrotizing enterocolitis.[14] The nutrient content of unfortified breast milk is insufficient to meet the requirements in preterm infants. Approximately 30% to 50% of very low birth weight (VLBW) infants who are fed unfortified human milk or term infant formulas have decreased bone mineral content compared with a fetus of comparable weight or gestational age.[15-17] VLBW infants fed unfortified milk achieve only a third of the intrauterine calcium-phosphorous accrual rates when consuming 180 to 200 mL/kg/d.[18] As a consequence, preterm and VLBW infants fed unfortified milk have abnormalities in calcium-phosphorous balance and increase in serum alkaline phosphatase activity compared with infants fed fortified preterm formula.[16]

It is the combined responsibility of all members of the heath care team to ensure increased opportunities for the availability of maternal breast milk. Furman and coworkers[19] conducted a prospective observational study of 119 mothers of singleton VLBW infants. Over 70% intended to breastfeed, but only 34% continued lactating beyond 40 weeks corrected gestational age. Significant correlates of lactation beyond 40 weeks corrected age included initiating milk expression within 6 hours of delivery, expressing milk greater than or equal to five times per day, and kangaroo care. These correlates remained significant after controlling for maternal age, race, marital status, and education beyond high school. Education on lactation for pregnant mothers at risk for premature delivery should begin in the antenatal period.[19] For infants unable to receive breast milk, formula enriched with additional phosphorus, calcium, and protein and used during the early neonatal period has been shown to improve bone mineralization at discharge over standard formula, even when caloric composition is the same.[20]

Postdischarge Nutritional Deficiencies

Postdischarge nutritional deficiencies in premature infants represent a grossly understudied area. Greater awareness of the long-term nutritional, metabolic, immune, and neurocognitive benefits of breast milk and has prompted increased advocacy for prolonged breastfeeding. The recently published World Health Organization Multicenter Growth Reference Study international growth charts used breastfed full-term infants as the standard for growth during the first year.[21] For premature infants, it is unclear what should be the optimal postdischarge growth standard. The commonly used Infant Health and Development Program growth charts have limited use because they used data from the 1980s and only followed 867 infants.[22] Although the updated Fenton growth chart includes several large meta-analyses, growth data for 40 weeks onward was collected in term, not premature, infants.[23] Premature infants differ significantly from term infants even after correcting for gestation age. Approximately 90% of preterm infants are less than the tenth percentile for corrected gestation age at the time of discharge.[9]

Nutritional status at discharge remains an uncontrolled variable in virtually every long-term study of premature infants. Data on how to feed these premature infants postdischarge are conflicting. Some studies suggest, whereas others do not, more favorable growth profiles and rates of bone mineralization with the use of enriched formula postdischarge.[24–27] A common misperception is that infants fed enriched formula are getting more calories. The relatively few studies examining caloric intake suggest that infants fed regular formulas ad libitum generally consume more calories.[28,29] For example, Koo and Hockman[30] in a randomized, double-blind comparison study involving 89 preterm infants found that those fed formula for term infants (20 kcal/oz) had greater weight gain and accrued more lean mass, fat mass, and bone mineral density during the first year than those who were fed a nutrient-enriched formula (22 kcal/oz). Although there is a paucity of data, small studies done on premature infants fed exclusively unfortified human milk postdischarge suggest they may be a population particularly vulnerable to nutrient deficiencies. Wauben and colleagues[31] found premature infants exclusively fed breast milk to have decreased bone mineral content at 6 months corrected age when compared with formula-fed infants. These differences correlated with lower calcium, phosphorus, and protein intakes in postbreastfed compared with post–formula-fed infants. Fortification of at least half of the milk for 12 weeks after hospital discharge may be an effective strategy in addressing early discharge nutrient deficits and poor growth without unduly influencing human milk feeding when intensive support is provided.[32] Schanler[33] evaluated preterm infants fed unfortified formula and found decreased bone mineral content 1 year postdischarge that later improved by 2 years.[34,35] Infant iron deficiency anemia and clinically significant zinc deficiency has also been reported in small studies.[34,35] Infants consuming lower volumes benefit the most from nutrient-enriched formula postdischarge.[36,37]

SPECIFIC NUTRIENT DEFICIENCIES

This section discusses specific nutrient deficiencies that the premature infant can develop and also other nutrients whose supplementation may be beneficial to premature infants. These nutrients include minerals, trace elements, vitamins, long-chain polyunsaturated fatty acids (LCPUFAs), and carnitine.

Calcium and Phosphorus

Preterm infants have increased calcium requirements compared with term infants because they miss part or all of the third trimester, which is an important period for fetal accretion of calcium. Nonsupplemented human milk cannot meet the calcium needs of a preterm infant.[16,18] To account for these higher requirements preterm infant formulas contain more calcium and phosphorous than term infants formulas. The calcium content of human milk can be increased by supplementing with human milk fortifiers.

The calcium/phosphorus ratio in infant formulas may be an important determinant of calcium absorption and retention. In human milk, the calcium/phosphorus ratio is approximately 2.[38] Based on the American Academy of Pediatrics Committee on Nutrition recommendations (2003), the recommended calcium/phosphorus ratio is 1.9.[36] The Committee on Nutrition of the Preterm Infant of the European Society of Pediatric Gastroenterology and Nutrition (1987) recommended that preterm formulas have a calcium/phosphorus ratio between 1.4 and 2.[39]

Adequate intake of calcium, phosphorus, and vitamin D is required to prevent osteopenia of prematurity. Osteopenia of prematurity tends to remain asymptomatic but severely affected infants may develop rickets, difficulty in weaning from the ventilator, poor linear growth, and hypotonia.[38] Osteopenia of prematurity is common in VLBW infants and gestation age less than 28 weeks. The major risk factors are extreme prematurity, prolonged feeding intolerance, parenteral nutrition, inadequate calcium and phosphate intake,[40] chronic lung disease, and prolonged immobility.[38]

Screening for osteopenia of prematurity should begin at about 6 weeks postnatal age in at-risk infants and should continue at 1- to 2-week intervals to allow early identification of the biochemical changes.[38] The biochemical screening tools are serum concentrations of calcium, inorganic phosphate, and alkaline phosphatase. None of these measurements by themselves, however, is adequately sensitive for diagnostic purposes. One study showed that a combination of serum alkaline phosphatase greater than 900 IU/L and inorganic phosphate less than 1.8 mmol/L in a group of preterm infants yielded a sensitivity of 100% and a specificity of 70% in detecting low bone mineral density at 3 months corrected gestational age.[41]

The major goal in the treatment of osteopenia of prematurity is to provide sufficient calcium, phosphate, and vitamin D[42] to achieve intrauterine rates of bone mineralization. This requires 200 mg/kg/d of calcium and 90 mg/kg/d of phosphorus enterally. Early trophic enteral feeding significantly enhances achievement of full-volume feeds, calcium/phosphate intake, and retention. In addition to the use of preterm infant formulas and human milk fortifiers, extremely preterm infants may need additional calcium and phosphorus after discharge until they reach 3.5 to 4 kg.[38] Infants with osteopenia, rickets, and fractures require additional therapy with calcium and phosphorus supplements until normalization of serum alkaline phosphatase concentration or at least 6 months postnatal age.[38]

Iron

Premature infants have limited iron stores, which are prone to rapidly being depleted within the first few weeks of postnatal growth. The risk factors for developing iron deficiency include inadequate intake and frequent phlebotomy.[43] Increased erythropoiesis, rapid catch-up growth, and use of erythropoietin further deplete iron stores.[44–46] The hemoglobin nadir is lower and occurs earlier in preterm and VLBW infants.[47] As the body preferentially distributes iron to red blood cells, decreased hemoglobin is a late finding of iron deficiency.[48] Supplementing preterm and VLBW infants tolerating 100 mL/kg/d of enteral feeds with iron was found to be safe, feasible, and reduced the incidence of iron deficiency and late blood transfusions.[49]

Because iron deficiency seems particularly amenable to intervention, several groups have studied iron status of premature infants postdischarge over the last few decades. Catch-up growth is associated with increased iron requirements. Studies done in the 1960s and 1970s showed that supplementing preterm infants with iron 2 mg/kg/d prevented iron deficiency anemia in premature infants at 6 to 12 months corrected gestational age.[46,50,51] More recently, Schiza and colleagues[52] found over 10% of predominantly formula-fed premature infants (32–36 weeks gestation) had decreased iron stores (ferritin <12 μg/L) between 3 and 12 months postdischarge. Anemia is a late finding of iron deficiency, a point at which brain iron stores may already be severely depleted and the effects on development may be irreversible.[48,53] The earlier studies suggesting efficacy of supplemental iron of 2 mg/kg/d in preventing iron deficiency anemia in preterm infants for the entire first year of life must be interpreted with caution because iron deficiency may exist without anemia. In addition, recommendations based on studies conducted during postdischarge follow-up of larger preterm infants fed iron-fortified formula may not be applicable to VLBW at greater risk for iron deficiency because of limited reserves at birth and inadequate iron in breast milk.

Zinc

Zinc is perhaps the most widely studied microelement in infant feeding because it is a component of several enzymes involved in intermediary metabolism ranging from growth to cell differentiation and metabolism of proteins, carbohydrates, and lipids.[54] The clinical features of zinc deficiency include anorexia, failure to thrive, irritability, periorificial and extensor dermatitis, stomatitis, glossitis, nail dystrophy, diarrhea, and increased susceptibility to infection.[55] Many ex-preterm infants have subtle zinc deficiency, which may benefit from extra zinc.[56] Zinc deficiency has been described in breastfed preterm infants (gestation <34 weeks).[55] This may be explained by the relative inability of breast milk to supply the zinc needs of the preterm infant. Affected infants tend to be boys usually presenting at about 3 months postnatal age, which coincides with the nadir for plasma zinc concentrations (6–12 weeks).[55] Male infants may disproportionately be more affected because of more rapid weight gain. Current recommended intakes for enterally fed infants are from 500 to 1000 μg/kg/d. Recommended zinc intakes for the parenterally fed neonate range from 150 to 400 μg/kg/d.[57]

Copper

Copper is an essential trace mineral that functions as a cofactor in many important enzymes, such as ceruloplasmin, elastase, cytochrome oxidase, and superoxide dismutase.[58] Copper deficiency is associated with hypochromic anemia resistant to iron supplementation, neutropenia, osteoporosis, and difficulty in gaining weight.[54] Preterm infants have decreased serum copper and hepatic stores compared with full-term infants.[59] The serum copper concentrations in full-term infants rapidly increase to reach adult levels. Preterm infants continue to have serum low serum copper, however, during the first 4 to 6 postnatal months.[60] This difference in serum copper concentrations is dependent on the rate of growth (ie, infants growing rapidly have relatively decreased serum copper concentrations compared with infants with slower growth).[61] Copper requirements increase during phases when there is rapid growth.

The World Health Organization has recommended a minimum intake of 60 μg/kg/d for infants,[62] whereas the new recommended daily allowance for copper is 200 μg/d.[63] The copper content in breast milk, preterm infant formulas, and formula for full-term infants is 0.2 to 0.4 mg/L, 1 to 2 mg/dL, and 0.4 to 0.6 mg/L, respectively. In comparison, breast milk has the least amount of copper; however, it is more bioavailable than infant formula.[64,65]

Selenium

Selenium is a constituent part of selenoenzymes, including glutathione peroxidase, which has a role in protecting against oxidative damage. Glutathione peroxidase participates in antioxidant defense and helps scavenge free radicals and protect the body against oxidative insult.[66] Serum glutathione peroxidase levels have been used to assess short-term selenium status, whereas erythrocyte glutathione peroxidase levels have been used as an indicator of longer-term status. Serum selenium levels are also used frequently to assess selenium status.

Premature infants have lower tissue and plasma selenium concentrations than term infants.[67] No data exist on the fetal concentrations of selenium, but a selenium intake of at least 1 μg/kg/d is recommended to achieve intrauterine tissue accretion.[54] The evaluation of selenium status in preterm infants is difficult. In one study preterm infants were fed either human milk (24 ng selenium/mL); preterm formula (7.8 ng selenium/mL); or preterm formula supplemented with selenium (34.8 ng selenium/mL). Although selenium intakes of infants fed the selenium-supplemented formula were greater than those of infants in the other two groups, there were no differences found in plasma or erythrocyte selenium or glutathione peroxidase.[67] Risk for developing selenium deficiency may be increased, however, in disorders associated with oxidative stress. Preterm infants with respiratory distress syndrome receiving parenteral nutrition without selenium had decreased serum concentrations of selenium compared with infants supplemented with 3 μg/kg of selenium in parenteral fluids and prevented the fall in the concentration seen in nonsupplemented infants.[68]

Darlow and colleagues[69] assessed the effects of selenium supplementation in a multicenter, randomized, double-blind study of VLBW infants. Supplementation was associated with increased serum concentrations of selenium at postnatal age 28 days and 36 weeks corrected gestation age. These observations have been confirmed by most studies on selenium with preterm infants. It is still unclear, however, whether selenium is effective in preventing or ameliorating respiratory distress syndrome, bronchopulmonary dysplasia, retinopathy of prematurity, and other disorders associated with oxidative stress. In a meta-analysis that included three studies, selenium supplementation of very preterm infants was associated with a reduction in one or more episodes of sepsis.[70] Supplementation was not associated, however, with improved survival, a reduction in chronic lung disease, or retinopathy of prematurity. Because these data were dominated by data from a large trial conducted in New Zealand (a country with low selenium concentrations), the findings may not apply to preterm infants in geographic areas with higher selenium concentrations.[70]

The amount of selenium recommended for supplementation in preterm infants is variable. In the United States, 2 μg/kg/d given parenterally is recommended. A large clinical trial conducted in New Zealand, however, suggested 3 μg/kg/d to maintain concentrations at the umbilical cord blood levels.[69] To increase the concentrations above umbilical cord blood levels and closer to range in breastfed full-term infants, 5 to 7 μg/kg/d is recommended.[54] An expert panel organized by the Food and Drug Administration and American Society for Nutritional Sciences[71] recommended a minimum selenium concentration of 1.8 μg/100 kcal and a maximum of 5 μg/100 kcal in preterm formulas.

OTHER MINERALS

The iodine content of breast milk is dependent on maternal intake of iodine, which in turn is related to geographic location.[72] Transient hypothyroidism has been reported in preterm infants obtaining less than 30 μg/kg/d of iodine.[72] The recommended intake of iodine is 30 to 60 μg/kg/d.[73] In healthy preterm infants fed human milk, deficiencies of chromium, manganese, or molybdenum have not been reported.[73]

Water-soluble Vitamins

Like in all humans, the preterm infant has a limited reserve of water-soluble vitamins and needs a constant supply to avoid deficiencies. Preterms have higher recommended intakes based on reduced vitamin stores and increased protein requirements.[73] These increased requirements can be met in two ways. Preterm formulas contain larger amounts of water-soluble vitamins than term formulas and meet the increased needs for these vitamins. Breastfed preterm infants can have these needs met by using a vitamin-containing human milk fortifier.[73] It is important to note that standard infant multivitamin supplements do not contain all of these water-soluble vitamins.[73]

Fat-soluble Vitamins

Vitamin A promotes normal growth and differentiation of epithelial tissues. In the developing world, supplementing newborn infants with vitamin A within 48 hours of birth significantly reduces infant mortality, with the greatest benefit to those of low birth weight.[74]

The preterm infant is born with lower stores of vitamin A than term infants. Term infants absorb vitamin A when it is provided enterally.[75] In VLBW infants, vitamin A given orally in conjunction with early feeds can achieve comparable plasma concentrations of retinol as vitamin A given intramuscularly.[75] Extremely low birth weight (<1000 g) infants do not absorb vitamin A to significantly increase plasma concentrations even when large doses are provided.[75] These infants may benefit from three-times-a-week intramuscular injections of vitamin A with a reduction in death or oxygen requirement at 1 month of age.[76] This relatively small benefit needs to be balanced with the need to give frequent intramuscular injections to these infants.

Overt vitamin D deficiency is rare in the preterm infant in the United States. The main cause of metabolic bone disease of prematurity is a deficiency of calcium and phosphorus and not vitamin D.[42] All preterm formulas and human milk fortifiers provide between 200 and 400 IU/day of vitamin D.[73]

Vitamin E is an antioxidant vitamin whose requirement increases with the level of LCPUFA in the diet. Vitamin E deficiency has induced hemolytic anemia among preterm infants. This has occurred with the use of formulas that contained high quantities of LCPUFA with inadequate vitamin E.[77] These formulas also contained supplemental iron, which functioned as a pro-oxidant.[77] Today's formulas are designed to provide a minimum of 0.7 IU of vitamin/100 kcal at least of vitamin E and 1 IU/g of linoleic acid.[73] The use of large doses of vitamin E to prevent retinopathy of prematurity or bronchopulmonary dysplasia is not recommended.[73]

Hemorrhagic disease of the newborn is most commonly seen in exclusively breastfed infants, and is a manifestation of vitamin K deficiency. A preventive intramuscular injection of vitamin K (1 mg for children >1 kg and 0.3 mg/kg for children <1 kg) is recommended.[73] Breast milk has a low vitamin K content, which can be supplemented by the use of vitamin-containing human milk fortifiers. Preterm formulas contain adequate vitamin K to meet the daily needs of the infant.

LCPUFAs

Preterm infants exhibit poorer developmental outcomes in a wide range of domains than infants born at term.[78–82] LCPUFAs, such as docosahexaenoic acid and arachidonic acid, are rapidly accumulated into the tissues of the central nervous system during the third trimester and early postnatal life. Biochemical studies have shown that term infants who receive a full complement of all LCPUFAs through breast milk have higher concentrations of LCPUFAs in their blood cells and higher concentrations of docosahexaenoic acid in the brain than do infants fed formulas that do not contain LCPUFAs.[83] Several randomized controlled trials have reported that preterm infants fed LCPUFA-enriched formulas have enhanced visual development, including improved retinal sensitivity and visual acuity, compared with those fed unsupplemented formulas.[84–88] Such data have led to many intervention trials involving LCPUFA-enriched formulas for preterm infants with developmental end points. The addition of LCPUFAs to preterm formulas has shown conflicting results with regard to neurodevelopment. Some studies have suggested strong benefits of LCPUFA supplementation,[89,90] whereas other studies have shown no effect.[88,91,92] A more recent study that had an adequate sample size showed benefit in premature girls but not in boys who were supplemented with high-dose docosahexaenoic acid.[93]

These formulas seem to be safe. Further studies are needed to determine the extent of the benefit of supplemental LCPUFAs on the neurodevelopment and health outcomes of infants born preterm.

Carnitine

Carnitine plays an important role in fatty acid oxidation by facilitating the transport of long-chain fatty acids into the mitochondria.[94,95] Preterm infants have very low stores of skeletal muscle carnitine and are considered at high risk of carnitine deficiency. Infants on full feeds with breast milk or infant formula receive adequate amounts of carnitine. The risk for developing carnitine deficiency is increased in infants receiving parenteral nutrition without carnitine supplements. Studies have shown that parenteral supplementation of carnitine may increase serum carnitine concentrations[96–98] and improve lipid tolerance,[95,97] weight gain, and nitrogen retention[96] in preterm infants who received 10 to 20 mg/kg/d of carnitine. One study that used a higher dose of carnitine (48 mg/kg/d) showed slower growth rates in preterm infants compared with those receiving lower amounts.[98] A Cochrane database review that included all randomized trials involving parenteral supplementation of carnitine in neonates for improvements in growth or lipid tolerance found no evidence supporting routine supplementation with carnitine.[99] This review is limited by the fact that most of the studies included were short-term studies. Carnitine supplementation may be important for infants requiring long-term parenteral nutrition with minimal or no enteral nutrition.

SUMMARY

Infants born prematurely are prone to nutrient deficiencies at birth that are exacerbated by the time of discharge from the neonatal intensive care unit, and understudied thereafter. General guidelines are available for postdischarge feeding practices and follow-up.[36] More comprehensive nutritional care should be provided depending on the risk and specific needs of each infant.

REFERENCES

1. Kretchmer N, Beard JL, Carlson S. The role of nutrition in the development of normal cognition. Am J Clin Nutr 1996;63(6):997S–1001S.
2. Barker DJ, Gluckman PD, Godfrey KM, et al. Fetal nutrition and cardiovascular disease in adult life. Lancet 1993;341(8850):938–41.

3. Hovi P, Andersson S, Eriksson JG, et al. Glucose regulation in young adults with very low birth weight. N Engl J Med 2007;356(20):2053–63.
4. Ong KK, Ahmed ML, Emmett PM, et al. Association between postnatal catch-up growth and obesity in childhood: prospective cohort study. BMJ 2000; 320(7240):967–71.
5. Rotteveel J, van Weissenbruch MM, Twisk JW, et al. Infant and childhood growth patterns, insulin sensitivity, and blood pressure in prematurely born young adults. Pediatrics 2008;122(2):313–21.
6. Singhal A, Cole TJ, Fewtrell M, et al. Is slower early growth beneficial for long-term cardiovascular health? Circulation 2004;109(9):1108–13.
7. Singhal A, Cole TJ, Lucas A. Early nutrition in preterm infants and later blood pressure: two cohorts after randomised trials. Lancet 2001; 357(9254):413–9.
8. Cooke RJ, Ainsworth SB, Fenton AC. Postnatal growth retardation: a universal problem in preterm infants. Arch Dis Child Fetal Neonatal Ed 2004;89(5): F428–30.
9. Ehrenkranz RA, Younes N, Lemons JA, et al. Longitudinal growth of hospitalized very low birth weight infants. Pediatrics 1999;104(2 Pt 1):280–9.
10. Sakurai M, Itabashi K, Sato Y, et al. Extrauterine growth restriction in preterm infants of gestational age. Pediatrics Int 2008;50(1):70–5.
11. Ziegler EE, O'Donnell AM, Nelson SE, et al. Body composition of the reference fetus. Growth 1976;40(4):329–41.
12. Hulzebos CV, Sauer PJ. Energy requirements. Semin Fetal Neonatal Med 2007; 12(1):2–10.
13. Embleton NE, Pang N, Cooke RJ. Postnatal malnutrition and growth retardation: an inevitable consequence of current recommendations in preterm infants? Pediatrics 2001;107(2):270–3.
14. Schurr P, Perkins EM. The relationship between feeding and necrotizing entero-colitis in very low birth weight infants. Neonatal Netw 2008;27(6):397–407.
15. Koo WW, Sherman R, Succop P, et al. Sequential bone mineral content in small preterm infants with and without fractures and rickets. J Bone Miner Res 1988; 3(2):193–7.
16. Schanler RJ, Abrams SA, Garza C. Mineral balance studies in very low birth weight infants fed human milk. J Pediatr 1988;113(1 Pt 2):230–8.
17. Schanler RJ, Abrams SA, Garza C. Bioavailability of calcium and phosphorus in human milk fortifiers and formula for very low birth weight infants. J Pediatr 1988; 113(1 Pt 1):95–100.
18. Abrams SA. In utero physiology: role in nutrient delivery and fetal develop-ment for calcium, phosphorus, and vitamin D. Am J Clin Nutr 2007;85(2): S604–7.
19. Furman L, Minich N, Hack M. Correlates of lactation in mothers of very low birth weight infants. Pediatrics 2002;109(4):e57.
20. Lapillonne A, Salle BL, Glorieux FH, et al. Bone mineralization and growth are enhanced in preterm infants fed an isocaloric, nutrient-enriched preterm formula through term. Am J Clin Nutr 2004;80(6):1595–603.
21. Available at: http://www.who.int/childgrowth/mgrs/en/. Accessed April 16, 2009.
22. Guo SS, Roche AF, Chumlea WC, et al. Growth in weight, recumbent length, and head circumference for preterm low-birthweight infants during the first three years of life using gestation-adjusted ages. Early Hum Dev 1997;47(3): 305–25.

23. Fenton TR. A new growth chart for preterm babies: Babson and Benda's chart updated with recent data and a new format. BMC Pediatr 2003;3:13.
24. Henderson G, Fahey T, McGuire W. Nutrient-enriched formula versus standard term formula for preterm infants following hospital discharge. Cochrane Database Syst Rev 2007;(4):CD004696.
25. Chan GM. Growth and bone mineral status of discharged very low birth weight infants fed different formulas or human milk. J Pediatr 1993;123: 439–43.
26. Bishop NJ, King FJ, Lucas A. Increased bone mineral content of preterm infants fed with a nutrient enriched formula after discharge from hospital. Arch Dis Child 1993;68(Spec No 5):573–8.
27. Lucas A, Bishop NJ, King FJ, et al. Randomised trial of nutrition for preterm infants after discharge. Arch Dis Child 1992;67:324–7.
28. Lucas A, King F, Bishop NB. Postdischarge formula consumption in infants born preterm. Arch Dis Child 1992;67(6):691–2.
29. Cooke RJ, Griffin IJ, McCormick K, et al. Feeding preterm infants after hospital discharge: effect of dietary manipulation on nutrient intake and growth. Pediatr Res 1998;43(3):355–60.
30. Koo WW, Hockman EM. Posthospital discharge feeding for preterm infants: effects of standard compared with enriched milk formula on growth, bone mass, and body composition. Am J Clin Nutr 2006;84(6):1357–64.
31. Wauben IP, Atkinson SA, Shah JK, et al. Growth and body composition of preterm infants: influence of nutrient fortification of mother's milk in hospital and breastfeeding post-hospital discharge. Acta Paediatr 1998;87(7): 780–5.
32. O'Connor DL, Khan S, Weishuhn K, et al. Growth and nutrient intakes of human milk-fed preterm infants provided with extra energy and nutrients after hospital discharge. Pediatrics 2008;121(4):766–76.
33. Schanler RJ, Burns PA, Abrams SA, et al. Bone mineralization outcomes in human milk-fed preterm infants. Pediatr Res 1992;31(6):583–6.
34. Iwai Y, Takanashi T, Nakao Y, et al. Iron status in low birth weight infants on breast and formula feeding. Eur J Pediatr 1986;145(1–2):63–5.
35. Kienast A, Roth B, Bossier C, et al. Zinc-deficiency dermatitis in breast-fed infants. Eur J Pediatr 2007;166(3):189–94.
36. Schanler RJ. Post-discharge nutrition for the preterm infant. Acta Paediatr Suppl 2005;94(449):68–73.
37. Carver JD, Wu PY, Hall RT, et al. Growth of preterm infants fed nutrient-enriched or term formula after hospital discharge. Pediatrics 2001;107:683–9.
38. Bass JK, Chan GM. Calcium nutrition and metabolism during infancy. Nutrition 2006;22:1057–66.
39. Committee on Nutrition of the Preterm Infant. European Society of Paediatric Gastroenterology and Nutrition (ESPGAN). Nutrition and feeding of preterm infants. Oxford(England): Blackwell Scientific Publications; 1987.
40. Masel JP, Tudehope D, Cartwright D, et al. Osteopenia and rickets in the extremely low birth weight infant: a survey of the incidence and a radiological classification. Australas Radiol 1982;26:83–96.
41. Backstrom MC, Kouri I, Kuusela AL, et al. Bone isoenzyme of serum alkaline phosphatase and serum inorganic phosphate in metabolic bone disease of prematurity. Acta Paediatr 2000;89:867–73.
42. Johnson CB. Neonatal rickets: metabolic bone disease of prematurity. Neonatal Netw 1991;9:13–7.

43. Rao R, Georgieff MK. Iron therapy for preterm infants. Clin Perinatol 2009;36(1): 27–42.
44. Haga P. Plasma ferritin concentrations in preterm infants in cord blood and during the early anaemia of prematurity. Acta Paediatr Scand 1980;69(5):637–41.
45. Halvorsen S, Seip M. Erythrocyte production and iron stores in premature infants during the first months of life: the anemia of prematurity-etiology, pathogenesis, iron requirement. Acta Paediatr 1956;45(6):600–17.
46. Lundstrom U, Siimes MA, Dallman PR. At what age does iron supplementation become necessary in low-birth-weight infants? J Pediatr 1977;91(6):878–83.
47. Halliday HL, Lappin TR, McClure G. Iron status of the preterm infant during the first year of life. Biol Neonate 1984;45(5):228–35.
48. Rao R, Georgieff MK. Iron in fetal and neonatal nutrition. Semin Fetal Neonatal Med 2007;12(1):54–63.
49. Franz AR, Mihatsch WA, Sander S, et al. Prospective randomized trial of early versus late enteral iron supplementation in infants with a birth weight of less than 1301 grams. Pediatrics 2000;106(4):700–6.
50. Gorten MK, Cross ER. Iron metabolism in premature infants: prevention of iron deficiency. J Pediatr 1964;64:509–20.
51. James JA, Combes M. Iron deficiency in the premature infant: significance, and prevention by the intramuscular administration of iron-dextran. Pediatrics 1960; 26:368–74.
52. Schiza V, Giapros V, Pantou K, et al. Serum transferrin receptor, ferritin, and reticulocyte maturity indices during the first year of life in 'large' preterm infants. Eur J Haematol 2007;79(5):439–46.
53. Lozoff B, Georgieff MK. Iron deficiency and brain development. Semin Pediatr Neurol 2006;13(3):158–65.
54. Trindade CE. [Minerals in the nutrition of extremely low birth weight infants]. J Pediatr (Rio J) Mar;81(Suppl 1):S43–S51[in Portuguese].
55. Aggett PJ. Trace elements of the micropremie. Clin Perinatol 2000;27(1):119–29.
56. Friel JK, Andrews WL, Matthew JD, et al. Zinc supplementation in very-low-birth-weight infants. J Pediatr Gastroenterol Nutr 1993;17:97–104.
57. Riefen RM, Zlotkin S. Microminerals. In: Tsang RC, Lucas A, Uauy R, et al, editors. Nutritional needs of the preterm infant. Baltimore(MD): Williams & Wilkins; 1993. p. 195–207.
58. Cousins RJ. Absorption, transport, and hepatic metabolism of copper and zinc: special reference to metallothionein and ceruloplasmin. Physiol Rev 1985;65(2): 238–309.
59. McMaster D, Lappin TR, Halliday HL, et al. Serum copper and zinc levels in the preterm infant: a longitudinal study of the first year of life. Biol Neonate 1983;44: 108–13.
60. L'Abbé MR, Friel JK. Copper status of very low birth weight infants during the first 12 months of infancy. Pediatr Res 1992;32:183–8.
61. Manser JI, Crawford CS, Tyrala EE, et al. Serum copper concentrations in sick and well preterm infants. J Pediatr 1980;97:795–9.
62. Salim S, Farquharson J, Arneil GC, et al. Dietary copper intake in artificially fed infants. Arch Dis Child 1986;61(11):1068–75.
63. Institute of Medicine. Dietary reference intakes for vitamin A, vitamin K, arsenic, boron, chromium, copper, iodine, iron, manganese, molybdenum, nickel, silicon, vanadium, and zinc. Washington, DC: National Academies Press; 2001. p.155–398.

64. Lönnerdal B, Hoffman B, Hurley LS. Zinc and copper binding proteins in human milk. Am J Clin Nutr 1982;36(6):1170–6.
65. Lönnerdal B. Copper nutrition during infancy and childhood. Am J Clin Nutr 1998;67(Suppl):1046S–53S.
66. Litov RE, Combs GF Jr. Selenium in pediatric nutrition. Pediatrics 1991;87(3): 339–51.
67. Smith AM, Chan GM, Moyer-Mileur LJ, et al. Selenium status of preterm infants fed human milk, preterm formula, or selenium-supplemented preterm formula. J Pediatr 1991;119(3):429–33.
68. Amin S, Chen SY, Collipp PJ, et al. Selenium in premature infants. Nutr Metab 1980;24:331–40.
69. Darlow BA, Winterbourn CC, Irider TE, et al. The effect of selenium supplementation on outcome in very low birth weight infants: a randomized controlled trial. The New Zealand Neonatal Study Group. J Pediatr 2000; 136:473–80.
70. Darlow BA, Austin NC. Selenium supplementation to prevent short-term morbidity in preterm neonates. Cochrane Database Syst Rev 2003;(4):CD003312.
71. Klein CJ. Nutrient requirements for preterm-infant formulas: 10. Minerals: calcium and phosphorus. J Nutr 2002;132(6 Suppl 1):S1490.
72. Delange F, Dalhem A, Bourdoux P, et al. Increased risk of primary hypothyroidism in preterm infants. J Pediatr 1984;105(3):462–9.
73. Nutritional Needs of Preterm Infant. In: Kleinman RE, editor. Pediatric Nutrition Handbook. 6th edition. Elk Grove (IL): American Academy of Pediatrics; 2009. p. 76–112.
74. Rahmathallah L, Tielsch JM, Thulasiraj RD, et al. Impact of supplementing newborn infants with vitamin A on early infant mortality: community based randomized trial in southern India. BMJ 2003;327:254–7.
75. Mactier H, Weaver LT. Vitamin A and preterm infants: what we know, what we don't know, and what we need to know. Arch Dis Child Fetal Neonatal Ed 2005;90:F103–8.
76. Darlow BA, Graham PJ. Vitamin A supplementation to prevent mortality and short and long-term morbidity in very low birthweight infants. Cochrane Database Syst Rev 2007;(4):CD000501.
77. Williams ML, Shoot RJ, O'Neal PL, et al. Role of dietary iron and fat on vitamin E deficiency anemia of infancy. N Engl J Med 1975;292:887–90.
78. Martinez M. Tissue levels of polyunsaturated fatty acids during early human development. J Pediatr 1992;120(Suppl):S129–38.
79. Bhutta AT, Cleves MA, Casey PH, et al. Cognitive and behavioral outcomes of school-aged children who were born preterm. JAMA 2002;288:728–37.
80. Peterson BS, Vohr B, Kane MJ, et al. A functional magnetic resonance imaging study of language processing and its cognitive correlates in prematurely born children. Pediatrics 2002;110:1153–62.
81. Gray RF, Indurkhya A, McCormick MC. Prevalence, stability, and predictors of clinically significant behavior problems in low birth weight children at 3, 5, and 8 years of age. Pediatrics 2004;114:736–43.
82. Wolke D, Meyer R. Cognitive status, language attainment, and prereading skills of 6-year-old very preterm children and their peers: the Bavarian Longitudinal Study. Dev Med Child Neurol 1999;41:94–109.
83. Makrides M, Neumann MA, Byard RW, et al. Fatty acid composition of brain, retina, and erythrocytes in breast- and formula-fed infants. Am J Clin Nutr 1994;60:189–94.

84. Birch D, Birch E, Hoffman DR, et al. Retinal development of very low birthweight infants fed diets differing in n–3 fatty acids. Invest Ophthalmol Vis Sci 1992;33: 2365–76.

85. Birch E, Birch D, Hoffman DR, et al. Dietary essential fatty acid supply and visual acuity development. Invest Ophthalmol Vis Sci 1992;33:3242–53.

86. Carlson SE, Werkman SH, Rhodes PG, et al. Visual-acuity development in healthy preterm infants: effect of marine-oil supplementation. Am J Clin Nutr 1993;58:35–42.

87. Carlson SE, Werkman SH, Tolley EA. Effect of long-chain n–3 fatty acid supplementation on visual acuity and growth of preterm infants with and without bronchopulmonary dysplasia. Am J Clin Nutr 1996;63:687–97.

88. O'Connor DL, Hall R, Adamkin D, et al. Growth and development in preterm infants fed long-chain polyunsaturated fatty acids: a prospective randomized controlled trial. Pediatrics 2001;108:359–71.

89. Clandinin MT, Van Aerde JE, Merkel KL, et al. Growth and development of preterm infants fed infant formulas containing docosahexaenoic acid and arachidonic acid. J Pediatr 2005;146:461–8.

90. Fang PC, Kuo HK, Huang CB, et al. The effect of supplementation of docosahexaenoic acid and arachidonic acid on visual acuity and neurodevelopment in larger preterm infants. Chang Gung Med J 2005;28:708–15.

91. Fewtrell MS, Morley R, Abbott RA, et al. Double-blind, randomized trial of long-chain polyunsaturated fatty acid supplementation in formula fed to preterm infants. Pediatrics 2002;110:73–82.

92. Fewtrell MS, Abbott RA, Kennedy K, et al. Randomized, double-blind trial of long-chain polyunsaturated fatty acid supplementation with fish oil and borage oil in preterm infants. J Pediatr 2004;144:471–9.

93. Makrides RA, Gibson AJ, McPhee CT, et al. Neurodevelopmental outcomes of preterm infants fed high-dose docosahexaenoic acid: a randomized controlled trial. JAMA 2009;301(2):175–82.

94. Borum P. Carnitine in neonatal nutrition. J Child Neurol 1995;10:S25–31.

95. McDonald C, MacKay M, Curtis J. Carnitine and cholestasis: nutritional dilemmas for the parenteral nourished newborn. Support Line 2003;25:10–6.

96. Scaglia F, Longo N. Primary and secondary alteration of neonatal carnitine metabolism. Semin Perinatol 1999;23:152–61.

97. Bonner C, DeBrie K, Hug G. Effects of parenteral L-carnitine supplementation on fat metabolism and nutrition in premature neonates. J Pediatr 1995;126:287–92.

98. Sulkers E, Lafeber H, Degenhart H. Effects of high carnitine supplementation on substrate utilization in low-birth-weight infants receiving total parenteral nutrition. Am J Clin Nutr 1990;52:889–94.

99. Cairns P, Stalker D. Carnitine supplementation of parenterally fed neonates. Cochrane Database Syst Rev 2000;(4):CD000950.

100. Clandinin MT, Chappell JE, Heim T, et al. Fatty acid utilization in perinatal de novo synthesis of tissues. Early Hum Dev 1981;5(4):355–66.

101. Battaglia FC, Regnault TR. Placental transport and metabolism of amino acids. Placenta 2001;22(2-3):145–61.

102. Li YQ, Yan H, Bai B. Change in iron transporter expression in human term placenta with different maternal iron status. Eur J Obstet Gynecol Reprod Biol 2008;140(1):48–54.

103. Demarini S. Calcium and phosphorous nutrition in preterm infants. Acta Paediatr Suppl 2005;94(449):87–92.

104. Siddappa AM, Rao R, Long JD, et al. The assessment of newborn iron stores at birth: a review of the literature and standards for ferritin concentrations. Neonatology 2007;92(2):73–82.
105. Sweet DG, Savage GA, Tubman R, et al. Cord blood transferring receptors to assess fetal iron status. Arch Dis Child Fetal Neonatal Ed. 2001;85(1):F46–8.
106. Makhoul IR, Sammour RN, Diamond E, et al. Selenium concentrations in maternal and umbilical cord blood at 24–42 weeks of gestation: basis for optimization of selenium supplementation to premature infants. Clin Nutr 2004; 23(3):373–81.
107. Elizabeth KE, Krishnan V, Vijayakumar T. Umbilical cord blood nutrients in low birth weight babies in relation to birth weight and gestation age. Indian J Med Res 2008;128(2):128–33.
108. Leonce J, Brockton N, Robinson S, et al. Glucose production in the human placenta. Placenta 2006;27(Suppl A):S103–8.
109. Innis SM. Essential fatty acid transfer and fetal development. Placenta 2005; 26(Suppl A):S70–5.

Nutritional Deficiencies in Children on Restricted Diets

Midge Kirby, MS, RD, CD, CSP*, Elaine Danner, RD, CD, CNSD

KEYWORDS

- Deficiencies • Restricted • Diets • Gluten
- Allergies • Vegetarian

Nutrient deficiencies in infants and children, commonly associated with poverty in developing countries, are caused by multiple factors, including maternal undernutrition; low-calorie, nutrient-poor complementary foods; and high incidence of infections. Estimates show that up to 40% of children less than 5 years of age living in poverty can be affected by protein energy malnutrition.[1] Specific micronutrient deficiencies considered major public health problems worldwide include those for iron, iodine, vitamin A, zinc, and selenium.[2] In the United States, such clinical nutrient deficiencies do not exist to the same degree, although diets may not always be optimal. The Feeding Infants and Toddlers Study, the first national study comparing nutrient intake of infants and toddlers with the new Dietary Reference Intakes (DRIs) concluded that healthy infants and toddlers in the United States had adequate intakes of most nutrients. However, there were inadequate intakes of vitamin E in 58% of toddlers from 12 to 24 months, low fat intakes for 29% of toddlers, low fiber intake, and high intake of vitamin A and zinc compared with recommended intake.[3] For children aged 2 to 11 years, the American Dietetic Association suggests potential inadequate dietary intake of vitamin E, folate, calcium, iron, magnesium, potassium, and fiber.[4] Finally, in adolescents, dietary deficiencies of vitamins A and C, calcium, iron, riboflavin, and thiamin have been noted.[5]

A review of the literature over the past 30 years demonstrates that clinical nutrient deficiencies in the United States are not absent, and particular pediatric populations may be at higher risk: children on medically prescribed diets, such as gluten-free, allergen-free, ketogenic, or tube feedings; and children on restricted diets because of developmental or behavioral disability and/or parent-selected dietary regimens. In contrast to deficiencies in developing countries, pediatric deficiencies in the United States are often not associated with poverty, but rather with caregiver nutritional

Clinical Nutrition, Children's Hospital of Wisconsin, 9000 W. Wisconsin Avenue, Milwaukee, WI 53201, USA
* Corresponding author.
E-mail address: mkirby@chw.org (M. Kirby).

Pediatr Clin N Am 56 (2009) 1085–1103
doi:10.1016/j.pcl.2009.07.003
0031-3955/09/$ – see front matter © 2009 Elsevier Inc. All rights reserved.

pediatric.theclinics.com

ignorance, nutrition misinformation, fad diets, alternative nutrition therapies, and cultural preferences. This article reviews the importance of macro- and micronutrients for infants and children, and discusses the incidence and risks of nutrient deficiencies in both medically prescribed restricted diets and parent/child-selected restricted diets.

NUTRIENTS

Nutrients can be grouped into macronutrients of carbohydrates, protein, and fat, which supply calories, and micronutrients of vitamins and minerals. The DRIs have established recommended intakes for both macro- and micronutrients.[6] These include acceptable calorie reference ranges, the acceptable macronutrient distribution range, adequate intake, and recommended dietary allowances for essential vitamins and minerals.

Nutrient deficiencies result from inadequate nutrients in relation to biologic need. This imbalance can be caused by inadequate intake, impaired nutrient absorption, or increased nutrient need. Certain nutrient deficiencies can rapidly result in impaired growth, while other deficiencies deplete body stores initially, then tissue concentrations, and ultimately impair metabolic pathways, which lead to clinical symptoms. Deficiencies of macronutrients can be classified as marasmus (a primary calorie deficit), kwashiorkor (a primary protein deficit), and marasmic kwashiorkor (both a calorie and protein deficit). Calorie deficit is a primary nutrient deficiency. However, there can also be deficiencies or imbalances of the macronutrients: carbohydrates, protein, and fat. The acceptable macronutrient distribution range for children and adolescents is:

Carbohydrates: 45% to 65% of total calories
Protein: 5% to 20% for ages 1 to 3 and 10% to 30% for ages 4 and older
Fat: 30% to 40% for ages 1 to 3 and 25% to 35% for ages 4 and older

Specific micronutrient deficiencies that may be more frequently seen in restricted diets will be discussed in more detail and include those related to iron, zinc, calcium, vitamin D, and B vitamins.

Iron

Iron is a critical component of several proteins, including hemoglobin, myoglobin, cytochromes, and numerous enzymes. The largest portion of the body's iron is in the erythrocytic hemoglobin used in the transport of oxygen. The requirements are particularly elevated during periods of rapid growth. For this reason, cow's milk, which is a poor source of iron, is not recommended for use in infants under 1 year of age (under 9 months in Canada). Breast-feeding or the use of an iron-fortified formula should be continued until this time. Iron-fortified infant cereals can provide a significant amount of iron in the infant's diet once solid foods are started. During the growth spurt of preadolescence and adolescence, the need for iron can increase significantly. For females, the recommended dietary allowance for iron increases from 8 mg/d for 9- to 13-year-olds to 15 mg/d for 14- to 18-year-olds. For girls who have not started menstruating by this age, the requirement is approximately 10.5 mg/d.[7] For males, the recommended dietary allowance for iron increases from 8 mg/d for 9- to 13-year-olds to 11 mg/d for 14- to 18-year-olds.

The two forms of dietary iron are heme iron and nonheme iron. Heme iron is highly bioavailable. Sources of heme iron include beef, pork, lamb, chicken, turkey, fish, and shellfish. Nonheme iron is not as readily absorbed by the body and is found in beans, soybeans, eggs; whole-grain, iron-fortified, or iron-enriched foods such as rice, pasta, breads, and cereals; cooked spinach, nuts, seeds, and dried fruits. The absorption of nonheme iron can be enhanced if consumed with foods that contain vitamin C or with foods high in heme iron. In 2004, over 50% of the iron in the United States diet was from grain products. This was primarily due to the enrichment of flour with iron and the increased consumption of enriched grains and fortified ready-to-eat breakfast cereals. Meat, poultry, and fish were the secondary sources of iron, providing approximately 16%, followed by vegetables at 10%.[8]

The most common manifestation of an iron deficiency is iron deficiency anemia. According to the third National Health and Nutrition Examination Survey (1988–1994), iron deficiency and iron deficiency anemia are still relatively common in toddlers and adolescent girls. Nine percent of toddlers aged 1 to 2 years and 9% to 11% of adolescent girls were iron deficient. Of these, iron deficiency anemia was found in 3% and 2% respectively.[9]

Zinc

Zinc is critical for proper growth and development and is required for the senses of taste and smell. It also is a catalyst for approximately 100 enzymes, has a role in protein synthesis, and supports immune function. The recommended dietary allowance for zinc increases with age dramatically from 3 mg/d for the age range of 7 months to 3 years to a maximum of 11 mg/d for 14- to 18-year-old males.

Sources include meat (especially red meat), some seafood, poultry, eggs, cheese, milk, whole grains, and beans. In 2004, over 37% of the zinc in the American diet came from meats, fish, and poultry. This was followed by grain products and then dairy products at 25% and 16% respectively.[8]

Overt zinc deficiency as seen in acrodermatitis enteropathica is uncommon, but mild zinc deficiency can impair immune function, increase susceptibility to infection, and decrease ability to fight infection.[10] Signs and symptoms might include poor growth, poor appetite, altered immune function, hair loss, skin and eye lesions, and delayed puberty.[7]

Calcium

Calcium is needed for formation of bones and teeth, for muscle contractions, for blood vessel contraction and vasodilatation, for transmission of nerve impulses, and for hormone and enzyme secretion. More than 99% of total body calcium is found in the skeleton. Adequate intake of calcium during childhood and adolescence is necessary for accretion of peak bone mass. This may be important in reducing the risk of fractures and in prevention of osteoporosis later in life. The adequate intake levels for calcium increase throughout infancy and childhood. For children aged 1 to 3 years, the adequate intake is 500 mg/d. This increases to 800 mg/d for children aged 4 to 8 years, and to 1300 mg/d for 9- to 18-year-olds. Individual calcium needs are affected by the rate of growth, the degree of absorption, and the availability of other nutrients, including vitamin D and phosphorus, as well as calories and protein. Dietary substances that may decrease calcium retention include caffeine, excessive phosphorus intake, oxalic and phytic acids, and protein.[11]

Sources of calcium include dairy products; calcium-set tofu; calcium-fortified milk alternatives; such vegetables as Chinese cabbage, broccoli, and kale; and calcium-fortified fruit juices. In 2004, over 70% of the calcium in the American diet came from dairy products, primarily milk, cheese, and yogurt. These were followed by vegetables at 7%.[8] Calcium intake tends to be lower when carbonated drinks and fruit juices/drinks replace milk as a beverage.

Studies show that the percentage of children who meet the recommended adequate intake level declines with age, reaching its lowest point between the ages of 12 and 19.[12] Females in this age range have the lowest intake with only approximately 10% meeting the adequate intake level. They are followed by males at only 25%.[13]

Vitamin D

Vitamin D facilitates the intestinal absorption of calcium and phosphorus and plays a role in cellular metabolism. The adequate intake for vitamin D is 5 μg/d or 200 IU/d in the absence of exposure to sunlight. Recently, the American Academy of Pediatrics issued a recommendation that all infants and children, including adolescents, have a minimum daily intake of 400 IU of vitamin D beginning soon after birth.[14]

Sources include the diet and vitamin D synthesized in the skin with exposure to sunlight. Two dietary forms of vitamin D are vitamin D_2 (ergocalciferol) and vitamin D_3 (cholecalciferol). Vitamin D is naturally found in very few foods other than butter, cream, egg yolk, salmon, herring, and liver. However, almost all fluid milk is fortified with vitamin D as are many ready-to-eat cereals. Dairy foods, other than milk, may be good sources of calcium, but they are not always fortified with vitamin D.

Vitamin D deficiency may result in rickets, osteomalacia, and osteoporosis. Additionally, a number of recent studies have indicated that there is a high incidence of vitamin D insufficiency in the United States and Canada. Epidemiologic studies indicate that this may result in increased risk of various cancers.

B-Complex Vitamins

B-complex vitamins include thiamin, riboflavin, niacin, folate, B_6, and B_{12}. Thiamin, riboflavin, and niacin function as coenzymes in energy metabolism. Folate functions as a coenzyme in nucleic and amino acid metabolism. Vitamin B_6 plays a role in various metabolic reactions, especially in protein metabolism. Vitamin B_{12} is essential for blood formation and neurologic function. During periods of growth and the accompanying increased energy needs, the requirements for these nutrients also increase.

In 2004, grain products, especially enriched flours and fortified ready-to-eat cereals, provided the largest percentages of thiamin, riboflavin, niacin, and folate to the United States diet: 58%, 38%, 42%, and 70% respectively. Meat, fish, and poultry supplied over 75% of the B_{12} and 36% of the B_6. Meat alone was the next largest source of thiamin (16%), and meat and poultry combined equally to provide a total of 33% of the niacin. Milk products were a major secondary source of riboflavin (26%) and B_{12} (20%). The next largest sources of folate were vegetables and legumes. Vegetables were a secondary contributor to B_6 but half of this was from white potatoes.[8]

Much of the nutrient content of whole grains is in the outer husk and germ and is lost in the milling process. In the United States, wheat products and fortified cereals are enriched with thiamin, riboflavin, niacin, folate, and iron. Since January 1, 1998, all enriched cereal grains (eg, enriched bread, pasta, flour, breakfast cereal, and rice) have been required to be fortified with folate at 1.4 mg/kg of grain.[15]

RESTRICTED DIETS AND NUTRIENT DEFICIENCIES

Restricted diets in infants, children, and adolescents can increase risk of nutrient deficiencies. Some diets are medically necessary, such as the gluten-free diet for management of celiac disease, allergy-restricted diets, ketogenic diet for seizure management, and tube feedings for nutrition support. Other restricted diets are parent- or child-selected, such as vegetarian diets, milk alternatives, and diets frequently seen with developmental disabilities.

Gluten-Free Diet and Celiac Disease

The cause of nutritional deficiencies seen in celiac disease may be twofold: a result of celiac disease, and/or a consequence of the gluten-free diet. The length of time that celiac disease has gone undiagnosed or untreated, the location and degree of damage to the small bowel, and the degree of malabsorption all have a bearing. Since the damage likely occurs in the proximal small bowel, deficiencies of iron, folate, and calcium may occur. Malabsorption of fat-soluble vitamins (A, D, E, and K), carbohydrates, fat, and other micronutrients may occur if more distal portions of the small intestine are affected. Deficiencies of Vitamins B_{12} and B_6, as well as zinc, selenium, and copper have all been seen in celiac disease.[16–18]

After the diagnosis of celiac disease, it is important to ensure that the gluten-free diet is adequate in all nutrients. In an Italian study, the diet of adolescents with celiac disease was compared with the diet of healthy adolescents. The group with celiac disease was further divided into two groups: those who were compliant with the gluten-free diet (53%) and those who were not (47%). Investigators found the diets of all three groups tended to be high in protein and fat with a resulting lower intake of carbohydrates. Comparing the two groups with celiac disease, the compliant group had a significantly higher intake of protein and a significantly lower intake of carbohydrates. The reverse was true with regard to fiber intake. The investigators concluded that strict compliance with a gluten-free diet may further worsen the imbalance of the adolescent diet and may place this group at nutritional risk.[19]

A 2005 study reviewed the adequacy of 3-day food records of 47 adults with celiac disease. These adults were recruited from the readership of a number of celiac disease publications and may have been more knowledgeable about the gluten-free diet. None of the women in the group consumed the recommended amounts of fiber, iron, or calcium and the men did not consume enough fiber or calcium. This led the investigator to conclude that nutrition therapy for celiac disease should not just focus on the foods permitted or forbidden on the gluten-free diet, but should also stress the nutritional quality of the diet.[20]

In addition to the inadequacy based on food choices, the gluten-free alternatives may not provide the same level of nutrients found in the gluten-containing foods. This is particularly evident with the grain-containing foods. Many of the gluten-free grains do not inherently contain thiamin, riboflavin, niacin, folate, and iron, nor are they required to be enriched/fortified as are many of the gluten-containing grains. However, some manufacturers are opting to do so. Food labels need to be scrutinized for gluten-containing ingredients to avoid, as well as for the addition of thiamin, riboflavin, niacin, folate, and/or iron. (**Fig. 1**) The "Nutrition Facts" portion of the label will also give the "% Daily value," which can be used as a tool for comparing products.

Wheat alternatives that are better sources of nutrients include amaranth, buckwheat, millet, brown rice, quinoa, sorghum, teff, and wild rice. Beans, such as garbanzo, fava, navy, and great northern, are also being milled into flour and used in place of wheat flour. Choosing grains and flours that are more nutritionally dense helps improve the quality of the diet. **Table 1** contains a comparison of enriched white flour to some of the gluten-free alternatives. However, most of these grains cannot compare with enriched white flour as sources of B vitamins. Therefore, a gluten-free multivitamin seems to be a prudent recommendation for patients with celiac disease.

Nutrition Facts	
Serving Size ¼ Cup (30 g)	
Servings Per Container About 65	
Amount Per Serving	
Calories 110	
	% Daily value
Total Fat 0 g	0%
Sodium 0 mg	0%
Total Carbohydrate 24 g	4%
Dietary Fiber 2 g	
Protein 3 g	
Iron	6%
Thiamin	10%
Riboflavin	6%
Niacin	8%
Folic Acid	10%
INGREDIENTS: White Rice Flour, Tapioca Starch, Teff, Niacin, Iron, Thiamin Mononitrate, Riboflavin, Folic Acid	

Fig. 1. Food label with "Nutrition Facts" and "% Daily value."

Allergy Diets

In 2007, approximately 4% of United States children under the age of 18 had a food allergy. Ninety percent of food allergies are caused by reaction to cow's milk, eggs, peanuts, tree nuts, wheat, soy, fish, and shellfish.[21] The mainstay of allergy treatment is the elimination of the offending protein. However, a food-avoidance diet can have

Table 1
Comparison of enriched white flour and alternative grains

Grain (100 g)	Fiber (g)	Calcium (mg)	Iron (mg)	Zinc (mg)	Thiamin (mg)	Riboflavin (mg)	Niacin (mg)	Folate (µg)
Wheat flour, white, all-purpose, enriched, unbleached	3	15	4.6	0.7	0.8	0.5	5.9	183
Rice flour, brown	5[a]	11	2.0	2.5[a]	0.4	0.1	6.3	16
Teff, uncooked	8[a]	180[a]	7.6[a]	3.6[a]	0.4	0.3	3.4	NA
Amaranth, uncooked	7[a]	159[a]	7.6[a]	2.9[a]	0.1	0.2	0.9	82
Buckwheat flour, whole-groat	10[a]	41[a]	4.1	3.1[a]	0.4	0.2	6.2[a]	54
Millet, raw	9[a]	8	3.0	1.7[a]	0.4	0.3	4.7	85
Quinoa, uncooked	7	47[a]	4.6[a]	3.1[a]	0.4	0.3	1.5	184[a]
Sorghum	6[a]	28[a]	4.4	NA	0.2	0.1	2.9	NA
Tapioca, pearl, dry	1	20[a]	1.6	0.1	0.0	0.0	0.0	4
Rice flour, white	2	10	0.4	0.8[a]	0.1	0.0	2.6	4
Potato flour	6[a]	65[a]	1.4	0.5	0.2	0.1	3.5	25

Abbreviation: NA, not available.
[a] Values equal to or exceeding those of enriched white flour.
Data from USDA National Data Laboratory. National Nutrient Database for Standard Reference. Available at: http://www.nal.usda.gov/fnic/foodcomp/search. Accessed March 19, 2009; with permission.

the potential risk of being nutritionally inadequate, especially if more than one food is being eliminated. It is recommended that reliable allergy testing be completed by an allergist before placing the child on a restricted diet.

Elimination of even one of the eight most common food allergens, especially dairy or wheat, can have a major impact on the adequacy of the diet. Individually, the elimination of soy, eggs, peanuts, tree nuts, fish, or shellfish should not compromise the nutritional quality of the child's diet. However, as the number of foods eliminated increases, so does the risk of nutrient inadequacy. Also, as the previous section showed, the removal of wheat-containing products does have a negative effect on a number of nutrients. Equally, the elimination of dairy products, which are the major source of calcium and vitamin D in the diet, can alter the level of these nutrients significantly.

Inadequate growth and nutritional deficiencies are more likely to occur in children who are allergic to cow's milk and in children with allergy to more than two foods.[22,23] A study of 34 children with known food allergy showed the nutrients most likely to be negatively affected are calcium, vitamin D, vitamin E, and zinc.[24]

If dairy products must be eliminated, calcium and vitamin D must be replaced by an alternative source. Additionally, other sources of protein, riboflavin, phosphorus, fat, and calories (if the child is under 24 months of age) may need to be included. For the infant, soy-based, hydrolyzed, or elemental infant formulas supply all the nutrients needed for growth, provided that the infant consumes an adequate amount. For a toddler and older child, a milk-free formula or such beverages as soymilk, which are fortified with calcium and vitamin D, should be used.

In a review of the diets of 127 United States children (9–18 years of age) who were not consuming dairy products, only 1 of the subjects had a calcium intake of 1300 mg/d or more, which is the adequate intake for this age group.[13] The investigators concluded that an intake of 1.5 servings of a calcium-fortified citrus juice resulted in a more adequate intake of calcium.

With the elimination of an offending food and potential loss of nutrients, suitable substitute foods that provide comparable nutrients must be identified. **Table 2** provides a reference for identifying critical nutrients provided by specific foods or food groups, and for substituting alternate foods to minimize risk of deficiencies.

Ketogenic Diet

The ketogenic diet is a high-fat diet used in the treatment of intractable seizures and for certain metabolic disorders, such as pyruvate dehydrogenase complex deficiency and glucose transporter type 1 deficiency.[32] The ketogenic diet has been shown to be

Table 2 Restricted diets and affected food groups	
Restricted Diet	**Primary Food Group(s) Affected**
Gluten-free diet	Grains
Milk allergy	Dairy
Wheat allergy	Grains
Ketogenic	Grains, dairy, fruits, vegetables
Vegetarian	Protein, dairy
Macrobiotic	Protein, dairy, fruits, vegetables
Milk alternative	Dairy, protein, fat
Gluten-free, casein-free	Grains, dairy

effective in some infants[33] and children.[34] The diet provides 70% to 90% of calories from fat, with the remaining calories provided by protein and carbohydrates. This macronutrient distribution differs significantly from the recommended acceptable macronutrient distribution range noted previously. The restrictive nature of the diet raises the risk of growth retardation and micronutrient deficiency when not appropriately supplemented. A study by Couch and colleagues[34] demonstrated stable height and weight for age percentiles after 6 months on the diet. However, a study by Williams and colleagues[35] demonstrated that, after 1.2 years on the diet, 86% of study participants had a decrease in their height-for-age percentile. Adequate micronutrient intake is also a concern. Zupec-Kania and Spellman[36] report inadequate micronutrient intake of 19 known essential micronutrients on a 4:1 ketogenic diet despite using nutrient-dense foods. They concluded that the ketogenic diet requires careful vitamin and mineral supplementation for nutrient adequacy.

Tube Feedings

Children with developmental disabilities have a higher risk of feeding difficulty, inadequate intake, and nutritional problems due to a variety of reasons, including oral motor and swallowing difficulty, altered nutritional needs, altered nutrient absorption and metabolism, drug-nutrient interactions, delay in feeding skills, altered appetite and thirst, and extended feeding times. Advances in medical technology, however, now allow for provision of nutrition support by nasogastric, gastrostomy, and jejunostomy feeding tubes, selecting from an increasing variety of formulas developed for various medical needs. For most infants and children, these formulas can provide adequate nutrition, thus preventing nutrient deficiency.[37] However, two situations that can increase the risk of nutrient deficiencies are (1) low volume of formula provided and (2) the use of home-blenderized tube feeding.

Generally, the volume of tube feeding formula delivered for a specific infant or child is planned to match the energy expenditure, promoting acceptable weight gain and linear growth. Developmentally disabled children with low calorie expenditure receive a lower volume of formula to provide energy balance. This can result in inadequate micronutrient intake. Jones and colleagues[38] describe a 3-year-old boy with cerebral palsy, developmental delay, and seizure disorder. The boy, who was receiving a tube feeding volume matched to his energy needs, developed scurvy and deficiencies of vitamin A and zinc. This case highlights the need for careful evaluation of tube feeding not only for adequate calorie and macronutrient intake, but also for adequate micronutrient intake.

Although there are available an increasing number of nutritionally adequate formulas designed for various pediatric medical conditions, some families prefer to prepare their own home-blenderized tube feeding from foods available in their home. Such tube feedings can be nutritionally adequate. However, the use of home-blenderized tube feeding requires nutrition education for caregivers with regard to formula recipes, proper food safety techniques, nutrient balance, and appropriate supplementation. Ongoing nutrient analysis of formula recipes as well as monitoring of the child's growth and nutritional status must be provided. Major concerns include not only adequate calorie, protein, and fat intake, but also macronutrient balance, adequate micronutrient intake, and adequate intake of sodium, other electrolytes, and fluid.

Vegetarian Diets

Carefully planned and monitored vegetarian diets can provide adequate nutrients for infants and children, according to the American Academy of Pediatrics,[32] the American Dietetic Association, and the Dietitians of Canada.[39] However, due to the critical nutrient needs in infancy and childhood, and to the restrictive aspects of some forms of vegetarianism, nutrients of concern whose adequacy needs to be assured include calories; protein; fat; vitamins A, D, and B_{12}; and the minerals iron, zinc, and calcium. Careful attention must be given especially to vegan diets that avoid all meat, fish, poultry, eggs, and dairy.

Calories

Calorie needs may not be met because of early satiety with the high bulk and fiber content and at times lower calorie density of vegetarian diets, especially in children less than 5 years of age.[40] Texture modifications, regularly scheduled snacks, and the inclusion of healthy fats can help to provide adequate calories for growth.

Protein

Protein intake from vegetarian diets focuses on the amino acid composition and the lower digestibility of the plant foods. Dietary protein provides amino acids, which are categorized into three groups: essential amino acids, which cannot be synthesized by humans and must be obtained from foods; nonessential amino acids, which can be synthesized by humans; and conditionally essential amino acids, which under certain circumstances, such as growth or illness, become essential. Animal foods are the best source of essential amino acids, while plant foods are often lacking in one or more essential amino acids: legumes and fruits are low in methionine and cysteine; cereals are low in threonine, and all plant foods are lower than animal foods in lysine.[32] Including a variety of plant foods helps balance the amino acid composition and optimizes protein intake. This concept of complementary proteins underscores the importance of including a variety of plant foods within a single day or even within a period of several hours to optimize protein intake.[41] To allow for the amino acid composition and the lower digestibility of plant foods, it has been recommended that protein intake be increased 30% to 35% for infants, 20% to 30% for children 2 to 6 years old, and 15% to 20% for children over 6.[41] When a variety of plant foods are carefully selected and calorie intake is adequate, vegetarian diets can meet protein needs of infants and children.

Fat

Fat intake is a concern especially for vegan infants and young children, for whom adequate fat is critical not only for energy but also for brain development, and to provide the essential fatty acids: linoleic (18:2 ω 6) and alpha-linolenic (18:3 ω 3). It is recommended that diets of breast-feeding vegan mothers and vegan children include sources of alpha-linolenic acid, such as canola oil, soy, flax, and walnuts, to enhance conversion of alpha-linolenic to docosahexanoic acid and eicosapentanoic acid, both of which are low in vegan diets.[41,42]

Vitamin A

Vitamin A intake may be a concern only for vegans, since preformed vitamin A is found only in animal foods, and vegans depend on beta-carotene and other carotenoids, which are converted to vitamin A. Three servings per day of deep yellow or orange vegetables or fruits are recommended.[39]

Vitamin D

Vitamin D deficiency and nutritional rickets has been associated with unsupplemented breast-feeding and strict vegetarian diets.[43] Lacto-ovo-vegetarian diets can provide adequate vitamin D from cow's milk. Vegan diets require vitamin D from fortified soy or rice milk, breakfast cereals, or supplements.

Vitamin B$_{12}$ (cobalamin)

Vitamin B$_{12}$ (cobalamin) adequacy is a concern primarily for vegan diets. Dairy products and eggs eaten regularly provide adequate vitamin B$_{12}$ for lacto-ovo-vegetarians. However, vegan diets, especially the more processed and hygienic diets in developed countries, cannot be relied upon to provide adequate B$_{12}$, and should be supplemented with either B$_{12}$ supplements, or B$_{12}$-fortified foods, such as certain brands of soy milk, breakfast cereals, meat analogs, or nutritional yeast grown on a vitamin B$_{12}$ medium. Weiss and colleagues[44] describe a 6-month-old breast-fed female diagnosed with severe vitamin B$_{12}$ deficiency with neurologic sequelae associated with a maternal strict vegetarian diet. Therefore, vitamin B$_{12}$ supplementation for pregnant and breast-feeding vegan mothers is recommended.

Iron

Iron deficiency for children on vegetarian diets is a concern for two reasons: (1) iron from plants is nonheme iron, which is less well absorbed than the heme iron found in animal products, and (2) many plant foods contain phytates, which bind with iron, decreasing its bioavailability. To compensate for these differences, the DRI recommends an 80% increase in dietary iron intake for vegetarians. In addition, iron absorption can be enhanced by combining a vitamin C–rich food with an iron-containing food, or by using special food preparation methods, such as leavening whole grain breads with yeast, to reduce the phytate content.[45]

Zinc

Zinc intake from vegetarian diets, especially vegan diets, is also a concern for infants and children due to the lower zinc content in plant foods, and the phytate content, which binds zinc, making it less available for absorption. The DRI recommends a 50% increase in dietary zinc intake for strict vegetarians.

Calcium

Calcium intake is a concern for vegans because the high oxalate content of certain vegetables, such as greens and broccoli, can inhibit absorption of calcium from foods. Calcium-enriched foods or supplements should be encouraged.

Special considerations for vegetarian infants

The American Academy of Pediatrics recommends vitamin D supplements for all breast-fed infants soon after birth and a source of iron by 6 months of age. In addition, breast-fed infants of mothers who do not include vitamin B$_{12}$–fortified foods or supplements regularly in their diet require a vitamin B$_{12}$ supplement.[39] Finally, adequate zinc intake should be provided when complementary foods are introduced.

Macrobiotic Diets

Macrobiotic diets, which are based on eating "in harmony with one's local environment,"[42] can be considered one subset of vegetarian diets. These diets can significantly vary in practice, but most rely heavily on brown rice, sea vegetables, root vegetables, and beans, with moderate intake of fruits, nuts, and seeds; and usual avoidance of meats, dairy foods, tropical fruits, potatoes, and processed sweeteners.[46] Several studies have identified serious concerns in macrobiotic infants and children: growth retardation;[47–49] kwashiorkor, marasmus, and rickets;[50] dietary deficiencies of calories, protein, calcium, vitamin D, riboflavin, and vitamin B$_{12}$;[51,52] vitamin D deficiency rickets;[53] severe megaloblastic anemia with neurologic sequelae;[44] and iron deficiency anemia due to low iron availability from plant foods.[49] Dietary modifications of a macrobiotic diet to improve nutrient intake include (1) increased fat as a source of calories; (2) adequate protein for growth; (3) adequate sources of calcium and vitamin D, such as fortified soymilk products; and (4) a reliable source of vitamin B_{12} from foods or supplement.

Milk Alternatives

Years of research and monitoring infant growth and nutritional status support breast milk as the optimum source of nutrition for infants, with complementary foods introduced at 6 months. When breast-feeding is not possible or requires supplementation, iron-fortified infant formula is recommended. When infants do not tolerate standard cow's milk–based formulas, nutritionally appropriate alternatives are available, such as soy formula, hypoallergenic formulas, and elemental formulas. For infants, cow's milk and goat's milk are inappropriate because of the their high renal solute load, high protein load, and inadequate micronutrients of iron, zinc, vitamin E, vitamin C, and folic acid.

Serious health consequences can result when alternative milk substitutes replace breast milk or formula. A review of the literature demonstrates that an alarming number of infants and toddlers develop serious nutritional deficiencies when caregivers discontinued breast milk or formula. Milk substitutes include nondairy creamers, which are extremely low in protein; vitamins A, C, B_1, and B_2; niacin; calcium; iron;[25] unfortified goat's milk, which is low in folic acid; or rice milk, which is low in protein, fat, and, when unfortified, low in vitamins A and D and in calcium. **Table 3** identifies 19 case reports of infants and toddlers developing kwashiorkor or severe protein energy malnutrition from using a nutritionally inferior milk alternative.[25–31] Rickets has also been noted in unsupplemented breast-feeding and with early transition to non–vitamin D–fortified beverages.[31,43] Severe iodine and carnitine deficiencies and osteopenia were described in a 7.5-month-old transitioned at 2.5 months of age from breast milk to an almond extract in water.[54] These case reports demonstrate the existence in affluent countries of severe nutrient deficiencies not associated with poverty, but rather with nutritional ignorance, suspected milk intolerance, cultural diets, and trends toward health food alternatives. It is critical for pediatric providers to carefully review infant and toddler feeding histories for early identification of inappropriate feeding practices.

Developmental and Behavioral Disabilities and Restricted Diets

Some of the more challenging feeding problems present in children with pervasive development delay (PDD) and/or autism spectrum disorder (ASD). These problems include refusal of certain food textures, color, and food presentation; a need for specific utensils; delayed feeding skills; and disruptive mealtime behaviors. The result is often mild to severe food selectivity. Schreck and colleagues[55] compared eating habits of autistic children with typically developing children, finding that 72% of the autistic group accepted approximately 50% of the food variety in most food groups with the exception of starches. Ahearn[56] also demonstrated food selectivity, and categorized the patterns of acceptance as complete food refusal, overly selective acceptance of primarily starch foods and some fruits, moderately selective acceptance, texture selectivity, and high overall acceptance. In 17 children with ASD, Cornish reports 7 ate 20 or more different foods, 7 ate 10 to 19 foods, and 3 ate fewer than 8 different foods.[57]

Severe food selectivity can result in nutrient deficiency, as demonstrated in the case report by Tamura and colleagues,[58] in which a previously healthy 5-year-old boy developed scurvy secondary to a 5-month self-restricted diet of biscuits, Pop-Tarts, cheese pizza, and water, while refusing fruits, vegetables, juices, and a vitamin-mineral

Table 3
Case reports of kwashiorkor related to milk alternatives

Age	Dietary Manipulation	Rationale for Dietary Change	References
3 mo	High-fat, low-protein nondairy creamer	Suspected intolerance to milk	[25]
4 mo	Rice Dream milk and Poly Vi Sol	Colic, feeding problems	[26]
5 mo	Juice, cereal, applesauce	Parental belief child did not need milk	[26]
5 mo	Brown rice emulsion, black strap molasses, chlorophyll, acidophilus extract, flaxseed oil, vitamins	Vegan family; chronic constipation	[26]
5.5 mo	High-fat, low-protein nondairy creamer	Suspected intolerance to milk	[25]
7 mo	High-fat, low-protein nondairy creamer for 1.5 mo with small amounts of cereal, fruits, vegetables	Suspected intolerance to milk and soy	[25]
7 mo	Rice Dream, small amounts of baby food, iron supplement	Formula intolerance noted at 2 mo of age; changed to rice beverage	[27]
8 mo	Rice flour, water, and baby food	Vomiting; perceived formula dislike	[26]
8 mo	Goat's milk, juice, herbal tea, graphite tablets, yogurt	Atopic dermatitis	[26]
8 mo	Cream soda supplemented with calcium powder; occasional strained vegetables and fruits	Physician prescribed because of diagnosed milk intolerance with vomiting; infant had been breast-fed for 1 mo, then fed cow's milk for 2 wk	[28]
8 mo	Daily intake: 8 jars baby food (primarily fruit) and 8 oz Similac formula	Nutritional ignorance	[26]
9 mo	Barley, water and cinnamon emulsion, foods	Chronic vomiting; milk protein allergy	[26]
11 mo	Potatoes and juice	Nutritional ignorance	[26]
14 mo	Rice Dream, vegetables, meat	Breast-fed for 8 mo; did not tolerate formula; started on rice beverage	[27]
17 mo	Rice milk, first-stage infant foods	Breast-fed for 4 months; hypoallergenic formula until 8 months of age; soy formula until 12 months of age; then enriched rice milk and restricted variety of foods because of eczema	[29]
17 mo	Rice milk; small amounts of baby foods or solid foods without meat	Chronic atopic dermatitis and positive radioallergosorbent test to multiple foods	[30]
18 mo	High-fat, low-protein nondairy creamer	Suspected intolerance to milk	[25]
22 mo	Plantains, lentils, other vegetables	Suspected allergy to milk with pulmonary congestion and diarrhea	[26]
22 mo	Rice milk with poor intake of solids	Breast-fed for 13 mo; then changed to rice milk because of chronic eczema and perceived milk intolerance	[31]

supplement. However, there are conflicting reports on the nutritional consequences of the food selectivity seen with PDD/ASD. Raiten and Massaro[59] analyzed food diaries of 40 autistic children and determined that their diets were nutritionally adequate. Williams and colleagues[60] presented the results of 100 surveys sent to families of children with ASD, reporting that although two thirds reported picky eating behaviors, over half reported adequate nutritional intake. On the other hand, Cornish's dietary analysis of 17 children ages 42 to 117 months with ASD demonstrated inadequate intakes for vitamins C, D, and B$_6$; riboflavin; niacin; calcium; and zinc in 53% of the children.[57] Finally, Bowers' review[61] of 26 food records demonstrated adequate intakes for energy and protein, but inadequate intake of micronutrients. These conflicting reports raise several thoughts:

It seems clear that this population demonstrates a higher incidence of food selectivity than typically developing children.

The selectivity is highly variable.

Appetite appears to be less of a problem and, when these children are allowed their preferred foods, adequate energy intake is often achieved.

Inadequate micronutrient intake may be associated less with selectivity within a specific food group than with complete avoidance of one or more food groups.

Some preferred foods eaten in large amounts and more readily available fortified foods can become sources of nutrients lacking due to avoidance of other foods.

However, food selectivity can be associated with nutrient deficiency, especially when foods become limited to fewer than 20, when complete food groups are omitted, and when selectivity involves children less than the age of 5 years. Often, a complete multivitamin-mineral supplement can address some of these concerns. However, the child with texture selectivity is often unwilling to accept these supplements, increasing the risk of deficiency.

Gluten-Free, Casein-Free Diet

The self-restricted diet noted in children with PDD/ASD can be complicated by the addition of a gluten-free, casein-free diet (GFCF), an elimination diet that has become a popular alternative therapy for this population. The diet is based on several proposed theories. These include:

The theory that opioid excess leads to altered central nervous system activity

The immune dysfunction theory, which suggests that gluten and/or casein act as proinflammatory stimuli in the gastrointestinal mucosa

The theory of decreased peptidase activity contributing to abnormal leaky gut[62]

Though these theories carry some possible rationale for the elimination diet, there is limited published literature of trials addressing the efficacy of these diets, and many of the studies are considered flawed.[62] Elder's double-blind repeated-measures crossover study[63] of 13 children and young adults ages 2 to 26 years with ASD comparing a regular diet and a GFCF diet showed no statistically significant differences in autism symptoms, although many parents chose to continue the diet.

The question then becomes what harm can there be in the use of this GFCF diet. First, eliminating gluten and casein requires major changes in food choices from the grain and dairy groups. The nutrients at risk are those mentioned earlier in this article in the discussion of celiac disease and milk allergy. Second, imposing this diet on a child who has self-restricted to a limited variety of foods increases the risk of nutrient deficiency. Third, the GFCF diet requires additional resources for purchasing alternative grains and dairy substitutes, some of which are not fortified. This increases the need for supplements, which are often difficult for the child with PDD/ASD to accept because of texture aversion.

Limited studies have been published comparing nutritional status of children on the GFCF diet with those on unrestricted diets. Cornish reported on nutrient analysis of 37 food records, 8 following a GFCF diet and 29 following the child's self-selected diet, finding no significant differences in energy, protein, and micronutrient intakes between the two groups.[64] However, individual children in both groups had inadequate intake of specific micronutrients, demonstrating the individual food selectivity that occurs with this population. Arnold and colleagues[65] demonstrated lower plasma levels of essential amino acids in children with ASD on GFCF diets when compared with those autistic children on unrestricted diets and those children with developmental disabilities other than ASD; and Hediger and colleagues[66] demonstrated potential negative impact of the GFCF diet on bone development. With these cautions in mind, a nutritionally adequate GFCF diet can still be provided, but it requires caregiver education, monitoring of patient growth and nutrient intake, and individualization.

Vitamin/Mineral Supplementation

Depending on the situation, a vitamin and/or mineral supplement may be necessary to provide the nutrient(s) lacking in one of these diets. Clinicians must be aware of the great variations in the number of nutrients, the form of the nutrients, the amount of the nutrients, and the recommended dose in various supplements. The word *complete* to describe the pediatric multivitamin/mineral indicates that a wide variety of both vitamins and minerals are contained; it does not mean that the product contains 100% of the recommended dietary allowance for each nutrient. These authors reviewed nine vitamin and vitamin/mineral supplements designed for children: four chewable complete, one chewable with only vitamins, three gummy-type, and one liquid. The number of nutrients in these products ranged from 10 to 22. Likewise, there was a wide range of nutrient content—from 0 to 1.5 mg of thiamin, 0 to 400 μg of folic acid, and 0 to 18 mg of iron, for example. The form of vitamin A and vitamin D also varied. In general, the gummy-type products tended to have a fewer number of nutrients and lower amounts of most nutrients than the complete chewable-type. The four chewable complete products all contained iron and calcium, while none of the gummy-types did; three of the former also contained significantly more zinc than did the latter. These products do contain labeling similar to that for food (see **Fig. 1**) so that a comparison of products can be easily done paying close attention to those nutrients deemed to be lacking. Note that the daily value for calcium is based on 1000 mg. Therefore, if using labeling as a guide to intake, 9- to 18-year-olds need 130% of the daily value.

SUMMARY

Nutrient deficiencies exist. However, they may be the result of medically necessary diets or parent/child-selected diets rather than poverty. A diet history should be done on a regular basis and unusual eating habits, omission of food groups, and actual or perceived food allergies should trigger a more in-depth assessment of the child's nutritional status. Once the restricted diet is recognized, **Table 2** can help to determine which food groups are affected. **Table 4** can then help the clinician identify the affected nutrients and offer alternative food sources to provide these nutrients. Growth should be monitored because poor growth may be related to poor nutrition. Consideration should be given to the need for appropriate nutritional supplements. Lastly,

Table 4
Sources of nutrients—food groups and alternative sources

Food Group	Nutrient	Alternative Sources
Grains: breads, cereal, rice, pasta	Thiamin	Allowable grains,[a] allowable ready-to-eat cereals,[b] pork, ham
	Riboflavin	Milk and milk products, allowable grains,[a] allowable ready-to-eat cereals,[b] organ meats
	Niacin	Meat, fish, poultry, allowable grains,[a] allowable ready-to-eat cereals[b]
	Folate	Allowable grains,[a] allowable ready-to-eat cereals,[b] dark leafy vegetables, lentils, legumes
	Iron	Meat and poultry, allowable grains,[a] allowable ready-to-eat cereals,[b] eggs, legumes, lentils, spinach, raisins
	Magnesium	Green leafy vegetables, allowable whole grains, nuts and seeds, legumes, fish, meat, fruits, other vegetables
	Selenium	Organ meats, meats, seafood, allowable grains and cereals, nuts
Dairy: milk, yogurt, cheese	Calcium	Calcium-fortified milk alternatives and juices, dark green leafy vegetables, tofu, legumes, fish with bones (eg, sardines, herring)
	Protein	Meat, poultry, fish, eggs, meat substitutes, legumes, nuts, seeds
	Vitamin A	Liver, fish, dark green and deep yellow fruits and leafy vegetables
	Vitamin D	Vitamin D–fortified milk alternatives, juices and cereals, fish oils, fatty fish (salmon, tuna, sardines, mackerel), egg yolk
	Riboflavin	Enriched grains, fortified ready-to-eat cereals,[b] organ meats
	Phosphorus	Meat, fish, poultry, eggs, lentils, legumes, nuts, seeds
	Vitamin B$_{12}$	Meat, fish, vitamin B$_{12}$–fortified milk alternatives, fortified ready-to-eat cereals[b]
Protein: meats, poultry, fish, eggs, nuts, beans	Protein	Cheese, milk, yogurt, meat substitutes, legumes, nuts, seeds
	Iron	Whole grains and enriched grain products,[a] fortified ready-to-eat cereals,[b] legumes, lentils, spinach, raisins
	Zinc	Lentils, legumes, whole grains, fortified ready-to-eat cereals, milk and milk products, nuts
	Selenium	Grains and cereals, nuts
	Thiamin	Whole grains,[a] enriched grains, ready-to-eat cereals[b]
	Riboflavin	Milk and milk products, enriched grains, ready-to-eat cereals[b]
	Vitamin B$_6$	Fortified ready-to-eat cereals,[b] fortified soy-based meat alternatives, enriched grains, white potatoes, starchy vegetables
	Vitamin B$_{12}$	Milk, vitamin B$_{12}$–fortified milk alternatives, fortified ready-to-eat cereals[b]
	Niacin	Whole grains,[a] enriched grains, ready-to-eat cereals[b]

[a] See **Table 1** for alternative grains that are high in this nutrient or allowable grains that are enriched/or fortified with this nutrient.
[b] Check food label for "% Daily value."
Data from Standing Committee on the Scientific Evaluation of Dietary Reference Intakes and its Panel on Folate, Other B Vitamins, and Choline and Subcommittee on Upper Reference Levels of Nutrients, Food and Nutrition Board, Institute of Medicine. Dietary reference intakes for thiamin, riboflavin, niacin, vitamin B6, folate, vitamin 2, pantothenic acid, biotin, and choline. Washington (DC): The National Academies Press; 1998; and United States Department of Agriculture. USDA national nutrient database for standard reference, release 21. 2009;2009(3/19).

referral to a registered dietitian knowledgeable about infant, childhood, and adolescent nutrition should be done for those clients with very restricted diets, poor growth, and/or poor nutritional status.

REFERENCES

1. Matallinos-Katsaras E, Gorman KS. Efffects of undernutrition on growth and development. In: Kessler DB, Dawson P, editors. Failure to thrive and pediatric undernutrition. A Transdisciplinary Approach. Baltimore (MD): Paul H. Brookes Publishing Co., Inc; 1999. p. 38.
2. Allen LH. Causes of nutrition-related public health problems of preschool children: available diet. J Pediatr Gastroenterol Nutr 2006;43(Suppl 3):S8–12.
3. Devaney B, Ziegler P, Pac S, et al. Nutrient intakes of infants and toddlers. J Am Diet Assoc 2004;104(Suppl 1):s14–21.
4. Nicklas TA, Hayes D. American Dietetic A. Position of the American Dietetic Association: nutrition guidance for healthy children ages 2 to 11 years. J Am Diet Assoc 2008;108(6):1038–44.
5. Wahl R. Nutrition in the adolescent. Pediatr Ann 1999;28(2):107–11.
6. National Academy of Sciences. Institute of Medicine. Food and Nutrition Board. Dietary reference intakes: recommended intakes for individuals (PDF|87 KB); 2009(2/5):7. Available at: http://www.iom.edu/CMS/3788/21370/21372.aspx. Accessed March 1, 2009.
7. Otten JJ, Hellwig JP, Meyers LD, editors. Dietary reference intakes: the essential guide to nutrient requirements. Washington (DC): National Academy of Sciences; 2006. p. 331, 410.
8. Hiza HAB, Bente L. Nutrient content of the U.S. food supply, 1909–2004 a summary report. Home Economics Research Report No 57 2007. Available at: http://www.cnpp.usda.gov/publications/foodsupply/FoodSupply1909–2004Report.pdf. Accessed March 5, 2009.
9. Looker AC, Dallman PR, Carroll MD, et al. Prevalence of iron deficiency in the United States. JAMA 1997;277(12):973–6.
10. Fischer Walker C, Black RE. Zinc and the risk for infectious disease. Annu Rev Nutr 2004;24:255–75.
11. Mitchell MK. Nutrition across the life span. Philadelphia: W.B. Saunders Company; 2003.
12. Greer FR, Krebs NF, American Academy of Pediatrics Committee on Nutrition. Optimizing bone health and calcium intakes of infants, children, and adolescents. Pediatrics 2006;117(2):578–85.
13. Gao X, Wilde PE, Lichtenstein AH, et al. Meeting adequate intake for dietary calcium without dairy foods in adolescents aged 9 to 18 years (National Health and Nutrition Examination Survey 2001–2002). J Am Diet Assoc 2006;106(11): 1759–65.
14. Wagner CL, Greer FR, American Academy of Pediatrics Section on Breastfeeding, et al. Prevention of rickets and vitamin D deficiency in infants, children, and adolescents. Pediatrics 2008;122(5):1142–52.
15. A Report of the Standing Committee on the Scientific Evaluation of Dietary Reference Intakes and its Panel on Folate, Other B Vitamins, and Choline and Subcommittee on Upper Reference Levels of Nutrients, Food and Nutrition Board, Institute of Medicine. Dietary reference intakes for thiamin, riboflavin, niacin, vitamin B6, folate, vitamin 2, pantothenic acid, biotin, and choline. Washington (DC): The National Academies Press; 1998.

16. Haines ML, Anderson RP, Gibson PR. Systematic review: the evidence base for long-term management of coeliac disease. Aliment Pharmacol Ther 2008;28(9): 1042–66.

17. Barton SH, Kelly DG, Murray JA. Nutritional deficiencies in celiac disease. Gastroenterol Clin North Am 2007;36(1):93–108.

18. Reinken L, Zieglauer H. Vitamin B-6 absorption in children with acute celiac disease and in control subjects. J Nutr 1978;108(10):1562–5.

19. Mariani P, Viti MG, Montuori M, et al. The gluten-free diet: a nutritional risk factor for adolescents with celiac disease? J Pediatr Gastroenterol Nutr 1998;27(5): 519–23.

20. Thompson T, Dennis M, Higgins LA, et al. Gluten-free diet survey: Are Americans with coeliac disease consuming recommended amounts of fibre, iron, calcium and grain foods? J Hum Nutr Diet 2005;18(3):163–9.

21. Kuehn BM. Food allergies becoming more common. JAMA 2008;300(20):2358.

22. Isolauri E, Sutas Y, Salo MK, et al. Elimination diet in cow's milk allergy: risk for impaired growth in young children. J Pediatr 1998;132(6):1004–9.

23. Christie L, Hine RJ, Parker JG, et al. Food allergies in children affect nutrient intake and growth. J Am Diet Assoc 2002;102(11):1648–51.

24. Salman S, Christie L, Burks W, et al. Dietary intakes of children with food allergies: comparison of the food guide pyramid and the recommended dietary allowance. 10th edition [abstract]. J Allergy Clin Immunol 2002;109(1):S214.

25. Sinatra FR, Merritt RJ. Iatrogenic kwashiorkor in infants. Am J Dis Child 1981; 135(1):21–3.

26. Liu T, Howard RM, Mancini AJ, et al. Kwashiorkor in the United States: fad diets, perceived and true milk allergy, and nutritional ignorance. Arch Dermatol 2001; 137(5):630–6.

27. Katz KA, Mahlberg MJ, Honig PJ, et al. Rice nightmare: kwashiorkor in 2 Philadelphia-area infants fed Rice Dream beverage. J Am Acad Dermatol 2005;52(5 Suppl 1):s69–S72.

28. Schreiber R, Adelson JW. Kwashiorkor in an urban Canadian child. CMAJ 1985; 133(9):888–9.

29. Tosh A, Fischer PR. A toddler with developmental regression. Clin Pediatr (Phila) 2004;43(3):305–6.

30. Kuhl J, Davis MD, Kalaaji AN, et al. Skin signs as the presenting manifestation of severe nutritional deficiency: report of 2 cases. Arch Dermatol 2004;140(5): 521–4.

31. Carvalho NF, Kenney RD, Carrington PH, et al. Severe nutritional deficiencies in toddlers resulting from health food milk alternatives. Pediatrics 2001;107(4):e46.

32. American Academy of Pediatrics. In: Kleinman RE, editor. Pediatric nutrition handbook. Elk Grove (IL): American Academy of Pediatrics; 2009.

33. Nordli DR Jr, Kuroda MM, Carroll J, et al. Experience with the ketogenic diet in infants. Pediatrics 2001;108(1):129–33.

34. Couch SC, Schwarzman F, Carroll J, et al. Growth and nutritional outcomes of children treated with the ketogenic diet. J Am Diet Assoc 1999;99(12):1573–5.

35. Williams S, Basualdo-Hammond C, Curtis R, et al. Growth retardation in children with epilepsy on the ketogenic diet: a retrospective chart review. J Am Diet Assoc 2002;102(3):405–7.

36. Zupec-Kania BA, Spellman E. An overview of the ketogenic diet for pediatric epilepsy. Nutr Clin Pract 2008;23(6):589–96.

37. Johnson TE, Janes SJ, MacDonald A, et al. An observational study to evaluate micronutrient status during enteral feeding. Arch Dis Child 2002;86(6):411–5.

38. Jones M, Campbell KA, Duggan C, et al. Multiple micronutrient deficiencies in a child fed an elemental formula. J Pediatr Gastroenterol Nutr 2001;33(5):602–5.
39. American Dietetic Association, Dietitians of Canada. Position of the American Dietetic Association and Dietitians of Canada: vegetarian diets. J Am Diet Assoc 2003;103(6):748–65.
40. Sanders TA, Reddy S. Vegetarian diets and children. Am J Clin Nutr 1994;59(5 Suppl):1176S–81S.
41. Messina V, Mangels AR. Considerations in planning vegan diets: children. J Am Diet Assoc 2001;101(6):661–9.
42. Mangels AR, Messina V. Considerations in planning vegan diets: infants. J Am Diet Assoc 2001;101(6):670–7.
43. Edidin DV, Levitsky LL, Schey W, et al. Resurgence of nutritional rickets associated with breast-feeding and special dietary practices. Pediatrics 1980;65(2): 232–5.
44. Weiss R, Fogelman Y, Bennett M. Severe vitamin B12 deficiency in an infant associated with a maternal deficiency and a strict vegetarian diet. J Pediatr Hematol Oncol 2004;26(4):270–1.
45. Hunt JR. Bioavailability of iron, zinc, and other trace minerals from vegetarian diets. Am J Clin Nutr 2003;78(3 Suppl):633S–9S.
46. Messina V. Vegetarian diets for children. In: Samour PQ, King K, editors. Handbook of pediatric nutrition. 3rd edition. Sudbury (MA): Jones and Barlett Publishers; 2005. p. 143, 144–59.
47. Dagnelie PC, van Staveren WA, Vergote FJ, et al. Nutritional status of infants aged 4 to 18 months on macrobiotic diets and matched omnivorous control infants: a population-based mixed-longitudinal study. II. Growth and psychomotor development. Eur J Clin Nutr 1989;43(5):325–38.
48. Dagnelie PC, van Dusseldorp M, van Staveren WA, et al. Effects of macrobiotic diets on linear growth in infants and children until 10 years of age. Eur J Clin Nutr 1994;48(Suppl 1):S103–11 [discussion: S111–12].
49. Dagnelie PC, van Staveren WA, Hautvast JG. Stunting and nutrient deficiencies in children on alternative diets. Acta Paediatr Scand Suppl 1991;374:111–8.
50. Roberts IF, West RJ, Ogilvie D, et al. Malnutrition in infants receiving cult diets: a form of child abuse. Br Med J 1979;1(6159):296–8.
51. Dagnelie PC, van Staveren WA. Macrobiotic nutrition and child health: results of a population-based, mixed-longitudinal cohort study in The Netherlands. Am J Clin Nutr 1994;59(5 Suppl):1187S–96S.
52. van Dusseldorp M, Schneede J, Refsum H, et al. Risk of persistent cobalamin deficiency in adolescents fed a macrobiotic diet in early life. Am J Clin Nutr 1999;69(4):664–71.
53. Dagnelie PC, Vergote FJ, van Staveren WA, et al. High prevalence of rickets in infants on macrobiotic diets. Am J Clin Nutr 1990;51(2):202–8.
54. Kanaka C, Schutz B, Zuppinger KA. Risks of alternative nutrition in infancy: a case report of severe iodine and carnitine deficiency. Eur J Pediatr 1992; 151(10):786–8.
55. Schreck KA, Williams K, Smith AF. A comparison of eating behaviors between children with and without autism. J Autism Dev Disord 2004;34(4):433–8.
56. Ahearn WH, Castine T, Nault K, et al. An assessment of food acceptance in children with autism or pervasive developmental disorder-not otherwise specified. J Autism Dev Disord 2001;31(5):505–11.
57. Cornish E. A balanced approach towards healthy eating in autism. J Hum Nutr Diet 1998;11:501–9.

58. Tamura Y, Welch DC, Zic JA, et al. Scurvy presenting as painful gait with bruising in a young boy. Arch Pediatr Adolesc Med 2000;154(7):732–5.
59. Raiten DJ, Massaro T. Perspectives on the nutritional ecology of autistic children. J Autism Dev Disord 1986;16(2):133–43.
60. Williams PG, Dalrymple N, Neal J. Eating habits of children with autism. Pediatr Nurs 2000;26(3):259–64.
61. Bowers L. An audit of referrals of children with autistic spectrum disorder to the dietetic service. J Hum Nutr Diet 2002;15(2):141–4.
62. Christison GW, Ivany K. Elimination diets in autism spectrum disorders: any wheat amidst the chaff? J Dev Behav Pediatr 2006;27(2 Suppl):S162–71.
63. Elder JH, Shankar M, Shuster J, et al. The gluten-free, casein-free diet in autism: results of a preliminary double blind clinical trial. J Autism Dev Disord 2006;36(3): 413–20.
64. Cornish E. Gluten and casein free diets in autism: a study of the effects on food choice and nutrition. J Hum Nutr Diet 2002;15(4):261–9.
65. Arnold GL, Hyman SL, Mooney RA, et al. Plasma amino acids profiles in children with autism: potential risk of nutritional deficiencies. J Autism Dev Disord 2003; 33(4):449–54.
66. Hediger ML, England LJ, Molloy CA, et al. Reduced bone cortical thickness in boys with autism or autism spectrum disorder. J Autism Dev Disord 2008;38(5): 848–56.

Nutritional Deficiencies in Obesity and After Bariatric Surgery

Stavra A. Xanthakos, MD, MS[a,b,]*

KEYWORDS

- Obesity • Pediatric obesity • Nutritional deficiencies
- Bariatric surgery • Malabsorption

The presence of nutritional deficiencies in overweight and obesity may seem paradoxic in light of the evidence of excess caloric intake, but a growing body of literature has documented that several micronutrient deficiencies may be higher in prevalence in overweight and obese adults and children, particularly in those suffering from extreme obesity (body mass index [BMI] greater than $40kg/m^2$ in adults and greater than or equal to the 99th percentile in children). Consumption of excess calories does not automatically equate with overconsumption of fruits, vegetables and other unprocessed, high-quality nutrient-dense foods. Increased adiposity itself may influence the serum levels of some fat-soluble vitamins, such as vitamin D.[1] Compounding the problem, surgical treatments for severe obesity also have grown in frequency and may exacerbate pre-existing vitamin and mineral deficiencies or produce new ones, depending on dietary intake, adherence to recommended postoperative supplementation, and degree of malabsorption associated with the bariatric surgery procedure. Much of the recent data on nutritional deficits in obese individuals are from studies of adults undergoing preoperative evaluations for bariatric surgery, which indicate that baseline nutritional deficiencies are not negligible in extremely obese patients.

As the obesity epidemic continues unabated and the popularity of bariatric surgery rises for extremely obese adults and adolescents, clinicians must be aware of pre-existing nutritional deficiencies in overweight and obese patients. To optimize long-term health

This work was supported by Grant Number K23DK080888 from the National Institutes of Health.

[a] Division of Gastroenterology, Hepatology and Nutrition, Cincinnati Children's Hospital Medical Center, 3333 Burnet Avenue, MLC 2010, Cincinnati, OH 45229, USA
[b] Surgical Weight Loss Program for Teens, Cincinnati Children's Hospital Medical Center, Cincinnati, OH, USA
* Division of Gastroenterology, Hepatology and Nutrition, Cincinnati Children's Hospital Medical Center, 3333 Burnet Avenue, MLC 2010, Cincinnati, OH 45229.
E-mail address: stavra.xanthakos@cchmc.org

after bariatric surgery, it is important to screen for and recognize symptoms of deficiency, prescribe appropriate supplementation, and treat common and rare nutritional deficiencies that may emerge in the short term and in the long term postoperatively. Although not as common as in adults, the incidence of bariatric surgery also has increased dramatically in adolescents with severe obesity, rising fivefold between 1997 and 2003.[2] Therefore, pediatric practitioners may well encounter the postoperative bariatric patient in their practice and must be able to screen for and treat predictable nutritional deficiencies. The adolescent bariatric patient may be particularly at risk for nonadherence to recommended supplementation and requires close follow-up, given the longer anticipated life span with altered digestive physiology.[3] This article summarizes current knowledge of nutritional deficiencies in obese and overweight individuals, with a particular focus on those that commonly occur after bariatric surgery. Current algorithms for screening and supplementation also are reviewed.

MECHANISMS CONTRIBUTING TO NUTRITIONAL DEFICIENCIES IN OBESITY

Though commonly considered a state of overnutrition, obesity increasingly has been recognized as a risk factor for several nutrient deficiencies, including lower levels of antioxidants and certain fat-soluble vitamins.[4] More recently, studies of extremely obese adults undergoing bariatric surgery have identified a wider array of pre-existing nutritional deficiencies before surgery. The cause of these nutritional deficiencies in overweight and obese individuals is not completely known. In large part, however, they are thought to be caused by higher intake of higher-calorie processed foods associated with poor nutritional quality, particularly in highly developed countries in which there is an abundance of relatively cheap, energy-dense, but nutrient-poor food. About 27% to 30% of the daily caloric intake of American children and adults is comprised of low nutrient density food, with sweeteners and desserts contributing 18% to 24% of the total.[5,6] Unprocessed nutrient-dense foods include fruits and vegetables, dairy products, whole grains, nuts and legumes, and fish and protein sources, which contribute the bulk of vitamins and minerals obtained from a nonsupplemented diet. As intake of nutrient-poor food increases, the intake of unprocessed, nutrient-dense foods decreases proportionately.[5] Higher-fat diets (greater than 30% of total caloric intake) are associated with decreased intake of vitamins A, C, and folate.[7] Increased consumption of sweetened beverages also is associated with lower intake of milk, and therefore calcium and fortified vitamin D_3.[8] In the case of vitamin D_3, additional risk factors for deficiency may include reduced physical activity, leading to decreased sun exposure, increased storage of vitamin D_3 in excess adipose tissue, and ethnicity and skin tone.[9]

The rising rate of bariatric surgeries in extremely obese adults and adolescents also plays a role in increasing the risk of nutritional deficiencies associated with overweight and obese individuals.[2,10] The presence of nutritional deficiencies of selected micronutrients and macronutrients after bariatric surgery has been recognized for decades, but varies widely in prevalence and severity depending on type of bariatric surgery (**Fig. 1**).

Surgical weight loss procedures generally are classified as restrictive, malabsorptive, or a combination of both. Of the purely restrictive procedures, the vertical banded gastroplasty (VBG, **Fig. 1**D) and adjustable gastric band (AGB, **Fig. 1**E) create a 30 to 50 mL gastric pouch in the proximal stomach just under the gastroesophageal junction. The AGB is performed more often than the VBG. The vertical sleeve gastrectomy (VSG, **Fig. 1**G) is also a purely restrictive procedure, but it removes the greater curvature of the stomach, leaving a narrow gastric sleeve in continuity with the remainder of

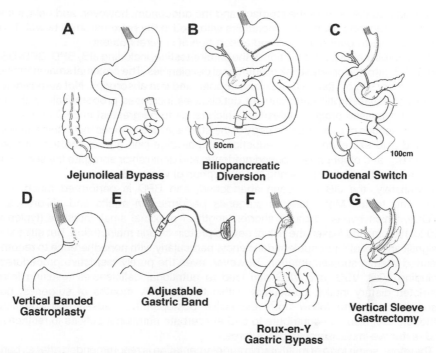

Fig. 1. Types of past and present bariatric surgery procedures. Jejunoileal bypass (*A*) largely has been abandoned because of the high risk of malabsorptive complications. Biliopancreatic diversion (*B*) also is performed less commonly. The most commonly performed procedures include the biliopancreatic diversion with duodenal switch (*C*), vertical-banded gastroplasty (*D*), the adjustable gastric band (*E*), the Roux-en-y gastric bypass (*F*), and the vertical sleeve gastrectomy (*G*). (*From* Xanthakos SA. Bariatric surgery for extreme adolescent obesity: indications, outcome, and physiologic effects on the gut–brain axis. Pathophysiology 2008;15:135; with permission.)

the small intestine. Initially performed as the first stage in a biliopancreatic diversion with duodenal switch procedure, it is gaining increased interest as a stand-alone procedure for surgical weight loss.

The purely malabsorptive jejunoileal bypass (JIB, **Fig.** 1A) that involved bypassing most of the small intestine largely has been abandoned because of numerous metabolic and nutritional complications. The biliopancreatic diversion (BPD, **Fig.** 1B) and biliopancreatic diversion with duodenal switch (BPD-DS, **Fig.** 1C) both involve restriction and malabsorption. In the BPD, up to 60% of the stomach is resected. The duodenal stump is closed, and the proximal ileum is transected and anastomosed to the distal small bowel about 50 cm proximal to the ileocecal valve. The distal ileal segment is anastomosed to the remaining stomach. The BPD-DS variant involves a gastric sleeve resection of the greater curvature of the stomach, but a small cuff of duodenum is preserved and anastomosed to the distal ileum. The proximal ileum is anastomosed to the distal small bowel about 100 cm from the ileocecal valve. This reduces the degree of micronutrient malabsorption compared with the BPD. The Roux-en-Y gastric bypass (RYGB, **Fig.** 1F), which currently is the most commonly performed procedure in both adults and children, is mainly restrictive, creating a 20 to 30 mL gastric pouch, which then is anastomosed to a Roux limb of proximal jejunum. It also bypasses the body of the stomach and the duodenum, however, and delays the mixing of biliary and pancreatic secretions with food in the proximal small bowel. This can contribute to poor digestion and absorption of several nutrients.

Procedures that bypass a portion of the small intestine, including JIB, BPD, BPD-DS, and RYGB carry the greatest risk of nutritional deficiencies. The proximal small intestine is the primary site of vitamin D, calcium, copper, and iron absorption. Not surprisingly, the risk of malabsorption and nutrient deficiencies increases proportionally with the length of bypassed proximal intestine, which tends to be greatest in BPD and JIB.[11] Gastric resection or bypass of the body of the stomach also reduces mechanical digestion and acid secretion. These reductions impair digestion and absorption of iron, vitamin B_{12}, and other protein-bound nutrients, and diminish or abrogate the secretion of intrinsic factor, further impairing the absorption of vitamin B_{12}.

Fortunately, the JIB has been abandoned, and BPD is performed much less commonly today. Most bariatric surgeries performed in adults and children are RYGBs, which bypass a much shorter length of proximal small intestine (typically 100 to 150 cm) and lessen the risk of severe protein calorie malnutrition, but still carry a significant risk of micronutrient deficiency, particularly with nonadherence to recommended vitamin supplementation. However, even the purely restrictive procedures, including AGB, VSG, and VBG can lead to nutritional deficiencies resulting from restricted dietary intake, particularly within the first few months of surgeries, but also over long-term follow up.[12] Excessive postoperative nausea and vomiting, although rare, also can contribute to and exacerbate nutritional deficits in restrictive and restrictive–malabsorptive procedures.

Therefore, some form of multivitamin supplementation is recommended after all bariatric procedures. Often the number of supplements is dictated by the type of procedure and the potential for malabsorption. After AGB, it is often typical to prescribe a single multivitamin and recommend additional elemental calcium supplementation, but single multivitamin supplementation does not appear to be sufficient to prevent iron and vitamin B_{12} deficiencies and anemia following the restrictive–malabsorptive procedures.[13] Recent comprehensive allied health nutritional guidelines from the American Society for Metabolic and Bariatric Surgery suggest laboratory measures to monitor pre-existing and postprocedure deficiencies, and suggested postoperative vitamin and mineral supplementation, including dosing and administration specifications.[14] All recommendations for supplementation are based on expert opinion and observational research demonstrating the emergence of predictable nutrient deficiencies after specific types of bariatric surgery. Prospectively controlled randomized trials to determine optimal types and amounts of supplementation are largely lacking. Therefore, available guidelines for supplementation are likely to change as new evidence becomes available. Supplementation practices currently vary widely across programs, but with emergence of guidelines, clinical practice may become more standardized, which will make it easier to compare nutritional outcomes across different programs and further refine guidelines.[15,16] A synopsis of screening and supplementation recommendations based on reported expert opinion and the current practice at the author's adolescent bariatric program is presented in **Table 1**.[14,17] However, despite supplementation practices already in place in the vast majority of bariatric programs, the prevalence of nutritional deficiencies among bariatric patients is still quite high as reviewed in the following sections, perhaps due to difficulties with adherence or because supplementation needs may vary among patients depending on adequacy of dietary intake and type of surgery. Evidence of poor adherence to medications and supplementation pre-operatively might also prompt choice of a purely restrictive bariatric procedure to reduce post-operative risk of significant nutritional deficits.

PREVALENCE AND CLINICAL SIGNIFICANCE OF NUTRITIONAL DEFICIENCIES IN OBESITY AND AFTER BARIATRIC SURGERY

Macronutrient Deficiencies

All types of bariatric surgery lead to very reduced total calorie intake, especially in the first 6 postoperative months, typically ranging from 700 to 900 kcal/d following RYGB.[18] This can contribute to the decreased intake of all macronutrients, especially protein, as patients may have difficulty achieving recommended protein intakes in the face of severely restricted caloric intake and in some cases temporary intolerance of protein-rich or dairy foods. Although patients are advised to consume at least 1 to 1.5 g of protein per kilogram, of ideal body weight (a minimum of 60 g of protein per day), some studies have indicated that protein intake in the first year after surgery may be much lower than recommended, often closer to 0.5 g/kg.[18,19] Baseline hypoalbuminemia appears to be uncommon in the United States, but was reported in up to 15.6% of subjects undergoing RYGB in Brazil.[18] Certainly, any pre-existing hypoalbuminemia could be worsened if adequate protein intake is not achieved during the periods of highest caloric restriction. Although the purely restrictive procedures and RYGB with 75 to 150 cm Roux limb lengths rarely cause hypoalbuminemia, BPD is more likely to lead to hypoalbuminemia, with reported prevalence of hypoalbuminemia ranging from 3% to 11%.[20–22] Longer Roux limb lengths in RYGB, however, can increase the risk of hypoalbuminemia.[23] Low protein intake can lead to increased hair loss and contribute to poor wound healing, which is especially critical if body-contouring surgeries are pursued by the patient at a later time.[24] Fortunately, significant protein calorie malnutrition or kwashiorkor rarely is seen, except in cases of extreme nonadherence to dietary recommendations.[25]

Micronutrient Deficiencies

Micronutrient deficiencies are the most likely long-term adverse events after bariatric surgery and can lead to wide-ranging symptoms, most commonly anemia (10% to 74%) and neurologic dysfunction (5% to 9%) (see **Table 1**).[26,27] Determining the true risk of developing micronutrient deficiencies is challenging, as there has been no consensus on the appropriate type and amount of vitamin and mineral supplementation across bariatric surgery programs; therefore supplementation practices vary widely.[15] Further, varying levels of adherence and dietary intake make it difficult to estimate the true risk of developing nutritional deficiencies. Nonetheless, it is clear that micronutrient deficiencies are relatively common in patients before and after all types of bariatric surgery; therefore, it is important to screen patients at baseline, and at a minimum, annually, for deficiencies. In women who become pregnant after bariatric surgery, it is critical to screen and treat nutritional deficits before and during pregnancies. A recommended screening and supplementation algorithm is presented in **Table 1**, but it is again important to emphasize that these suggestions are based on expert opinion and reported recommendations, rather than results of randomized–controlled trials. Importantly, supplements should not be enteric-coated or time-release formulations, as most bariatric patients have altered and diminished gastric phase digestion, particularly after RYGB, BPD, and VSG. Supplements and medications should dissolve readily in a glass of room temperature water within at most 30 minutes; liquid, suspension, or chewable preparations are ideal. In the early postoperative period (first month), liquid or chewable preparations often are tolerated better.

Iron

Iron deficiency is perhaps the most common and earliest nutritional deficiency to occur following bariatric surgery, occurring in up to 12% to 47% of patients,

Table 1
Recommended nutritional screening and supplementation after bariatric surgery

Nutrient	Biomarker(s)	Primary Symptoms of Deficiency
Baseline, 6-month, and annual screening after bariatric surgery		
Vitamin B_1	Serum thiamin	Ophthalmoplegia, nystagmus, ataxia, encephalopathy, rapid visual loss (Wernicke encephalopathy) Isolated peripheral neuropathy
Vitamin B_{12}	Serum vitamin B_{12}	Anemia, neurologic dysfunction, visual loss
Folate	Red blood cell folate Consider plasma homocysteine	Anemia
Iron	Serum, ferritin, TIBC, complete blood count with differential	Microcytic anemia
Vitamin D	Serum 25(OH) vitamin D, calcium, phosphorus, parathyroid hormone	Decreased bone mineral density Secondary hyperparathyroidism
Protein	Serum albumin	Edema, excessive alopecia, poor wound-healing
Additional annual screening after BPD and BPD-DS		
Vitamin A	Plasma retinol	Reduced night vision, visual impairment
Vitamin E	Plasma alpha-tocopherol	Neuropathy, ataxia
Vitamin K	Prothrombin time	Bleeding, easy bruising
Screen after any bariatric procedure if suggestive symptoms		
B6 (pyridoxine)	Plasma pyridoxal-5'-phosphate	Anemia, neurologic symptoms
Copper	Serum copper	Anemia, neuropathy
Zinc	Plasma zinc	Acrodermatitis enteropathica-like rash, taste alterations

General supplementation recommendations

Supplement	Daily recommendations	
Multivitamin (contains folic acid)	AGB/VSG	One daily
	RYGB	One to two daily
	BPD-DS	Two daily
Calcium citrate with vitamin D_3	AGB	1200–1500 mg/d
	RYGB and BPD-DS	1800 mg/d
Vitamin D_3	RYGB	Consider 1000 IU/d
	BPD-DS	2000 IU/d
Vitamin B_{12}	RYGB	Crystalline 500 μg/d orally or 1000 μg/mo intramuscularly
	BPD-DS	Monitor and start if needed
Elemental iron	RYGB and BDP-DS	65 mg elemental iron in menstruating females
Vitamin B_1	All procedures	Consider once daily in first 6 months
Vitamins A and K	BPD-DS	10,000 IU vitamin A and 300 μg/vitamin K

Abbreviations: AGB, adjustable gastric band; BPD, biliopancreatic diversion; BPD-DS, biliopancreatic diversion with duodenal switch; PTH, parathyroid hormone; RBC, red blood cell; RYGB: Roux-en-Y gastric bypass; TIBC, total iron binding capacity; VSG, vertical sleeve gastrectomy; 25 (OH) D, 25 hydroxy-vitamin D.

Recommend in most cases that routine supplementation begin at discharge from hospital so that the patient develops a routine early. The author's program begins with a multivitamin supplement and B complex preoperatively during preparatory weight management phase in all patients, and adds 1000 IU vitamin D_3, if preoperative vitamin D deficiency is found.

particularly after RYGB and BPD.[15,18,28] Menstruating and pregnant females are at greatest risk.[28,29] Anemia also can be exacerbated by chronic inflammation secondary to obesity.[30] Although often asymptomatic, iron deficiency can lead to anemia and fatigue, and in severe cases, it can present with pica.[28,31] It is important to emphasize, however, that baseline iron deficiency also has been reported in up to 44% of adults before bariatric surgery, which may contribute to iron deficiency postoperatively if not identified and treated.[32] In a cohort study of 379 consecutive patients presenting for RYGB, iron deficiency was also more prevalent in younger subjects (younger than 25 years) versus older subjects (older than 60 years) (79% versus 42% respectively).[32] Routine multivitamin supplementation does not appear to be sufficient to prevent iron deficiency after RYGB, and in most cases, supplemental iron is necessary.[28] It is not clear, however, if this is because preoperative deficiencies were not adequately identified and corrected before surgery, as baseline studies are often lacking in most retrospective studies. If refractory to oral iron supplementation and correction, parenteral iron therapy or even blood transfusions may be necessary, especially in menstruating and pregnant women.[29,33]

Calcium and vitamin D

Deficiency of vitamin D has gained widespread attention as deficiency of the hormone has been recognized increasingly as a risk factor for a multitude of diseases beyond development of rickets in childhood and osteomalacia in adulthood. In addition to reducing dietary calcium absorption, vitamin D deficiency may contribute to dysfunction of the innate immune system, and therefore play a role in increasing risk of cancers, diabetes mellitus, autoimmune diseases, and cardiovascular disease.[34] The optimal levels of 25-hydroxyvitamin D (25-OH D), the primary circulating form of the vitamin D, are debated, but deficiency is defined commonly as 25-OH D level less than 20 ng/mL (50 nmol/L) and insufficiency as 21 to 29 ng/mL (50 to 80 nmol/L). Widespread deficiency (40% to 100%) of 25-OH D has been noted in population-based studies in the United States and many other countries,[34–37] in part because of seasonal variation in sunlight exposure, increased use of sunscreens to prevent skin cancer, and changes in lifestyle favoring more indoor time.[34] Mean levels of 25-OH D have declined in national surveys of adults in the United States between 1988 through 1994 and 2000 through 2004.[38]

Accordingly, the 2008 American Academy of Pediatrics supplementation recommendations for vitamin D in childhood now include a recommendation that all infants, children, and adolescents have a minimum daily intake of 400 IU of vitamin D beginning soon after birth.[39] Expert opinion suggests that the intake be increased to 800 to 1000 IU for children and adults receiving inadequate sun exposure.[34] Adequate sun exposure is defined as twice-a-week exposure of arms and legs for 5 to 30 minutes between the hours of 10 AM and 3 PM, depending on the latitude, season, and skin pigmentation. Optimal supplementation for overweight and obese adults and children has not been determined, and current recommendations for the general population should be followed. Notably, vitamin D_2, which is more commonly found in over-the-counter multivitamins, is 70% less effective than vitamin D_3 in increasing and maintaining sufficient 25-OH D levels.[40]

Dietary intake also may play a role, although the predominant source of vitamin D remains synthesis in the skin after ultraviolet radiation exposure, with less than 10% of vitamin D originating from dietary intake.[41] Intake of vitamin D-fortified milk, which is a large source of vitamin D, declines as children age.[42] Further, milk intake declines as consumption of larger quantities of sweetened beverages increases, as observed in young African American and Caucasian girls followed longitudinally between ages 9 to

10 and 19 years.[43] Some studies have noted disparities in vitamin D intake in certain racial and ethnic groups, with Mexican American and African American adults consuming lower levels of vitamin D, potentially because of higher rates of lactose intolerance.[44] Because of frequently darker skin tones, these groups also may make lower levels of vitamin D after sun exposure.

Overweight and obese individuals tend to have lower mean levels of 25-OH D compared with lean subjects.[45] Potential explanations include decreased dietary intake of fortified milk products, more sedentary lifestyle, reduced exposure to bright sunlight, and sequestration of the lipid-soluble vitamin in increased adipose tissue stores. Low serum 25-OH D appears to be inversely proportional to increasing fat mass.[46,47] Marked seasonal variation in 25-OH D levels also may be present in adult obese subjects, independent of the degree of obesity. In one cross-sectional study of 248 obese subjects with BMI ranging from 30.1 to 68.9 kg/m^2, prevalence of 25-OH D deficiency was 3.8-fold higher during the winter when compared with summer months (91.2 versus 24.3%, $P<.001$).[48] In contrast, comparison of 41 age-, sex-, race/ethnicity- and seasonally matched preoperative obese adult patients with nonobese controls demonstrated that the prevalence of vitamin D deficiency (61%) and insufficiency (90%) was substantially higher than in controls (12% and 32% respectively), even after controlling for sunlight exposure and dietary intake of calcium and vitamin D.[49]

Accordingly, 25% to 80% of adult prebariatric patients may have baseline vitamin D deficiency.[32,50] Hispanic and African American patients undergoing bariatric surgery may have even higher rates of vitamin D deficiency (approximately 78%) than their Caucasian counterparts (36%).[51,52] In a study of 70 adult patients presenting for RYGB, mean 25-OH D levels also were correlated inversely with BMI, lending support to the theory that fat mass may influence bioavailability.[53] Of concern is that 45% of these individuals continued to have insufficient vitamin D levels, despite recommended postoperative supplementation. Optimal dosing of vitamin D after various types of bariatric surgery remains unclear. A recent expert guideline suggests supplementation of 2000 IU/d for patients after BPD-DS, with no additional vitamin D_3 for patients after RYGB or AGB, above that associated with the elemental calcium supplement.[14] Based on the experience at the author's adolescent bariatric surgery program, vitamin D deficiency appears to be very prevalent both before and after RYGB, necessitating additional vitamin D_3 supplementation, up to 1000 IU orally daily or 50,000 IU monthly in cases of severe deficiency (Xanthakos SA and Inge TH, 2009; unpublished data). One recent prospective randomized clinical study has indicated that doses up to 5000 IU appear to be safe and necessary in some adults patients after RYGB to maintain vitamin D sufficiency, yet not enough to prevent vitamin D insufficiency for others.[54] Supplementation of calcium with vitamin D at recommended levels for 6 months did not appear to suppress secondary hyperparathyroidism or bone resorption in 44 women 3 or more years after RYGB.[55] Further prospective studies will be necessary to determine the true prevalence and risk factors for vitamin D_3 deficiency before and after different types of bariatric surgery in extremely obese adults and adolescents, and optimal dosing strategies.

Despite high prevalence of vitamin D deficiency after bariatric surgery, serum calcium levels frequently are maintained in normal ranges. Elevated parathyroid hormone levels are far more common (up to 29% in RYGB and 63% after BPD), but it is unclear whether prevalence differs significantly from baseline.[56–58] Reported sequelae of vitamin D and resultant calcium deficiency after bariatric surgeries, particularly in surgeries that include a malabsorptive component, include high bone turnover and decreased bone mass.[57,59,60] Concomitant risk factors may lead to earlier presentation. Osteomalacia has been reported in a 42-year-old patient with a history of corticosteroid-dependent asthma, within 6/5 years of RYGB.[59] Up to 70% of patients develop secondary hyperparathyroidism after BPD[61]

A routine multivitamin typically contains 400 IU of vitamin D (most often ergocalciferol or D_2) and 100 to 200 mg of calcium carbonate. Calcium with vitamin D supplements vary considerably in the amount and type of calcium and vitamin D. A typical calcium with vitamin D supplement often contains 500 to 600 mg per dose of calcium (carbonate or citrate) and 400 to 500 IU of vitamin D (ergocalciferol [D_2] or cholecalciferol [D_3]). Calcium citrate is easier to absorb, particularly in conditions with reduced stomach acid, and it is preferable for patients after bariatric surgery. Taken three times a day, calcium citrate plus vitamin D supplements can provide up to 1500 to 1800 mg of calcium and 1200 to 1500 IU of vitamin D. Although these amounts of calcium and vitamin D are likely to be sufficient for patients after the purely restrictive procedures, patients after RYGB may require additional supplemental vitamin D_3, and patients after BPD-DS should be prescribed supplemental vitamin D_3, as outlined in **Table 1**.

Other Fat-soluble Vitamins: Vitamins A, K, and E

Several large cross-sectional studies of obese and overweight children indicate that they may have lower concentrations of antioxidant vitamins retinol and beta-carotene (vitamin A) and alpha-tocopherol (vitamin E).[4,62] Studies of baseline nutritional deficits in adults presenting for bariatric surgery also indicate potential vitamin A and E deficiencies in the extremely obese. Up to a 12.5% prevalence of low levels of retinols and beta-carotene recently was described preoperatively in adults undergoing bariatric surgery, with increased severity postoperatively.[63,64] In cases of very severe deficiency, this can cause xerophthalmia and nyctalopia, with visual deterioration reported in one 39-year-old woman 3 years following RYGB.[65] Pre-existing vitamin E deficiency has been reported in up to 23% of RYGB patients.[66] Although less common, significant declines in vitamin E also have been reported after RYGB.[67] Vitamin E may be clinically significant because of its antioxidant function. Neuropathy has been reported in association with vitamin E deficiency after gastrectomy for gastric cancer, but reports of symptomatic deficiencies after bariatric surgery are lacking.[68] In general, however, fat-soluble vitamin deficiencies, including vitamins A (69%), E (7.1%), and K (68%), appear to be more common after BPD because of significant fat malabsorption.[69,70] Routine annual monitoring therefore is suggested only after BPD or BPD-DS procedures, but it should be considered after any bariatric surgery procedure if symptoms develop (see **Table 1**).

Vitamins B_{12}, B_1 (Thiamin), Folate, and Vitamin B_6

The B vitamins are generally important for neurologic and hematological function. Further, low folate and B_{12} levels can be associated with elevated plasma homocysteine levels, which may be a potential independent risk factor for oxidative stress and cardiovascular disease.[71] A recent meta-analysis of supplemental folate therapy, however, did not show any benefit in reducing cardiovascular disease, so evidence is still inconclusive.[72]

Overweight has been associated with a greater risk of decreased intake of folate in adolescents.[73] Prevalence of preoperative folic acid deficiency (up to 54%) has been noted in international studies before bariatric surgery. Recent US studies, however, report very low prevalence of folate deficiency (0% to 6%) at baseline, perhaps because of widespread folate fortification of foods in the United States.[51,70,74] Similarly, risk of folate deficiency appears to be very low after bariatric surgery in the United States, and addition of a routine multivitamin nearly always corrects any deficiencies.[28] This is likely because of additional dietary sources from fortified foods, the absorption of folate along the entire length of the small intestine, and bacterial synthesis of folate in the intestine.[75] Low folate levels after bariatric surgery therefore can indicate lack of adherence to multivitamin supplementation.[74]

In contrast with the low baseline risk of folate deficiency, low vitamin B_{12} levels have been reported before bariatric surgery in up to 18% of severely obese adults.[51] Vitamin B_{12} deficiency postoperatively is associated more commonly with RYGB (up to one third of patients),[28] but the rate is significantly reduced to approximately 4% of patients with vitamin B_{12} supplementation.[64,76] Multivitamin supplementation alone is not sufficient to prevent vitamin B_{12} deficiency.[28] Daily oral vitamin B_{12} (350 to 600 mg/day) is effective in correcting deficiency in 81% to 95% of patients,[77,78] and intramuscular monthly vitamin B_{12} injections are another option in patients who have trouble adhering to daily oral supplements.

Baseline vitamin B_1 or thiamin deficiency has been reported in up to 29% of patients undergoing bariatric surgery.[32] One study of 378 adults found that pre-existing thiamin deficiency may be highest in African American (31%) and Hispanic patients (47%), compared with Caucasian patients (7%). Thiamin deficiency is more common after procedures that involve gastric bypass because of decreased acidification of food and impaired absorption, but it also has been reported in isolated cases after purely restrictive procedures.[79,80] Asymptomatic thiamin deficiency has been reported in up to 18% of patients 1 year after RYGB. [64] Severe thiamin deficiency leading to peripheral neuropathy, and in some cases Wernicke encephalopathy, has been reported in both adults and adolescents after bariatric surgery.[81,82] Typically, this occurs around 6 weeks to 3 months after surgery, but it has been reported to occur as early as 2 weeks postoperatively.[83] Risk factors include excessive postoperative vomiting leading to reduced intake and nonadherence to multivitamin supplementation.[84] Rapid identification and treatment with intravenous supplementation can rapidly improve visual loss and promote resolution of neurologic sequelae, while delay in repletion can cause permanent disability.[81]

Vitamin B_6 (17.6%) and vitamin B_2 (13.6%) deficiencies also have been reported in patients 1 year after RYGB, but the true prevalence of pre-existing vitamin B_6 and vitamin B_2 deficiencies in obese patients is unknown, as these vitamins are not screened for commonly.[64]

Vitamin C (Ascorbic Acid)

Ascorbic acid or vitamin C deficiency has been noted in up to 36% of adult patients aged 20 to 66 years before bariatric surgery.[85] Ascorbic acid deficiency correlated with higher BMI, younger age, decreased intake of fruit and vegetables, and lack of vitamin supplementation. More recently, ascorbic acid deficiency has been reported in 34.5% of post-RYGB patients at 1 year postoperatively.[64] Like vitamin E, ascorbic acid has important antioxidant functions. Preliminary studies suggest that supplementation of vitamins C and E lowers markers of inflammation and may improve insulin sensitivity, but demonstration of significant adverse effects of vitamin C deficiency on clinical outcome after bariatric surgery remains lacking.[86] Routine screening is not recommended, and standard multivitamin supplementation should be sufficient to prevent deficiency postoperatively.

RARE BUT CLINICALLY SIGNIFICANT NUTRITIONAL DEFICIENCIES AFTER BARIATRIC SURGERY

Low serum zinc levels have been reported in preoperative (up to 28%) and postoperative bariatric patients (36% to 51%).[69,87] In most cases, these zinc deficiencies have been asymptomatic, but zinc deficiency with an acrodermatitis enteropathica-like rash has been reported in a patient who was completely nonadherent to recommended multivitamin supplementation after a distal RYGB procedure.[25] Cardiomyopathy presumably secondary to selenium deficiency has been reported 9 months following BPD.[88] Selenium also has antioxidant function. Copper deficiency following bariatric surgery has gained increased attention in recent years. Copper deficiency causing anemia and neurologic impairment has been reported in two patients following RYGB and copper deficiency also has been shown to increase in prevalence after BPD.[70,89] If unexplained anemia persists in patients after bariatric surgery, copper deficiency should be excluded. Zinc supplementation in high doses (50 mg/d or more) can interfere with intestinal absorption, and patients receiving prolonged zinc supplementation should be monitored for copper deficiency. Routine screening for these less common deficiencies is probably not cost-effective given their low incidence, but screening should be triggered by the onset of symptoms of unexplained anemia, neurologic impairment, unusual skin manifestations, or cardiac dysfunction.

NUTRITIONAL DEFICIENCIES AND PREGNANCY AFTER BARIATRIC SURGERY

The importance of routine nutritional screening and supplementation is heightened in pregnancy following bariatric surgery. In general, pregnancy after bariatric surgery appears to be very safe after the rapid weight loss phase has ended and a stable weight has been achieved.[90,91] Anemia is the most common problem during pregnancy after bariatric surgery; however, rare but severe fetal and maternal complications caused by nutrient deficiencies have been reported. A fetal cerebral hemorrhage was reported because of maternal vitamin K deficiency following vomiting after gastric band slippage.[92] Infantile visual impairment also has occurred secondary to maternal, and subsequently fetal, vitamin A deficiency.[93] Therefore, all nutrient deficiencies should be identified before pregnancy if possible and corrected before pregnancy. Additional vitamin and calcium supplementation is often necessary. In some cases, parenteral iron therapy or blood transfusions have been necessary to correct anemia.[29]

SUMMARY

Overweight and obese individuals are at risk for deficiencies in several micronutrients, including iron, and vitamins D, B_{12}, E, and C. Risk factors include predominantly nutrient-poor diets. Additional factors, however, may play a role in vitamin D deficiency, including reduced sun exposure and increased adipose stores. Bariatric surgery, an increasingly acceptable treatment for severe obesity in adults and adolescents, also can lead to several predictable nutritional deficiencies and can worsen preexisting ones. It is critical to screen for nutritional deficiencies in obese patients before bariatric surgery and at regular intervals after bariatric surgery, and to encourage adherence to supplementation.

At present there is a lack of evidence or expert recommendation to screen all overweight and obese children for nutritional deficiencies. Given the emerging data on the high prevalence of nutritional deficiencies associated with overweight and obesity, however, practice recommendations may evolve as further information becomes available. If signs or symptoms suggest a nutritional deficiency, screening for specific micronutrient deficits should be performed, independent of bariatric surgery status. Despite a very high prevalence of vitamin D deficiency in the general population, universal 25-OH D screening has not been recommended. Rather, supplemental vitamin D (400 IU/d) should be recommended for those children and adolescents who do not obtain at least 400 IU/d through fortified milk, cereals, and other foods.

Given the high prevalence of baseline nutritional deficiencies, the quality of the diet should be screened in all overweight and obese children, and a routine multivitamin and focused dietary consultation should be considered, if the child's diet is not balanced adequately.

REFERENCES

1. Gillis L, Gillis A. Nutrient inadequacy in obese and nonobese youth. Can J Diet Pract Res 2005;66:237–42.
2. Schilling PL, Davis MM, Albanese CT, et al. National trends in adolescent bariatric surgical procedures and implications for surgical centers of excellence. J Am Coll Surg 2008;206:1–12.
3. Rand CS, Macgregor AM. Adolescents having obesity surgery: a 6-year follow-up. South Med J 1994;87:1208–13.
4. Strauss RS. Comparison of serum concentrations of alpha-tocopherol and beta-carotene in a cross-sectional sample of obese and nonobese children (NHANES III). National Health and Nutrition Examination Survey. J Pediatr 1999;134:160–5.
5. Kant AK. Reported consumption of low-nutrient density foods by American children and adolescents: nutritional and health correlates, NHANES III, 1988 to 1994. Arch Pediatr Adolesc Med 2003;157:789–96.
6. Kant AK. Consumption of energy-dense, nutrient-poor foods by adult Americans: nutritional and health implications. The third National Health and Nutrition Examination Survey, 1988–1994. Am J Clin Nutr 2000;72:929–36.
7. Hampl JS, Betts NM. Comparisons of dietary intake and sources of fat in low- and high-fat diets of 18- to 24-year-olds. J Am Diet Assoc 1995;95:893–7.
8. Keller KL, Kirzner J, Pietrobelli A, et al. Increased sweetened beverage intake is associated with reduced milk and calcium intake in 3- to 7-year-old children at multi-item laboratory lunches. J Am Diet Assoc 2009;109:497–501.
9. Wachs TD. Multiple influences on children's nutritional deficiencies: a systems perspective. Physiol Behav 2008;94:48–60.
10. Santry HP, Gillen DL, Lauderdale DS. Trends in bariatric surgical procedures. JAMA 2005;294:1909–17.
11. Gracia JA, Martinez M, Aguilella V, et al. Postoperative morbidity of biliopancreatic diversion depending on common limb length. Obes Surg 2007;17:1306–11.
12. Nadler EP, Youn HA, Ren CJ, et al. An update on 73 US obese pediatric patients treated with laparoscopic adjustable gastric banding: comorbidity resolution and compliance data. J Pediatr Surg 2008;43:141–6.
13. Vargas-Ruiz AG, Hernandez-Rivera G, Herrera MF. Prevalence of iron, folate, and vitamin B_{12} deficiency anemia after laparoscopic Roux-en-Y gastric bypass. Obes Surg 2008;18:288–93.
14. Aills L, Blankenship J, Buffington C, et al. ASMBS allied health nutritional guidelines for the surgical weight loss patient. Surg Obes Relat Dis 2008;4:S73–108.
15. Brolin RE, Leung M. Survey of vitamin and mineral supplementation after gastric bypass and biliopancreatic diversion for morbid obesity. Obes Surg 1999;9:150–4.
16. Pournaras DJ, le Roux CW. After bariatric surgery, what vitamins should be measured, and what supplements should be given? Clin Endocrinol (Oxf) 2009 [Epub ahead of print].
17. Xanthakos SA, Inge TH. Nutritional consequences of bariatric surgery. Curr Opin Clin Nutr Metab Care 2006;9:489–96.

18. Bavaresco M, Paganini S, Lima TP, et al. Nutritional course of patients submitted to bariatric surgery. Obes Surg 2008 [Epub ahead of print].
19. Moize V, Geliebter A, Gluck ME, et al. Obese patients have inadequate protein intake related to protein intolerance up to 1 year following Roux-en-Y gastric bypass. Obes Surg 2003;13:23–8.
20. Kalfarentzos F, Papadoulas S, Skroubis G, et al. Prospective evaluation of biliopancreatic diversion with Roux-en-Y gastric bypass in the superobese. J Gastrointest Surg 2004;8:479–88.
21. Wylezol M, Gluck M, Zubik R, et al. Biliopancreatic diversion in Poland. J Physiol Pharmacol 2005;56(Suppl 6):117–26.
22. Skroubis G, Anesidis S, Kehagias I, et al. Roux-en-Y gastric bypass versus a variant of biliopancreatic diversion in a non-superobese population: prospective comparison of the efficacy and the incidence of metabolic deficiencies. Obes Surg 2006;16:488–95.
23. Kalfarentzos F, Dimakopoulos A, Kehagias I, et al. Vertical banded gastroplasty versus standard or distal Roux-en-Y gastric bypass based on specific selection criteria in the morbidly obese: preliminary results. Obes Surg 1999;9:433–42.
24. Agha-Mohammadi S, Hurwitz DJ. Nutritional deficiency of postbariatric surgery body contouring patients: what every plastic surgeon should know. Plast Reconstr Surg 2008;122:604–13.
25. Lewandowski H, Breen TL, Huang EY. Kwashiorkor and an acrodermatitis enteropathica-like eruption after a distal gastric bypass surgical procedure. Endocr Pract 2007;13:277–82.
26. Brolin RE, LaMarca LB, Kenler HA, et al. Malabsorptive gastric bypass in patients with superobesity. J Gastrointest Surg 2002;6:195–203 [discussion: 204–5].
27. Berger JR. The neurological complications of bariatric surgery. Arch Neurol 2004; 61:1185–9.
28. Brolin RE, Gorman JH, Gorman RC, et al. Are vitamin B_{12} and folate deficiency clinically important after Roux-en-Y gastric bypass? J Gastrointest Surg 1998;2: 436–42.
29. Gurewitsch ED, Smith-Levitin M, Mack J. Pregnancy following gastric bypass surgery for morbid obesity. Obstet Gynecol 1996;88:658–61.
30. von Drygalski A, Andris DA. Anemia after bariatric surgery: more than just iron deficiency. Nutr Clin Pract 2009;24:217–26.
31. Kushner RF, Gleason B, Shanta-Retelny V. Reemergence of pica following gastric bypass surgery for obesity: a new presentation of an old problem. J Am Diet Assoc 2004;104:1393–7.
32. Flancbaum L, Belsley S, Drake V, et al. Preoperative nutritional status of patients undergoing Roux-en-Y gastric bypass for morbid obesity. J Gastrointest Surg 2006;10:1033–7.
33. Varma S, Baz W, Badine E, et al. Need for parenteral iron therapy after bariatric surgery. Surg Obes Relat Dis 2008;4:715–9.
34. Holick MF. Vitamin D deficiency. N Engl J Med 2007;357:266–81.
35. Nesby-O'Dell S, Scanlon KS, Cogswell ME, et al. Hypovitaminosis D prevalence and determinants among African American and white women of reproductive age: third National Health and Nutrition Examination Survey, 1988–1994. Am J Clin Nutr 2002;76:187–92.
36. Hintzpeter B, Mensink GB, Thierfelder W, et al. Vitamin D status and health correlates among German adults. Eur J Clin Nutr 2008;62:1079–89.
37. Siddiqui AM, Kamfar HZ. Prevalence of vitamin D deficiency rickets in adolescent school girls in western region, Saudi Arabia. Saudi Med J 2007;28:441–4.

38. Looker AC, Pfeiffer CM, Lacher DA, et al. Serum 25-hydroxyvitamin D status of the US population: 1988–1994 compared with 2000–2004. Am J Clin Nutr 2008;88:1519–27.
39. Wagner CL, Greer FR. Prevention of rickets and vitamin D deficiency in infants, children, and adolescents. Pediatrics 2008;122:1142–52.
40. Armas LA, Hollis BW, Heaney RP. Vitamin D_2 is much less effective than vitamin D_3 in humans. J Clin Endocrinol Metab 2004;89:5387–91.
41. Misra M, Pacaud D, Petryk A, et al. Vitamin D deficiency in children and its management: review of current knowledge and recommendations. Pediatrics 2008;122:398–417.
42. Bowman SA. Beverage choices of young females: changes and impact on nutrient intakes. J Am Diet Assoc 2002;102:1234–9.
43. Striegel-Moore RH, Thompson D, Affenito SG, et al. Correlates of beverage intake in adolescent girls: the National Heart, Lung, and Blood Institute Growth and Health Study. J Pediatr 2006;148:183–7.
44. Moore CE, Murphy MM, Holick MF. Vitamin D intakes by children and adults in the United States differ among ethnic groups. J Nutr 2005;135:2478–85.
45. Yetley EA. Assessing the vitamin D status of the US population. Am J Clin Nutr 2008;88:558S–64S.
46. Buffington C, Walker B, Cowan GS Jr, et al. Vitamin D deficiency in the morbidly obese. Obes Surg 1993;3:421–4.
47. Vilarrasa N, Maravall J, Estepa A, et al. Low 25-hydroxyvitamin D concentrations in obese women: their clinical significance and relationship with anthropometric and body composition variables. J Endocrinol Invest 2007;30:653–8.
48. Ernst B, Thurnheer M, Schmid SM, et al. Seasonal variation in the deficiency of 25-hydroxyvitamin D_3 in mildly to extremely obese subjects. Obes Surg 2009; 19:180–3.
49. Goldner WS, Stoner JA, Thompson J, et al. Prevalence of vitamin D insufficiency and deficiency in morbidly obese patients: a comparison with nonobese controls. Obes Surg 2008;18:145–50.
50. Ernst B, Thurnheer M, Schmid SM, et al. Evidence for the necessity to systematically assess micronutrient status prior to bariatric surgery. Obes Surg 2009;19:66–73.
51. Gemmel K, Santry HP, Prachand VN, et al. Vitamin D deficiency in preoperative bariatric surgery patients. Surg Obes Relat Dis 2009;5:54–9.
52. Carlin AM, Rao DS, Meslemani AM, et al. Prevalence of vitamin D depletion among morbidly obese patients seeking gastric bypass surgery. Surg Obes Relat Dis 2006;2:98–103 [discussion: 104].
53. Mahlay NF, Verka LG, Thomsen K, et al. Vitamin D status before Roux-en-Y and efficacy of prophylactic and therapeutic doses of vitamin D in patients after Roux-en-Y gastric bypass surgery. Obes Surg 2009;19:590–4.
54. Goldner WS, Stoner JA, Lyden E, et al. Finding the optimal dose of vitamin D following Roux-en-Y gastric bypass: a prospective, randomized pilot clinical trial. Obes Surg 2009;19:173–9.
55. Goode LR, Brolin RE, Chowdhury HA, et al. Bone and gastric bypass surgery: effects of dietary calcium and vitamin D. Obes Res 2004;12:40–7.
56. Ybarra J, Sanchez-Hernandez J, Gich I, et al. Unchanged hypovitaminosis D and secondary hyperparathyroidism in morbid obesity after bariatric surgery. Obes Surg 2005;15:330–5.
57. Hamoui N, Kim K, Anthone G, et al. The significance of elevated levels of parathyroid hormone in patients with morbid obesity before and after bariatric surgery. Arch Surg 2003;138:891–7.

58. Newbury L, Dolan K, Hatzifotis M, et al. Calcium and vitamin D depletion and elevated parathyroid hormone following biliopancreatic diversion. Obes Surg 2003;13:893–5.
59. Collazo-Clavell ML, Jimenez A, Hodgson SF, et al. Osteomalacia after Roux-en-Y gastric bypass. Endocr Pract 2004;10:195–8.
60. Compher CW, Badellino KO, Boullata JI. Vitamin D and the bariatric surgical patient: a review. Obes Surg 2008;18:220–4.
61. Balsa JA, Botella-Carretero JI, Peromingo R, et al. Role of calcium malabsorption in the development of secondary hyperparathyroidism after biliopancreatic diversion. J Endocrinol Invest 2008;31:845–50.
62. de Souza Valente da Silva L, Valeria da Veiga G, Ramalho RA. Association of serum concentrations of retinol and carotenoids with overweight in children and adolescents. Nutrition 2007;23:392–7.
63. Pereira S, Saboya C, Chaves G, et al. Class III obesity and its relationship with the nutritional status of vitamin A in pre- and postoperative gastric bypass. Obes Surg 2009;19:738–44.
64. Clements RH, Katasani VG, Palepu R, et al. Incidence of vitamin deficiency after laparoscopic Roux-en-Y gastric bypass in a university hospital setting. Am Surg 2006;72:1196–202 [discussion: 1203–4].
65. Lee WB, Hamilton SM, Harris JP, et al. Ocular complications of hypovitaminosis A after bariatric surgery. Ophthalmology 2005;112:1031–4.
66. Boylan LM, Sugerman HJ, Driskell JA. Vitamin E, vitamin B_6, vitamin B_{12}, and folate status of gastric bypass surgery patients. J Am Diet Assoc 1988;88:579–85.
67. Coupaye M, Puchaux K, Bogard C, et al. Nutritional consequences of adjustable gastric banding and gastric bypass: a 1-year prospective study. Obes Surg 2009;19:56–65.
68. Rino Y, Suzuki Y, Kuroiwa Y, et al. Vitamin E malabsorption and neurological consequences after gastrectomy for gastric cancer. Hepatogastroenterology 2007;54:1858–61.
69. Slater GH, Ren CJ, Siegel N, et al. Serum fat-soluble vitamin deficiency and abnormal calcium metabolism after malabsorptive bariatric surgery. J Gastrointest Surg 2004;8:48–55 [discussion: 54–5].
70. de Luis DA, Pacheco D, Izaola O, et al. Clinical results and nutritional consequences of biliopancreatic diversion: three years of follow-up. Ann Nutr Metab 2008;53:234–9.
71. Wald DS, Law M, Morris JK. Homocysteine and cardiovascular disease: evidence on causality from a meta-analysis. BMJ 2002;325:1202–8.
72. Bazzano LA, Reynolds K, Holder KN, et al. Effect of folic acid supplementation on risk of cardiovascular diseases: a meta-analysis of randomized controlled trials. JAMA 2006;296:2720–6.
73. Vitolo MR, Canal Q, Campagnolo PD, et al. Factors associated with risk of low folate intake among adolescents. J Pediatr (Rio J) 2006;82:121–6.
74. Mallory GN, Macgregor AM. Folate status following gastric bypass surgery (the great folate mystery). Obes Surg 1991;1:69–72.
75. Russell RM, Dhar GJ, Dutta SK, et al. Influence of intraluminal pH on folate absorption: studies in control subjects and in patients with pancreatic insufficiency. J Lab Clin Med 1979;93:428–36.
76. Kalfarentzos F, Skroubis G, Kehagias I, et al. A prospective comparison of vertical banded gastroplasty and Roux-en-Y gastric bypass in a non-superobese population. Obes Surg 2006;16:151–8.

77. Schilling RF, Gohdes PN, Hardie GH. Vitamin B_{12} deficiency after gastric bypass surgery for obesity. Ann Intern Med 1984;101:501–2.
78. Rhode BM, Tamin H, Gilfix BM, et al. Treatment of vitamin B_{12} deficiency after gastric surgery for severe obesity. Obes Surg 1995;5:154–8.
79. Sola E, Morillas C, Garzon S, et al. Rapid onset of Wernicke's encephalopathy following gastric restrictive surgery. Obes Surg 2003;13:661–2.
80. Bozbora A, Coskun H, Ozarmagan S, et al. A rare complication of adjustable gastric banding: Wernicke's encephalopathy. Obes Surg 2000;10:274–5.
81. Singh S, Kumar A. Wernicke's encephalopathy after obesity surgery: a systematic review. Neurology 2007;68:807–11.
82. Towbin A, Inge TH, Garcia VF, et al. Beriberi after gastric bypass surgery in adolescence. J Pediatr 2004;145:263–7.
83. Al-Fahad T, Ismael A, Soliman MO, et al. Very early onset of Wernicke's encephalopathy after gastric bypass. Obes Surg 2006;16:671–2.
84. Aasheim ET, Hofso D, Hjelmesaeth J, et al. Peripheral neuropathy and severe malnutrition following duodenal switch. Obes Surg 2008;18:1640–3.
85. Riess KP, Farnen JP, Lambert PJ, et al. Ascorbic acid deficiency in bariatric surgical population. Surg Obes Relat Dis 2009;5:81–6.
86. Rizzo MR, Abbatecola AM, Barbieri M, et al. Evidence for anti-inflammatory effects of combined administration of vitamin E and C in older persons with impaired fasting glucose: impact on insulin action. J Am Coll Nutr 2008;27: 505–11.
87. Madan AK, Orth WS, Tichansky DS, et al. Vitamin and trace mineral levels after laparoscopic gastric bypass. Obes Surg 2006;16:603–6.
88. Boldery R, Fielding G, Rafter T, et al. Nutritional deficiency of selenium secondary to weight loss (bariatric) surgery associated with life-threatening cardiomyopathy. Heart Lung Circ 2007;16:123–6.
89. Griffith DP, Liff DA, Ziegler TR, et al. Acquired copper deficiency: a potentially serious and preventable complication following gastric bypass surgery. Obesity (Silver Spring) 2009;17:827–31.
90. Guelinckx I, Devlieger R, Vansant G. Reproductive outcome after bariatric surgery: a critical review. Hum Reprod Update 2009;15:189–201.
91. Roehrig HR, Xanthakos SA, Sweeney J, et al. Pregnancy after gastric bypass surgery in adolescents. Obes Surg 2007;17:873–7.
92. Van Mieghem T, Van Schoubroeck D, Depiere M, et al. Fetal cerebral hemorrhage caused by vitamin K deficiency after complicated bariatric surgery. Obstet Gynecol 2008;112:434–6.
93. Huerta S, Rogers LM, Li Z, et al. Vitamin A deficiency in a newborn resulting from maternal hypovitaminosis A after biliopancreatic diversion for the treatment of morbid obesity. Am J Clin Nutr 2002;76:426–9.

Nutrition Management of Pediatric Patients Who Have Cystic Fibrosis

Suzanne H. Michel, MPH, RD, LDN[a],*, Asim Maqbool, MD[b],
Maria D. Hanna, MS, RD, LDN[a], Maria Mascarenhas, MBBS[b]

KEYWORDS

- Cystic fibrosis - Nutrition - Vitamins - Minerals - Energy
- Protein - Fatty acids - Pancreatic - Enzymes

Cystic fibrosis (CF) is a common autosomal recessive genetic disorder, most often seen in people of northern European decent and in lesser frequency in other racial groups. Current US data indicate that CF occurs in approximately 1 in 2500 births and affects approximately 30,000 individuals. The gene, which is on chromosome 7, is called the CF transmembrane regulator and controls the flow of sodium and chloride ions across the cell membrane. Prior to the availability of newborn screening in the United States, the diagnosis of CF usually was not made until an infant or child developed pulmonary disease or gastrointestinal symptoms, often with failure to thrive and nutrient deficiencies. Poor weight gain and vitamin and mineral deficiencies usually are corrected with the use of pancreatic enzyme replacement therapy (PERT) and vitamin and mineral supplements.[1] Multivitamin supplements designed for infants, children, and adults who have CF are available in the United States (**Table 1**).

Pancreatic damage can start in utero, with approximately 80% of babies being pancreatic insufficient (PI) at diagnosis. Management of patients who are PI includes use of PERT. For infants, PERT is initiated at 2000 to 5000 lipase units per feeding and, as with all patients who are PI, adjusted to a maximum of 2500 lipase units per kilogram per meal not to exceed 10,000 lipase units per kilogram per day.[1] Patients who are pancreatic sufficient (PS) may go on to become PI; therefore, careful monitoring of pancreatic function is recommended, especially for those patients with

[a] Department of Clinical Nutrition, The Children's Hospital of Philadelphia, University of Pennsylvania School of Medicine, 34th Street and Civic Center Boulevard, 9NW, Room 82, Philadelphia, PA 19104-4399, USA
[b] Division of Gastroenterology, Hepatology, and Nutrition, The Children's Hospital of Philadelphia, University of Pennsylvania School of Medicine, 34th Street and Civic Center Boulevard, 7NW, Philadelphia, PA 19104-4399, USA
* Corresponding author.
E-mail address: michelsu@email.chop.edu (S.H. Michel).

Pediatr Clin N Am 56 (2009) 1123–1141
doi:10.1016/j.pcl.2009.06.008
0031-3955/09/$ – see front matter © 2009 Elsevier Inc. All rights reserved.

pediatric.theclinics.com

Table 1
Comparison of cystic fibrosis–specific vitamin and mineral supplements in United States to non–cystic fibrosis-specific products[a]

Age	SourceCF[b,c] Drops, Chewables, and Softgels	ADEK Chewables[b,d]	AquADEKS[b,e] Drops and Softgels	Vitamax[b,f] Drops and Chewables	Poly-Vi-Sol Drops[g] and Centrum Chewables and Tablet
Vitamin A (IU): retinol and beta carotene					
0–12 mo	4627 (1 mL) 75% BC	—	5751 (1 mL) 87% BC	3170 (1 mL) 0% BC	1500 (1 mL) 0% BC
1–3 y	9254 (2 mL) 75% BC	—	11502 (2 mL) 87% BC	6340 (2 mL) 0% BC	3000 (2 mL) 0% BC
4–8 y	16,000/chewable 88% BC	9000/chewable 60% BC	Ages 4–10 y: 18,167/1 softgel 92% BC	5000/chewable 50% BC	3500/chewable 29% BC
>9 y	32,000/2 softgels 88% BC	18,000/2 chewables 60% BC	Ages 10 and up: 36,334/2 softgels 92% BC	10,000/2 chewables 50% BC	7000/2 tablets 29% BC
Vitamin E (IU)[h]					
0–12 mo	50 (1 mL)	—	50 (1 mL)[i]	50 (1 mL)	5 (1 mL)
1–3 y	100 (2 mL)	—	100 (2 mL)[i]	100 (2 mL)	10 (2 mL)
4–8 y	200/chewable	150/chewable	Ages 4–10 y: 150/1 softgel[i]	200/chewable	30/chewable
>9 y	400/2 softgels	300/2 chewables	Ages 10 and up: 300/2 softgels[i]	400/2 chewables	60/2 tablets
Vitamin D (IU)					
0–12 mo	500 (1 mL)	—	400 (1 mL)	400 (1 mL)	400 (1 mL)
1–3 y	1000 (2 mL)	—	800 (2 mL)	800 (2 mL)	800 (2 mL)
4–8 y	1000/chewable	400/chewable	Ages 4–10 y: 800/1 softgel	400/chewable	400/chewable
>9 y	2000/2 softgels	800/2 chewables	Ages 10 and up: 1600/2 softgels	800/2 chewables	800/2 tablets

Vitamin K (µg)					
0–12 mo	400 (1 mL)	—	400 (1 mL)	300 (1 mL)	0
1–3 y	800 (2 mL)	—	800 (2 mL)	600 (2 mL)	0
4–8 y	800/chewable	150/chewable	Ages 4–10 y: 700/1 softgel	200/chewable	10/chewable
>9 y	1600/2 softgels	300/2 chewables	Ages 10 and up: 1400/2 softgels	400/2 chewables	50/2 tablets
Zinc (mg)					
0–12 mo	5 (1 mL)	—	5 (1 mL)	7.5 (1 mL)	0
1–3 y	10 (2 mL)	—	10 (2 mL)	15 (2 mL)	0
4–8 y	15/chewable	7.5/chewable	Ages 4–10 y: 10/softgel	7.5/chewable	15/chewable
>9 y	30/2 softgels	15/2 chewables	Ages 10 and up: 20/2 softgels	15/2 chewables	22/2 tablets

Abbreviation: BC, beta carotene.

a The content of this Table was confirmed December 2008. Products also contain a full range of water-soluble vitamins; see SourceCF.com for content.

b CF-specific products.

c SourceCF Liquid, Chewables, and Softgels are registered trademarks of SourceCF Inc, a subsidiary of Eurand Pharmaceuticals, Inc.

d ADEK Chewables is a registered trademark of Axcan Pharma, Inc.

e AquADEKs Liquid and Softgels are registered trademarks of Yasoo Health Inc.

f Vitamax Drops and Chewables are registered trademarks of Shear/Kershman Labs, Inc.

g Poly-Vi-Sol Drops is a registered trademark of Mead Johnson and Company. Centrum Chewables and Tablets are registered trademarks of Wyeth Consumer Care.

h α-Tocopherol.

i Contains mixed tocopherols.

genetic mutations known to be associated with PI.[1] Clinical symptoms of PI include maldigestion with subsequent malabsorption, diarrhea, weight loss, poor growth, and nutrient deficiencies. Liver disease and small bowel disease can add to nutritional problems seen in CF. Patients with and without PI require careful nutrition management to avoid nutrition deficiencies. These deficiencies include fat- and water-soluble vitamins, minerals, essential fatty acids (EFAs), and trace elements. Deficiency states of a specific nutrient can occur due to decreased intake, maldigestion, increased losses, increased needs, oxidative stress, and possible metabolic abnormalities at the cellular level. For a comprehensive review of international nutrition recommendations, see the international foundation articles listed in **Box 1**.

ENERGY AND PROTEIN

Nutritional status, as measured by height and weight, is linked to survival.[2,3,4] There is an association between body mass index percentile and forced expiratory volume in 1 second (FEV_1).[5] Therefore, optimal energy intake is pivotal to the overall well-being of patients who have CF. Defining energy needs of patients with CF is a challenge. Individual variables include differences in maldigestion and resultant malabsorption,[6] pulmonary exacerbation,[7] pulmonary function,[8] fat-free mass,[9] gender,[6] pubertal status,[10] genetic mutation,[6,11] and age[12] and medical complications, including liver disease or CF-related diabetes. These variables make defining specific individual energy requirements challenging. Daily calorie recommendations provided by various CF societies range from 110% to 200%[5,13] of that recommended for individuals who do not have CF. To achieve the recommended energy goal, patients with CF often require a greater fat intake (35%–40% of energy).[14] A formula that incorporates level of activity, pulmonary function, and degree of malabsorption was included in the Cystic Fibrosis Foundation nutrition consensus report for use by clinicians in CF centers (**Table 2**). Formulas for calculating the energy needs of children with mild to moderate CF were evaluated, and the estimated energy requirement of the Dietary Reference Intake at the active level best estimated the energy needs of this particular group.[15,16] It is suggested that formulas be used as a starting point for calculating energy needs, but gain in weight and height, velocity of weight and height gain, and fat stores may provide a more objective measure of energy balance.[13,15] Energy intake is adjusted based on these objective measures.

Box 1
Foundation nutrition guidelines for children who have cystic fibrosis

Consensus report on nutrition for pediatric patients with cystic fibrosis, 2002.[14]

Nutrition in patients with cystic fibrosis: a European Consensus, 2002.[68]

Nutritional management of cystic fibrosis. UK Cystic Fibrosis Trust Nutrition Working Group, 2002.[156]

Consensus statement: guide to bone health and disease in cystic fibrosis, 2005.[51]

Australasian clinical practice guidelines for nutrition in cystic fibrosis, 2006.[13]

Antioxidants in cystic fibrosis. Conclusions from the CF Antioxidant Workshop, Bethesda, Maryland, November 11–12, 2003.[39]

Evidence-based practice recommendations for nutrition-related management of children and adults with cystic fibrosis and pancreatic insufficiency: results of a systematic review, 2008.[5]

Cystic Fibrosis Foundation evidence-based guidelines for management of infants with cystic fibrosis, submitted for publication[1]

Table 2
Determination of energy requirements according to the US Cystic Fibrosis Foundation

1. Calculate BMR in kcal from body weight in kg using World Health Organization equations[a]

Age range in years	Females	Males
0–3	61.0 wt − 51	60.9 wt − 54
3–10	22.5 wt + 499	22.7 wt + 495
10–18	12.2 wt + 746	17.5 wt + 651
18–30	14.7 wt + 496	15.3 wt + 679

2. Calculate the DEE by multiplying the BMR by activity plus disease coefficients

AC	Disease coefficients	DEE
Confined to bed: BMR × 1.3	FEV_1 > 80% predicted: 0	BMR × (AC + 0)
Sedentary: BMR × 1.5	FEV_1 40%–79% predicted: 0.2	BMR × (AC + 0.2)
Active: BMR × 1.7	FEV_1 < 40% predicted: 0.3 to 0.5[b]	BMR × (AC + 0.3)

3. Calculate total DERs from DEE and degree of steatorrhea

If a stool collection is not available to determine the fraction of fat intake, an approximate value of 0.85 may be used in the calculation. For PS patients and PI patients with a COA > 93% of intake, DER = DEE. For example: a patient with a COA of 0.78, the factor is 0.93/0.78 or 1.2. If the COA is not known the factor is 1.1.

Example: 10 year-old boy. Weight = 32 kg; AC = active; FEV_1% predicted = 85%; COA = not available.

12.2 (32) + 746 = 1136
1136 × (1.7 + 0) = 1931
1931 × 1.1 = 2124 calories per day

Abbreviations: AC, activity coefficients; BMR, basal metabolic rate; COA, coefficient of fat absorption; DEE, daily energy expenditure; DER, daily energy requirement.
[a] *From* World Health Organization. Energy and protein requirements [appendix B]. WHO Tech Rep Ser 1985;924(724):115–6.
[b] May range up to 0.5 with very severe lung disease.
Data from Ramsey BW, Farrell PM, Pencharz P. Nutritional assessment and management in cystic fibrosis: a consensus report. Am J Clin Nutr 1992;55:108–16.

Limited information is available describing specific dietary protein requirements for children who have CF. Studies assessing protein catabolism and protein deposition provide varying results, which may reflect differences in nutritional status and health of the subjects prior to the studies and caloric intake during the studies.[17,18] Protein intake is correlated with overall calorie intake, and in general, patients with CF who consume adequate calories also consume adequate protein.[13,19,20] Subgroups who do not meet energy or protein intake recommendations require nutrition intervention.[20,21] Studies providing oral or enteral supplements to increase overall energy and protein intake have provided conflicting results.[5,20,22]

FAT-SOLUBLE VITAMINS: A, E, D, AND K

The term, vitamin A, refers to a family of compounds important for cellular integrity, growth, immune function, and vision that is comprised of preformed retinoid and provitamin A carotenoids. Excessive retinol intake and elevated serum levels have raised concerns regarding potential toxicity to the liver and adverse impact on bone.[23,24] Vitamin A status is assessed by serum retinol status, by measuring serum retinol-binding protein, and by functional testing. Serum retinol is depressed during acute inflammatory states but is not associated with disease severity.[25,26] There are no prospective randomized controlled trials demonstrating benefits of vitamin A supplementation on clinically relevant outcomes in CF.[27] To prevent deficiency states traditionally associated with CF, CF-specific multivitamins containing preformed, water-miscible retinol have been commercially available since 1993. Investigators have demonstrated elevated serum retinol in children, adolescents, and young adults with CF.[28] In response to concerns surrounding elevated serum retinol levels, several CF-specific multivitamins have lowered the retinol content and increased beta carotene (see **Table 1**).

Although serum retinol and retinol-binding protein are informative with respect to vitamin A adequacy, they are less informative regarding states of excess. Measurement of serum retinyl esters as a function of total serum retinol may be more informative for risk of toxicity and may be prudent to measure in this population.[29] Specific markers of hepatic injury and fibrosis also may need to be investigated in individuals with elevated serum vitamin A markers. Prospective studies of serum and tissue markers using newer, noninvasive techniques may be required to better determine vitamin A status across compartments and their relationships and to be able to better describe whole body status, from deficiency through adequacy to toxicity.[30] Regular surveillance to ensure adequacy and to avoid potential adverse effects may be indicated.

Vitamin E

Vitamin E includes eight chemically similar compounds, the most common being α-tocopherol; it is necessary for normal development, cell membrane stability, and prevention of hemolysis and important for its role as an antioxidant. Vitamin E requires bile, pancreatic juices, and dietary fat for optimal absorption, thereby putting patients with CF at risk for vitamin E deficiency if they do not receive adequate supplementation. Oxidative stress and a diet high in polyunsaturated fatty acids (PUFAs) may increase vitamin E needs in CF.[31] Reports of vitamin deficiency and its subsequent neurologic consequences in persons with CF have appeared in the literature[32,33] but are less common since the development of CF-specific multivitamins containing increased amounts of vitamin E. Low levels of vitamin E have been reported in PS patients.[34,35] Vitamin deficiency is present at the time of diagnosis in infants identified through newborn screening,[36] which, in some patients, continues into childhood.[37] Early, prolonged vitamin E deficiency can have a detrimental effect on cognitive function.[38] Therefore, the importance of initiating fat-soluble vitamin supplementation, especially vitamin E, at the time of diagnosis is paramount.[1] Vitamin E's role as an antioxidant in CF has been reviewed.[39] Varying results are reported describing the effect of vitamin E on lung function in patients with CF.[25,40,41] Serum/plasma vitamin E level is dependent on serum lipid levels and can be interpreted as a ratio to total cholesterol[42] or as a ratio to total lipids.[43] Extremes in lipid levels may influence interpretation of vitamin E results. To avoid detrimental effects of deficiency, vitamin E as contained in CF-specific multivitamins is started at diagnosis. Serum levels, best measured when patients are fasting, are assessed at least annually and vitamin E supplementation is adjusted as indicated.[14,44]

Vitamin D

Vitamin D is well known in association with bone health, but its role in maintaining health and preventing disease is still being explored.[45,46] Vitamin D deficiency is common in CF and found in infants diagnosed by newborn screening and in children and young adults.[37,47,48] Factors affecting vitamin D status in the general population and in CF include season, skin color, lack of exposure to sunlight, geographic location, use of sunscreen, and inadequate dietary intake from supplements and foods, such as fatty fish and fortified foods.[45,46,49] In CF, additional factors include decreased absorption from PI and hepatobiliary dysfunction; increased catabolism due to medications, such as glucocorticoids; decreased capacity to convert the circulating serum 25-hydroxyvitamin D (25[OH]D) to the bioactive form, 1,25-(OH)2D; and decreased sunlight exposure during times of illness or treatment with some antibiotics.[50,51] Patients with reduced fat mass have decreased storage and may have decreased circulating vitamin D–binding protein.[51,52] Inadequate vitamin D intake led the American Academy of Pediatrics to increase the recommendation for vitamin D supplementation for infants and children.[53]

The total concentration of 25(OH)D (ie, 25[OH]D2 plus 25[OH]D3) reflects stores and is the accepted measure of vitamin D status.[49] Currently there is no universally accepted definition for vitamin D deficiency. For patients who have CF, it is defined as 25(OH)D level less than 30 ng/mL (75 nmol/L).[51] Treatment recommendations outlined in the Cystic Fibrosis Foundation Bone consensus report[51] may not correct low vitamin D levels.[54,55] Two forms of vitamin D are available in the United States, vitamin D_2 (ergocalciferol) and vitamin D_3 (cholecalciferol). Vitamin D_3 is considered to have greater bioefficacy.[56,57] Suggested daily dose for toddlers and children who do not have CF or regular sun exposure is 1000 to 2000 international units of vitamin D_3.[45,46] In addition, treatment using sensible sun exposure and artificial UV-B light also has been explored.[45,49,58,59] Cod liver oil, with its risk for vitamin A toxicity, is not recommended.[46] The exact amount of vitamin D required to achieve normal blood levels for children with CF is not known. It may be prudent to start at doses recommended for persons who do not have CF, then repeat 25(OH)D levels in 2 to 3 months while they are still on therapy to monitor the adequacy of the treatment.[60]

Vitamin K

Maldigestion and resultant malabsorption from PI, bile salt deficiency, liver disease, bowel resection, or bacterial overgrowth; antibiotics; excessive vitamin E supplementation; and a diet inadequate in vitamin K–rich foods place children with CF at risk for vitamin K deficiency.[61,62,63] The best-known role of vitamin K is in coagulation; it also plays a role in bone metabolism.[61] Cerebral hemorrhage has been reported in CF infants prior to diagnosis and treatment.[64] Vitamin K deficiency may decrease bone formation and is associated with low bone mass; its aggressive supplementation improves markers of bone formation.[65,66] Assessing vitamin K status is a challenge. Circulating vitamin K_1 levels reflect recent dietary or supplement intake.[63] Prothrombin (or factor II) and osteocalcin (OC) are vitamin K–dependent proteins. Prothrombin is a delayed marker of hepatic vitamin K deficiency, as only 50% of its concentration is needed to maintain normal prothrombin time. Protein induced by vitamin K absence (PIVKA II) and undercarboxylated OC are more sensitive markers of vitamin K deficiency but not always clinically available.[61,67] Vitamin K supplementation recommendations range from 0.3 to 0.5 mg daily[14] to 1 mg daily to 10 mg weekly.[68] The optimal dose of vitamin K for children with CF is yet to be defined. Using markers of bone health to assess adequacy, suggested doses of vitamin K range from 1 mg daily to 10 mg weekly.[61,63,65,67,69,70] There are no known cases of vitamin K toxicity.[61]

WATER-SOLUBLE VITAMINS

Unlike for the fat-soluble vitamins, there are no specific water-soluble vitamin intake recommendations for patients with CF, perhaps due to the belief and some evidence that patients with CF who consume a balanced diet do not develop overt deficiencies.[71] Additionally, in the United States, multivitamins designed for patients with CF contain a full complement of water-soluble vitamins that may prevent clinical evidence of deficiencies. There is limited work regarding the more subtle cellular activity of the water-soluble vitamins and CF. Acute illness; complications, such as liver or renal disease; and medication may compromise water-soluble vitamin nutrition. In 2001, McCabe reported three cases of riboflavin deficiency in children with CF who presented with angular stomatitis.[72] All of the children described were acutely ill and required supplemental riboflavin. In preliminary work, supplemental 5-methyltetrahydrofolate (the active form of folic acid) and vitamin B_{12} were given to a small group of persons who had CF.[73] Those subjects receiving the supplement demonstrated improved inflammatory response. Plasma ascorbic acid decreases with age, although the explanation for this is unclear.[74,75] Additional research is needed to define the water-soluble needs of patients with CF.

MINERALS: SODIUM CHLORIDE, CALCIUM, AND MAGNESIUM

The relationship of salty skin to characteristics typical of CF was noted as early as 1650.[76] Salt, as sodium and chloride, has played a key role in the diagnosis and management of CF. Patients with CF lose excessive salt through their skin: this is the basis for the pilocarpine-stimulated sweat test to diagnosis CF. There is some evidence that genotype may influence overall sodium and chloride losses in sweat, thereby possibly having an impact on dietary salt needs.[77,78,79] Currently, there is no conclusive evidence to adjust dietary sodium intake based on sweat test results. The body maintains a delicate system to maintain electrolyte balance, yet in CF, the endocrine and metabolic adaptations to salt depletion have not been well studied.[80] There are many reports of hypoelectrolytemia in the literature.[78,79,81] Human milk and baby formulas do not contain sufficient salt to meet the needs of infants who have CF. Electrolyte depletion in infants was noted when salt was removed from commercially available infant foods.[82] Older patients with CF also are at risk for electrolyte abnormalities,[83] resulting in lower serum osmolality during periods of excessive sweating, which may blunt the trigger to drink and cause what is referred to as "voluntary dehydration."[84] Electrolyte abnormalities should be considered in CF patients presenting with overt symptoms of salt depletion and with failure to thrive and anorexia. Patients admitted with metabolic acidosis with hypoelectrolytemia without renal disease may have undiagnosed CF. To avoid electrolyte abnormalities, patients with CF are recommended to consume a high salt diet. For infants, that includes the addition of salt to the diet. Two- to 4-mEq sodium/kg is generally recommended.[85] In CF care, 0.125 teaspoon of salt is recommended for newborns and for stable, growing infants, increased to 0.25 teaspoon at 6 months of age.[1] Care must be taken to assure that parents correctly dose salt to avoid complications of excessive sodium intake. Older patients are encouraged to eat a high-salt diet. For those persons active in warm environments, the addition of 0.25 teaspoon of salt to 12 oz of typical sports drinks may avoid voluntary dehydration.[86]

Calcium and magnesium are important in CF because of their role in bone health. Many variables have an impact on their adequacy, including vitamin D and K deficiency, inadequate dietary intake, and trapping in fat soaps due to malabsorption caused by PI, bile salt deficiency, and liver disease.[51] The calcium intake of children with CF needs to be monitored on a regular basis to optimize dietary intake for age[51,87,88] and to prevent hypocalcemia in patients placed on vitamin D supplementation. Monitoring of serum magnesium levels is important for patients with CF with renal insufficiency, low bone mineral density, or CF-related diabetes or when using medications, such as aminoglycosides, that can cause renal tubular damage, and immunosuppressants, such as tacrolimus for transplant patients.[89,90,91,92]

TRACE ELEMENTS: ZINC, IRON, SELENIUM, AND COPPER

Zinc is a mineral involved in more than 300 functions in the body, including many related to pulmonary health, immunity, and growth.[93] Signs and symptoms of zinc deficiency are nonspecific and include lack of appetite, alterations in taste, growth failure, and disturbed immune function.[94,95] Zinc homeostasis is sensitive and maintained through the intestinal absorption of exogenous and endogenous zinc. Absorption is affected by the nutrient content of the diet and fat malabsorption,[96,97] placing persons who have CF at risk for zinc deficiency. Prior to initiation of PERT, infants with CF and PI are at risk for developing zinc deficiency due to malabsorption and increased endogenous losses.[98,99] Cases of acrodermatitis enteropathica-like rash due to zinc deficiency in infants and children prior to diagnosis with CF continue to be reported.[100,101] Lack of a clinically informative laboratory method and reference values to identify zinc deficiency makes diagnosing deficiency challenging. Reference values for zinc are dependent on the population and methods used to assess zinc levels.[102,103] Symptoms of zinc deficiency may occur while plasma levels are within normal reference ranges. The majority of zinc stores are intracellular and investigators suggest red blood cell zinc as a better indicator of zinc status.[104] In zinc supplementation trials, patients with CF and decreased serum zinc concentrations seem to benefit the most from supplementation.[102,105,106] Empiric zinc supplementation for 6 months has been recommended for children with CF exhibiting growth failure, vitamin A deficiency, or night blindness refractory to vitamin A therapy.[14,44]

Anemia is frequently seen in patients with CF and is associated with poorer lung function and vitamin deficiency.[107] The incidence of iron deficiency anemia ranges from 33% in children to 74% in older patients with CF.[108,109,110] Anemia can be due to true iron deficiency or anemia of chronic disease.[111] The etiology of iron deficiency may be related to decreased dietary intake, increased losses in sputum and the gastrointestinal tract, and possibly the severity of suppurative lung disease.[112,113] Evidence indicates that iron deficiency is not related to PERT.[112] It has been shown that *Pseudomonas aeruginosa* actively acquires iron from the proteins in the host airway, secretes siderophores (iron-chelating compounds) to acquire iron, and produces inflammatory cytokines, which results in anemia of chronic disease.[112,113] Iron deficiency is difficult to diagnose in patients with CF and has to be differentiated from anemia of chronic disease. Obtaining soluble transferrin receptor levels is recommended in addition to checking iron, transferrin, and ferritin levels.[109] There is some controversy regarding supplementation because some investigators believe that providing iron allows pseudomonas bacteria to grow. It is generally accepted, however, that if a true iron deficiency exists, it should be treated, whereas in anemia of chronic disease, the underlying inflammation needs to be treated and iron supplements withheld.

Selenium is a known antioxidant. Low selenium levels have been seen in patients with CF,[39,114,115] and supplementation with selenium containing PERT resulted in increased plasma selenium levels and gluthathione peroxidase activity.[114] Possible reasons for low levels include abnormalities in dietary intake, absorption, and metabolism and increased needs due to increased oxidative stress. Supplementation trials of selenium alone have not been shown to be effective,[116] although a trial in which selenium was one of many antioxidants given showed improved plasma levels and an increase in predicted FEV_1.[31]

Not much is known about copper metabolism in patients with CF. Persistent anemia unresponsive to iron supplements may be related to copper deficiency. Variable results have been found for serum copper and ceruloplasmin levels in patients with CF. Because inflammation can raise copper and ceruloplasmin levels, checking these levels in the presence of inflammation renders them less reliable. Reduced levels of copper enzyme activity (cytochrome oxidase and copper-zinc superoxide dismutase) have been seen in monocytes and neutrophils in patients with CF, suggesting a functional deficiency.[117,118,119]

POLYUNSATURATED AND ESSENTIAL FATTY ACIDS, CHOLINE, GLUTATHIONE, AND COENZYME Q10

Individuals who have CF are prone to PUFA abnormalities. Linoleic acid (LA) (ω-6) and α- linolenic acid (ω-3) are the EFAs; humans cannot synthesize them and are reliant on dietary sources to ensure adequacy and prevent deficiency. EFA and long-chain PUFAs have a variety of structural and functional roles throughout the life cycle, including cell signaling, gene expression via peroxisome proliferator-activated receptors, and proinflammatory activity via the eicosanoid pathways. EFA deficiency (EFAD) was first described in CF in 1962.[120] EFAD was present at the time of diagnosis, with classic clinical manifestations of alopecia, easy bruisability, desquamating skin rashes, and suboptimal growth. Although these symptoms may still occur, biochemical evidence of EFAD can be present in otherwise apparently well-nourished individuals.[121] The etiology is most likely multifactorial and may include fat malabsorption[122] and abnormal membrane release and metabolism.[123,124] EFAD has been found in association with ceramide deficiency,[125] CF genotype, and pancreatic status.[126,127] EFAD is typically associated with a blunted inflammatory response in otherwise healthy individuals; however, patients with CF, paradoxically, develop a more pronounced inflammatory effect.[128]

The two most frequently described PUFA abnormalities in CF are LA (the ω-6 EFA) deficiency and decrease in docosahexaenoic acid (DHA).[129,130] Serum LA status has been associated with clinically important outcomes of growth and pulmonary status.[131,132] Similar associations have not been observed with the triene:tetraene ratio,[133] suggesting serum LA status may be a more relevant indicator of EFA status in patients with CF. LA supplementation studies have demonstrated that improvement of LA status or "normalization" or "approching level of those in healthy individuals" is possible.[134] DHA is important in retinal and brain development and down-regulates the eicosanoid-mediated inflammatory response compared to arachidonic acid, which has a proinflammatory influence. Several short-term DHA supplementation trials have been performed to date. The supplements have been well tolerated without adverse health effects and were associated with an improvement of serum and tissue DHA status and a decrease of arachidonic acid:DHA ratio.[135,136,137] Furthermore, investigators have demonstrated that patients with CF supplemented with DHA have improved leukotriene B4 and other anti-inflammatory eicosanoids and cytokines.[138,139] Associations between DHA status, supplementation, and clinically significant outcomes (eg, pulmonary function and growth), however, have not been reported. Prevention of deficiency and attainment of adequacy is the first goal in the nutritional management of EFA deficiency and PUFA abnormalities in patients with CF. Alternatively, the goal could be attainment of serum PUFA profiles associated with optimal clinical outcomes, as proposed by Christophe and Robberecht,[140] but more research is required.

Choline

Choline is an essential nutrient and has myriad structural and functional roles, including cell membrane function, as a methyl donor intersecting with the folate, homocysteine-methionine, and DNA repair pathways. Choline is an essential nutrient with a dietary requirement.[141] Subjects with CF are prone to choline deficiency and to altered membrane phospholipid status.[142] This may be related to increase membrane turnover[142] and to dietary phospholipid malabsorption.[143] Supplementation with choline or its metabolites has been associated with improved serum choline status and profiles approaching that of healthy control subjects.[144]

Glutathione

Glutathione (GSH) is involved in several cellular processes, including cell differentiation, proliferation, apoptosis, redox reactions as an antioxidant, phospholipid metabolism, and immune system function. As such, GSH is often expressed as a ratio reflecting its redox state to GSH disulphide (GSSG). Alterations of GSH:GSSG occur during inflammation.[145] GSH concentrations in lung epithelial lining fluid (ELF) are decreased in patients with CF compared to healthy subjects and in other tissue compartments.[146,147] This may have an impact on viscosity and the inflammatory response in these different tissues compartments, particularly in the ELF. Low GSH concentrations maybe related to CF transmembrane regulator abnormalities and increased consumption due to increased oxidative stress and inflammation. Additionally, as seen in the CF mouse model, exposure to *Pseudomonas aeruginosa* is met with decreased export of GSH to the ELF, which in part may explain the difficulty in clearing such infections in patients with CF.[148] Choline supplementation trials in CF have shown improvements of GSH and the ratio of GSH to GSSG.[144] Oral intake of *N*-acetylcysteine has shown increased blood neutrophil GSH concentrations and decreased sputum elastase activity.[149] Aerosolized delivery of GSH and related compounds can result in bronchospasm.[150] Aerosolized GSH, however, has been associated with decreased prostaglandin E2 (proinflammatory) concentrations in bronchial fluids and improved post-treatment lung function in patients with CF.[151] *S*-nitrosoglutathione, another GSH entity normally found in pulmonary tissue, causes airway smooth muscle relaxation and improved ciliary function and is decreased in subjects with CF.[152] Clinical trials of aerosolized *S*-nitrosoglutathione have been performed in CF[153] but are not indicated for routine clinical use at this time.[39]

Coenzyme Q10

Also referred to as ubiquinone, coenzyme Q10 (COQ10) is a lipid-soluble, mitochondrial membrane–based constituent of the electron transport chain, which aids in maintaining vitamin E in a reduced state, thus contributing to the body's antioxidant system. The majority of COQ10 is synthesized along cholesterol synthesis pathways, with approximately 25% obtained from dietary sources of animal protein. Total plasma concentrations of COQ10 were found decreased in subjects with CF as compared to healthy controls.[154] Deficiency in subjects with CF seems to be related more to inadequate intake and malabsorptive losses than to oxidative stress or increased turnover.[155] A subsequent longitudinal study in subjects with CF reported decreased total serum COQ10 concentrations more frequently in subjects with CF and PI compared to those with CF and PS. Low levels of COQ10 are associated with total lipids, beta carotene, and α-tocopherol.[154] Prospective supplementation studies are required to further define effects on tissue compartment status, oxidative stress status, and clinical outcomes.

SUMMARY

Nutrition continues to be a challenge in the care of patients with CF. In the past, the goal was to provide adequate calories to insure survival; now, the goals are to optimize nutrient intake to promote normal growth and nutritional status, avoid overt and subtle nutrient deficiencies, and modulate inflammation. Compared to the general population, there is little evidence to support precise nutrition recommendations for patients with CF, although efforts have been made to use available evidence to set care standards (see **Box 1**). More research is required to address these concerns and gaps in current knowledge.

REFERENCES

1. Borowitz D, Robinson KA, Rosenfeld M, et al. CFF practice guidelines for the management of infants with cystic fibrosis during the first two years of life. J Pediatr, in press.
2. Corey M, McLaughlin FJ, Williams M, et al. A comparison of survival, growth, and pulmonary function in patients with cystic fibrosis in Boston and Toronto. J Clin Epidemiol 1988;41(6):583–91.
3. Beker LT, Russek-Cohen E, Fink RJ. Stature as a prognostic factor in cystic fibrosis survival. J Am Diet Assoc 2001;101(4):438–42.
4. Sharma R, Florea VG, Bolger AP, et al. Wasting as an independent predictor of mortality in patients with cystic fibrosis. Thorax 2001;56:746–50.
5. Stallings VA, Stark LJ, Robinson KA, et al. Clinical Practice Guidelines on Growth and Nutrition Subcommittee, Ad Hoc Working Group. Evidence-based practice recommendations for nutrition-related management of children and adults with cystic fibrosis and pancreatic insufficiency: results of a systematic review. J Am Diet Assoc 2008;108(5):832–9.
6. Allen JR, McCauley JC, Selby AM, et al. Differences in resting energy expenditure between male and female children with cystic fibrosis. J Pediatr 2003;142:15–9.
7. Reilly JJ, Ralston JM, Paton JY, et al. Energy balance during acute respiratory exacerbation in children with cystic fibrosis. Eur Respir J 1999;13:804–9.
8. Fried MD, Durie PR, Tsui LC, et al. The cystic fibrosis gene and resting energy expenditure. J Pediatr 1991;119(6):913–6.
9. Stallings VA, Tomezsko JL, Schall JI, et al. Adolescent development and energy expenditure in females with cystic fibrosis. Clin Nutr 2005;24:737–45.
10. Barclay A, Allen JR, Blyler E, et al. Resting energy expenditure in females with cystic fibrosis: is it affected by puberty? Eur J Clin Nutr 2007;61:1207–12.
11. Magoffin A, Allen JR, McCauley J, et al. Longitudinal analysis of resting energy expenditure in patients with cystic fibrosis. J Pediatr 2008;152:703–8.
12. Bines JE, Truby HD, Armstrong DS, et al. Energy metabolism in infants with cystic fibrosis. J Pediatr 2002;140:527–33.
13. Australasian clinical practice guidelines for nutrition in cystic fibrosis. 2005. Available at: http://.cysticfibrosis.org.au/pdf/CF_Nutrition_Guidelines.pdf. Accessed July 28, 2009.
14. Borowitz D, Baker RD, Stallings V. Consensus report on nutrition for pediatric patients with cystic fibrosis. J Pediatr Gastroenterol Nutr 2002;35(3):246–59.
15. Trabulsi J, Ittenbach RF, Schall JI, et al. Evaluation of formulas for calculating total energy requirements of preadolescent children with cystic fibrosis. Am J Clin Nutr 2007;85:144–51.

16. Institute of Medicine. Dietary reference intakes for energy, carbohydrate, fiber, fat, fatty acids, choldesterol, protein and amino acids. Washington, DC: National Academy Press; 2002.
17. Vaisman N, Clarke R, Rossi M, et al. Protein turnover and resting energy expenditure in patients with undernutrition and chronic lung disease. Am J Clin Nutr 1992;55:63–9.
18. Geukers VGM, Oudshoorn JH, Taminiau JAJM, et al. Short-term protein intake and stimulation of protein synthesis in stunted children with cystic fibrosis. Am J Clin Nutr 2005;81:605–10.
19. Kawchak DA, Zhoa H, Scanlin TF, et al. Longitudinal, prospective analysis of dietary intake in children with cystic fibrosis. J Pediatr 1996;129:119–29.
20. White H, Morton AM, Peckham DG, et al. Dietary intakes in adult patients with cystic fibrosis-do they achieve guidelines? J Cyst Fibros 2003;3:1–7.
21. Schall JI, Bentley T, Stallings VA. Meal patterns, dietary fat intake and pancreatic enzyme use in preadolescent children with cystic fibrosis. J Pediatr Gastroenterol Nutr 2006;43:651–9.
22. Poustie VJ, Russell JE, Watling RM, et al. Oral protein energy supplements for children with cystic fibrosis: CALICO multicentre randomized controlled trial. BMJ 2006;332:632–6.
23. Institute of Medicine. Dietary reference intakes for vitamin A, vitamin K, boron, chromium, copper, iodine, iron, manganese, molybdenum, nickel, vanadium, and zinc. Washington, DC: National Academy Press; 2001.
24. Michaelsson K, Lithell H, Vessby B, et al. Serum retinol levels and the risk of fracture. N Engl J Med 2003;348:287–94.
25. Hakim F, Kerem E, Rivlin J, et al. Vitamins A and E and pulmonary exacerbations in patients with cystic fibrosis. J Pediatr Gastroenterol Nutr 2007;45(3):347–53.
26. Duggan C, Colin AA, Agil A, et al. Vitamin A status in acute exacerbations of cystic fibrosis. Am J Clin Nutr 1996;64(4):635–9.
27. O'Neil C, Shevill E, Chang AB. Vitamin A supplementation for cystic fibrosis. Cochrane Database Syst Rev 2008;23(1):CD006751.
28. Maqbool A, Graham-Maar RC, Schall JI, et al. Vitamin A intake and elevated serum retinol levels in children and young adults with cystic fibrosis. J Cyst Fibros 2008;7(2):137–41 [Epub 2007 Sep 4].
29. James DR, Owen G, Campbell IA, et al. Vitamin A absorption in cystic fibrosis: risk of hypervitaminosis A. Gut 1992;33(5):707–10.
30. Tanumihardjo SA. Assessing vitamin A status: past, present and future. J Nutr 2004;134(1):290S–3S.
31. Wood LG, Fitzgerald DA, Lee AK, et al. Improved antioxidant and fatty acid status of patients with cystic fibrosis after antioxidant supplementation is linked to improved lung function. Am J Clin Nutr 2003;77:150–9.
32. Willison HJ, Muller DPR, Matthews S, et al. A study of the relationship between neurological function and serum vitamin E concentrations in patients with cystic fibrosis. J Neurol Neurosurg Psychiatry 1985;48:1097–102.
33. Cynamon HA, Milov DE, Valenstein E, et al. Effect of vitamin E deficiency on neurologic function in patients with cystic fibrosis. J Pediatr 1988;113:637–40.
34. Lancellotti L, D'Orazio C, Mastella G, et al. Deficiency of vitamins E and A in cystic fibrosis is Independent of pancreatic function and current enzyme and vitamin supplementation. Eur J Pediatr 1996;155:281–5.
35. Dorlochter L, Aksnes L, Fluge G. Faecal elastase-1 and fat-soluble vitamin profiles in patients with cystic fibrosis in Western Norway. Eur J Nutr 2002;41:148–52.

36. Sokol RJ, Reardon MC, Accurso FJ, et al. Fat-soluble-vitamin status during the first year of life in infants with cystic fibrosis identified by screening of newborns. Am J Clin Nutr 1989;50:1064–71.

37. Feranchak AP, Sontag MK, Wagener JS, et al. Prospective, long-term study of fat-soluble vitamin status in children with cystic fibrosis identified by newborn screen. J Pediatr 1999;135:601–10.

38. Koscik RL, Lai HC, Laxova A, et al. Preventing early, prolonged vitamin E deficiency: an opportunity for better cognitive outcomes via early diagnosis through neonatal screening. J Pediatr 2005;147:S51–6.

39. Cantin AM, White TB, Cross CE, et al. Antioxidants in cystic fibrosis. Conclusions from the CF antioxidant workshop, Bethesda, Maryland, November 11–12, 2003. Free Radic Biol Med 2007;42:15–31.

40. Bines JE, Truby HD, Armstrong DS, et al. Vitamin A and E deficiency and lung disease in infants with cystic fibrosis. J Paediatr Child Health 2005;41:663–8.

41. Oudshoorn JH, Klijn PH, Hofman Z, et al. Dietary supplementation with multiple micronutrients: no beneficial effects in pediatric cystic fibrosis patients. J Cyst Fibros 2007;6:35–40.

42. Huang SH, Schall JI, Zemel BS, et al. Vitamin E status in children with cystic fibrosis and pancreatic insufficiency. J Pediatr 2006;148:556–9.

43. Sokol RJ. Selection bias and vitamin E status in cystic fibrosis. J Pediatr 2007; 150(5):e85.

44. Tinley CG, Withers NJ, Sheldon CD, et al. Zinc therapy for night blindness in cystic fibrosis. J Cyst Fibros 2008;7:333–5.

45. Holick MF. Vitamin D deficiency. N Engl J Med 2007;357:266–81.

46. Cannell JJ, Hollis BW, Zasloff M, et al. Diagnosis and treatment of vitamin D deficiency. Expert Opin Pharmacother 2008;9(1):107–18.

47. Neville LA, Ranganathan SC. Vitamin D in infants with cystic fibrosis diagnosed by newborn screening. J Paediatr Child Health 2009;45(1–2):36–41.

48. Rovner AJ, Stallings VA, Schall JI, et al. Vitamin D insufficiency in children, adolescents, and young adults with cystic fibrosis despite routine oral supplementation. Am J Clin Nutr 2007;86:1694–9.

49. Brannon PM, Yetley EA, Bailey RL, et al. Overview of the conference "Vitamin D and health in the 21st Century: an update". Am J Clin Nutr 2008;88(Suppl): 483S–90S.

50. Lark RK, Lester GE, Ontjes DA, et al. Diminished and erratic absorption of ergocalciferol in adult cystic fibrosis patients. Am J Clin Nutr 2001;73:602–6.

51. Aris RM, Merkel PA, Bachrach LK, et al. Consensus statement: guide to bone health and disease in cystic fibrosis. J Clin Endocrinol Metab 2005;90:1888–96.

52. Speeckaert MM, Wehlou C, Vandewalle S, et al. Vitamin D binding protein, a new nutritional marker in cystic fibrosis patients. Clin Chem Lab Med 2008;46(3): 365–70.

53. Wagner LW, Greer FR, The Section on Breastfeeding and Committee on Nutrition. Prevention of rickets and vitamin D deficiency in infants, children, and adolescents. Pediatrics 2008;122:1142–52.

54. Green D, Carson K, Leonard A, et al. Current treatment recommendations for correcting vitamin D deficiency in pediatric patients with cystic fibrosis are inadequate. J Pediatr 2008;153:554–9.

55. Virella-Lowell I, Bowman C, Wagner C, et al. Successful supplementation of vitamin D in cystic fibrosis. Pediatr Pulmonol 2006;29(Suppl):396.

56. Armas LAG, Hollis BW, Heaney RP. Vitamin D2 is much less effective than vitamin D3 in humans. J Clin Endocrinol Metab 2004;89:5387–91.

57. Houghton LA, Vieth R. The case against ergocalciferol (vitamin D2) as a vitamin supplement. Am J Clin Nutr 2006;84:694–7.
58. Gronowitz E, Larko O, Gilljam M, et al. Ultraviolet B radiation improves serum levels of vitamin D in patients with cystic fibrosis. Acta Paediatr 2005;94:547–52.
59. Khazai NB, Judd S, Jeng L, et al. Treatment and prevention of vitamin D insufficiency in cystic fibrosis patients: comparative efficacy of ergocalciferol, cholecalciferol and UV light. J Clin Endocrinol Metab 2009;94:2037–43.
60. Aris R. Update on bone mineralization in CF. Pediatr Pulmonol 2008;31(Suppl): 173–5.
61. Conway SP. Vitamin K in cystic fibrosis. J R Soc Med 2004;97(Suppl 44):48–51.
62. Booth SL, Golly I, Sacheck J, et al. Effect of vitamin E supplementation on vitamin K status in adults with normal coagulation status. Am J Clin Nutr 2004; 80(1):143–8.
63. Drury D, Grey VL, Ferland G, et al. Efficacy of high dose phylloquinone in correcting vitamin K deficiency in cystic fibrosis. J Cyst Fibros 2008;7:457–9.
64. Hamid B, Khan A. Cerebral hemorrhage as the initial manifestation of cystic fibrosis. J Child Neurol 2007;22(1):114–5.
65. Nicolaidou P, Stavrinadis I, Loukou I, et al. The effect of vitamin K supplementation on biochemical markers of bone formation in children and adolescents with cystic fibrosis. Eur J Pediatr 2006;165:540–5.
66. Fewtrell MS, Benden C, Williams JE, et al. Undercarboxylated osteocalcin and bone mass in 8–12 year old children with cystic fibrosis. J Cyst Fibros 2008; 7(4):307–12.
67. Mosler K, von Kries R, Vermeer C, et al. Assessment of vitamin K deficiency in CF—how much sophistication is useful? J Cyst Fibros 2003;2:91–6.
68. Sinaasappel M, Stern M, Littlewood J, et al. Nutrition in patients with cystic fibrosis: a European Consensus. J Cyst Fibros 2002;1:51–75.
69. Urquhart DS, Fitzpatrick M, Cope J, et al. Vitamin K prescribing patterns and bone health surveillance in UK children with cystic fibrosis. J Hum Nutr Diet 2007;20:605–10.
70. van Hoorn JHL, Hendriks JJE, Vermeer C, et al. Vitamin K supplementation in cystic fibrosis. Arch Dis Child 2003;88:974–5.
71. Solomons NW, Wagonfeld JB, Rieger C, et al. Some biochemical indices of nutrition in treated cystic fibrosis patients. Am J Clin Nutr 1981;34:462–74.
72. McCabe H. Riboflavin deficiency in cystic fibrosis: three case reports. J Hum Nutr Diet 2001;14:365–70.
73. Scambi C, DeFranceschi L, Guarini P, et al. Preliminary evidence for cell membrane amelioration n children with cystic fibrosis by 5-MTHF and vitamin B12 supplementation: a single arm trial. PLoS One 2009;4(3):e4782.
74. Winklhofer-Roob BM, Ellemunter H, Fruhwirth M, et al. Plasma vitamin C concentrations in patients with cystic fibrosis: evidence of associations with lung inflammation. Am J Clin Nutr 1997;65:1858–66.
75. Back EI, Frindt C, Nohr D, et al. Antioxidant deficiency in cystic fibrosis: when is the right time to take action? Am J Clin Nutr 2004;80:374–84.
76. Taussig LM. Cystic fibrosis. New York: Thieme-Stratton, Inc; 1984.
77. Leoni GB. A specific cystic fibrosis mutation (T3381) associated with the phenotype of isolated hypotonic dehydration. J Podiatr 1995;127:281–3.
78. Fustik S, Pop-Jordanova N, Slaveska N, et al. Metabolic alkalosis with hypoelectrolytemia in infants with cystic fibrosis. Pediatr Int 2002;44:289–92.
79. Yalcin E. Clinical features and treatment approaches in cystic fibrosis with pseudo-Bartter syndrome. Ann Trop Paediatr 2005;25:119–24.

80. Legris GJ, Dearborn D, Stern RC. Sodium space and intravascular volume: dietary sodium effects in cystic fibrosis and healthy subjects. Pediatrics 1998;101: 48–56.
81. Kessler WR, Anderson DH. Heat prostration in fibrocystic disease of the pancreas and other conditions. Pediatrics 1951;8:648–56.
82. Laughlin JJ, Brady MS, Eigen H. Changing feeding trends as a cause of electrolyte depletion in infants with cystic fibrosis. Pediatrics 1981;68:203–7.
83. Orenstein DM, Henke KG, Costill DL, et al. Exercise and heat stress in cystic fibrosis patients. Pediatr Res 1983;17:267–9.
84. Bar-Or O, Blimkie CJR. Voluntary dehydration and heat intolerance in cystic fibrosis. Lancet 1992;339:696–9.
85. Chan DS. Recommended daily allowance of maintenance parenteral nutrition in infants and children. Am J Health Syst Pharm 1995;52:651–3.
86. Kriemler S, Wilk B, Schurer W, et al. Preventing dehydration in children with cystic fibrosis who exercise in the heat. Med Sci Sports Exerc 1993;31:774–9.
87. Heaney RP, Weaver CM. Newer perspectives on calcium nutrition and bone quality. J Am Coll Nutr 2005;24(Suppl 6):574S–81S.
88. Schulze KJ, Cutchins C, Rosenstein BJ, et al. Calcium acquisition rates do not support age-appropriate gains in total body bone mineral content in prepuberty and late puberty in girls with cystic fibrosis. Osteoporos Int 2006;17(5):731–40.
89. von Vigier RO, Truttmann AC, Zindler-Schmocker K, et al. Aminoglycosides and renal magnesium homeostasis in humans. Nephrol Dial Transplant 2000;15: 822–6.
90. Greer RM, Buntain HM, Potter JM, et al. Abnormalities of the PTH-vitamin D axis and bone turnover markers in children, adolescents and adults with cystic fibrosis: comparison to healthy controls. Osteoporos Int 2003;14:404–11.
91. Glass S, Plant ND, Spencer DA. The effects of intravenous tobramycin on renal tubular function in children with cystic fibrosis. J Cyst Fibros 2005;4:221–5.
92. Gupta A, Eastham KM, Wrightson N, et al. Hypomagnesemia in cystic fibrosis patients referred for lung transplant assessment. J Cyst Fibros 2007;6:360–2.
93. Prasad AS. Zinc deficiency in women, infants, and children. J Am Coll Nutr 1996; 15:113–20.
94. Mocchegiani E, Provinciali M, Di Stefano G, et al. Role of the low zinc bioavailability on cellular immune effectiveness in cystic fibrosis. Clin Immunol Immunopathol 1995;75:214–24.
95. Cantin AM. Potential for antioxidant therapy of cystic fibrosis. Curr Opin Pulm Med 2004;10:531–6.
96. Krebs NF. Overview of zinc absorption and excretion in the human gastrointestinal tract. J Nutr 2000;130(Suppl 5S):1374S–7S.
97. Easley D, Krebs N, Jefferson M, et al. Effect of pancreatic enzymes on zinc absorption in cystic fibrosis. J Pediatr Gastroenterol Nutr 1998;26:136–9.
98. Krebs NF, Sontag M, Accurso FJ, et al. Low plasma zinc concentrations in young infants with cystic fibrosis. J Pediatr 1998;133:761–4.
99. Krebs NF, Westcott JE, Arnold TD, et al. Abnormalities in zinc homeostasis in young infant with cystic fibrosis. Pediatr Res 2000;48:256–61.
100. Crone J, Huber WD, Eichler I, et al. Acrodermatitis enteropathica-like eruption as the presenting sign of cystic fibrosis-case report and review of the literature. Eur J Pediatr 2002;161:475–8.
101. Bernstein ML, McCusker MM, Grant-Kels JM. Cutaneous manifestations of cystic fibrosis. Pediatr Dermatol 2008;25:150–7.

102. Abdulhamid I, Beck FW, Millard S, et al. Effect of zinc supplementation on respiratory tract infections in children with cystic fibrosis. Pediatr Pulmonol 2008;43: 281–7.

103. Maqbool A, Schall JI, Zemel BS, et al. Plasma zinc and growth status in preadolescent children with cystic fibrosis. J Pediatr Gastroenterol Nutr 2006;43: 95–101.

104. Akanli L, Lowenthal DB, Gjonaj S, et al. Plasma and red blood cell zinc in cystic fibrosis. Pediatr Pulmonol 2003;35:2–7.

105. Van Biervliet S, Van Biervliet JP, Robberecht E. Serum zinc in patients with cystic fibrosis at diagnosis and after one year of therapy. Biol Trace Elem Res 2006; 112:205–11.

106. Van Biervliet S, VandeVelde S, Van Biervliet JP, et al. The effect of zinc supplements in cystic fibrosis patients. Ann Nutr Metab 2008;52:152–6.

107. von Drygalski A, Biller J. Anemia in CF: incidence, mechanisms, and association with pulmonary function and vitamin deficiency. Nutr Clin Pract 2008;23(5): 557–63.

108. Keevil B, Rowlands D, Burton I, et al. Assessment of iron status in CF patients. Ann Clin Biochem 2000;37(Pt 5):662–5.

109. Khalid S, McGrowder D, Kemp M, et al. The use of soluble transferring receptor to assess iron deficiency in adults with cystic fibrosis. Clin Chim Acta 2007; 378(1–2):194–200.

110. Fischer R, Simmerlein R, Huber RM, et al. Lung disease severity, chronic inflammation, iron deficiency and erythropoietin response in adults with CF. Pediatr Pulmonol 2007;42(12):1193–7.

111. Weiss G, Goodnough LT. Anemia of chronic disease. N Engl J Med 2005;352: 1011–23.

112. Reid DW, Withers NJ, Francis L, et al. Iron deficiency in CF. Relationship to lung disease severity and chronic pseudomonas aeruginosa infection. Chest 2002; 121(1):48–54.

113. Reid DW, Lam QT, Schneider H, et al. Airway iron and iron-regulatory cytokines in CF. Eur Respir J 2004;24(2):286–91.

114. Winklhofer-Roob BM, Tiran B, Tuchschmid PE, et al. Effects of pancreatic enzyme preparations on erythrocyte glutathione peroxidase activities and plasma selenium concentrations in CF. Free Radic Biol Med 1998;25(2): 242–9.

115. Michaike B. Selenium speciation in human serum of CF patients compared to serum from healthy persons. J Chromatogr A 2004;1058(1–2):203–8.

116. Portal B, Richard MJ, Coudray C, et al. Effect of double-blind cross-over selenium supplementation on lipid peroxidation markers in CF patients. Clin Chim Acta 1995;234(1–2):137–46.

117. Percival SS, Bowser E, Wagner M. Reduced copper enzyme activities in blood cells of children with CF. Am J Clin Nutr 1995;62:633–8.

118. Percival SS, Kauwell GPA, Bowser E, et al. Altered copper status I adult men with CF. J Am Coll Nutr 1999;18(6):614–9.

119. Best K, McCoy K, Gemma S, et al. Copper enzyme activities in CF before and after copper supplementation plus or minus zinc. Metabolism 2004;53(1):37–41.

120. Kuo PT, Huang NN, Bassett R. The fatty acid composition of the serum chylomicrons and adipose tissue of children with cystic fibrosis of the pancreas. J Pediatr 1962;60:394–403.

121. Roulet M, Frascarolo P, Rappaz I, et al. Essential fatty acid deficiency in well nourished young cystic fibrosis patients. Eur J Pediatr 1997;156:952–6.

122. Kalivianakis M, Minich DM, Bijleveld CM, et al. Fat malabsorption in cystic fibrosis patients receiving enzyme replacement therapy is due to impaired intestinal uptake of long-chain fatty acids. Am J Clin Nutr 1999;69(1):127–34.

123. Carlstedt-Duke J, Bronnegard M, Strandvik B. Pathological regulation of arachidonic acid release in cystic fibrosis: the putative basic defect. Proc Natl Acad Sci U S A 1986;83:9202–6.

124. Freedman SD, Katz MH, Parker EM, et al. A membrane lipid imbalance plays a role in the phenotypic expression of cystic fibrosis in cftr(-/-) mice. Proc Natl Acad Sci U S A 1999;96(24):13995–4000.

125. Guilbault C, Wojewodka G, Saeed Z, et al. Cystic fibrosis fatty acid imbalance is linked to ceramide deficiency and corrected by fenretinide. Am J Respir Cell Mol Biol 2009;41:100–6 2008 Dec 4 [Epub ahead of print].

126. Strandvik B, Gronowitz E, Enlund F, et al. Essential fatty acid deficiency in relation to genotype in patients with cystic fibrosis. J Pediatr 2001;139(5):650–5.

127. Freedman SD, Blanco PG, Zaman MM, et al. Association of cystic fibrosis with abnormalities in fatty acid metabolism. N Engl J Med 2004;350(6):560–9.

128. Strandvik B, Svensson E, Seyberth HW. Prostanoid biosynthesis in patients with cystic fibrosis. Prostaglandins Leukot Essent Fatty Acids 1996;55(6): 419–25.

129. Coste T, Armand M, Lebacq J, et al. An overview of monitoring and supplementation of omega 3 fatty acids in cystic fibrosis. Clin Biochem 2007;40:511–20.

130. Cawood AL, Carroll MP, Wootton SA, et al. Is there a case for n-3 fatty acid supplementation in cystic fibrosis? Curr Opin Clin Nutr Metab Care 2005;8: 153–9.

131. Shoff SM, Ahn HY, Davis L, et al. Temporal associations among energy intake, plasma linoleic acid, and growth improvement in response to treatment initiation after diagnosis of cystic fibrosis. Pediatrics 2006;117:391–400.

132. Walkowiak J, Lisowska A, Blaszczynski M, et al. Polyunsaturated fatty acids in cystic fibrosis are related to nutrition and clinical expression of the disease. J Pediatr Gastroenterol Nutr 2007;45:488–90.

133. Maqbool A, Schall JI, Garcia-Espana JF, et al. Serum linoleic acid status as a clinical indicator of essential fatty acid status in children with cystic fibrosis. J Pediatr Gastroenterol Nutr 2008;47(5):635–44.

134. Lloyd-Still JD, Johnson SB, Holman RT. Essential fatty acid status in cystic fibrosis and the effects of safflower oil supplementation. Am J Clin Nutr 1981; 34(1):1–7.

135. Lloyd-Still JD, Powers CA, Hoffman DR, et al. Bioavailability and safety of a high dose of docosahexaenoic acid triacylglycerol of algal origin in cystic fibrosis patients: a randomized, controlled study. Nutrition 2006;22:36–46.

136. Van Biervliet S, Devos M, Delhaye T, et al. Oral DHA supplementation in DeltaF508 homozygous cystic fibrosis patients. Prostaglandins Leukot Essent Fatty Acids 2008;78(2):109–15 [Epub 2008 Feb 13].

137. McKarney C, Everard M, N'Diaye T. Omega-3 fatty acids (from fish oils) for cystic fibrosis. Cochrane Database Syst Rev 2007;17(4):CD002201.

138. Kurlandsky LE, Bennink MR, Webb PM, et al. The absorption and effect of dietary supplementation with omega-3 fatty acids on serum leukotriene B4 in patients with cystic fibrosis. Pediatr Pulmonol 1994;18:211–7.

139. Panchaud A, Sauty A, Kernen Y, et al. Biological effects of a dietary omega-3 polyunsaturated fatty acids supplementation in cystic fibrosis patients: a randomized, crossover placebo-controlled trial. Clin Nutr 2006;25(3): 418–27.

140. Christophe A, Robberecht E. Directed modification instead of normalization of fatty acid patterns in cystic fibrosis: an emerging concept. Curr Opin Clin Nutr Metab Care 2001;4(2):111–3.

141. Institute of Medicine. Dietary reference intakes for thiamin, riboflavin, niacin, vitamin B6, folate, vitamin B12, pantothenic acid, biotin, and choline. Washington, DC: National Academy Press; 1998.

142. Ulane MM, Butler JD, Peri A, et al. Cystic fibrosis and phosphatidylcholine biosynthesis. Clin Chim Acta 1994;230(2):109–16.

143. Chen AH, Innis SM, Davidson AG, et al. Phosphatidylcholine and lysophosphatidylcholine excretion is increased in children with cystic fibrosis and is associated with plasma homocysteine, S-adenosylhomocysteine, and S-adenosylmethionine. Am J Clin Nutr 2005;81(3):686–91.

144. Innis SM, Davidson AG, Melynk S, et al. Choline-related supplements improve abnormal plasma methionine-homocysteine metabolites and glutathione status in children with cystic fibrosis. Am J Clin Nutr 2007;85(3):702–8.

145. Ballatori N, Krance SM, Notenboom S, et al. Glutathione dysregulation and the etiology and progression of human diseases. Biol Chem 2009;390(3):191–214 [Epub ahead of print].

146. Hull J, Vervaart P, Grimwood K, et al. Pulmonary oxidative stress response in young children with cystic fibrosis. Thorax 1997;52(6):557–60.

147. Roum JH, Buhl R, McElvaney NG, et al. Systemic deficiency of glutathione in cystic fibrosis. J Appl Physiol 1993;75(6):2419–24.

148. Day BJ, van Heeckeren AM, Min E, et al. Role for cystic fibrosis transmembrane conductance regulator protein in a glutathione response to bronchopulmonary pseudomonas infection. Infect Immun 2004;72(4):2045–51.

149. Tirouvanziam R, Conrad CK, Bottiglieri T, et al. High-dose oral N-acetylcysteine, a glutathione prodrug, modulates inflammation in cystic fibrosis. Proc Natl Acad Sci U S A 2006;103(12):4628–33.

150. Griese M, Ramakers J, Krasselt A, et al. Improvement of alveolar glutathione and lung function but not oxidative state in cystic fibrosis. Am J Respir Crit Care Med 2004;169(7):822–8.

151. Hartl D, Starosta V, Maier K, et al. Inhaled glutathione decreases PGE2 and increases lymphocytes in cystic fibrosis lungs. Free Radic Biol Med 2005; 39(4):463–72.

152. Grasemann H, Gaston B, Fang K, et al. Decreased levels of nitrosothiols in the lower airways of patients with cystic fibrosis and normal pulmonary function. J Pediatr 1999;135(6):770–2.

153. Snyder AH, McPherson ME, Hunt JF, et al. Acute effects of aerosolized S-nitrosoglutathione in cystic fibrosis. Am J Respir Crit Care Med 2002;165(7):922–6.

154. Laguna TA, Sontag MK, Osberg I, et al. Decreased total serum coenzyme-Q10 concentrations: a longitudinal study in children with cystic fibrosis. J Pediatr 2008;153(3):402–7.

155. Oudshoorn JH, Lecluse AL, van den Berg R, et al. Decreased coenzyme Q10 concentration in plasma of children with cystic fibrosis. J Pediatr Gastroenterol Nutr 2006;43(5):646–50.

156. Nutritional management of cystic fibrosis. UK Cystic Fibrosis Trust Nutrition Working Group. Available at: www.cftrust.org.uk. 2002. Accessed July 28, 2009.

Nutritional Deficiencies During Critical Illness

Nilesh M. Mehta, MD[a],*, Christopher P. Duggan, MD, MPH[b]

KEYWORDS

- Critical care • Children • Malnutrition
- Deficiency • Nutrition

Awareness of the deleterious consequences of malnutrition during critical illness and the will to prioritize nutritional therapy are necessary first steps toward addressing this problem. Careful attention to preexisting malnutrition, regular and accurate assessment of nutritional requirements, and accurate measurement of energy expenditure in some cases allow individually tailored nutritional prescriptions to be designed for critically ill children. A multidisciplinary effort at the bedside is required to overcome barriers and deliver the prescribe nutrients to the critically ill child successfully. Nutrition support teams (NSTs), evidence- or consensus-based guidelines, and regular audits and improvements of practice parameters may facilitate this essential goal of critical care.

The prevalence of malnutrition in hospitalized patients is a significant health care problem because it influences patient outcomes.[1–5] Malnourished hospitalized patients have a higher rate of infectious and noninfectious complications, increased mortality, a longer length of hospital stay, and increased hospital costs.[5] In hospitalized children, malnutrition is associated with altered physiologic responses and increased resource use, and it influences outcome during critical illness.[6,7] The prevalence of malnutrition in children admitted to the pediatric intensive care unit (PICU) has remained unchanged over the past 3 decades.[8,9] Critical illness itself may increase metabolic demand on the host in the early stages of the stress response, and nutrient intake may be limited. Thus, children admitted to the PICU are at risk for worsening nutritional status and anthropometric changes with increased morbidity.[10]

Despite its high prevalence and consequences, medical awareness of malnutrition is lacking. Only a small number of hospitalized patients are assessed for nutritional

[a] Division of Critical Care Medicine, Department of Anesthesia, Bader 634, Children's Hospital, Harvard Medical School, 300 Longwood Avenue, Boston, MA 02115, USA
[b] Clinical Nutrition Service, Division of Gastroenterology, Children's Hospital, Harvard Medical School, 300 Longwood Avenue, Boston, MA 02115, USA
* Corresponding author.
E-mail address: nilesh.mehta@childrens.harvard.edu (N.M. Mehta).

Pediatr Clin N Am 56 (2009) 1143–1160
doi:10.1016/j.pcl.2009.06.007
0031-3955/09/$ – see front matter © 2009 Elsevier Inc. All rights reserved.

pediatric.theclinics.com

status or referred for nutritional support.[11] Careful nutritional evaluation at admission to the PICU is essential for identification of children at risk for further nutritional deterioration and should allow interventions to optimize nutrient intake. The epidemiology and causes of malnutrition in critically ill children are described here, as are the importance of nutritional assessment of children in the PICU and measures to prevent their nutritional deterioration.

EPIDEMIOLOGY AND RISK FACTORS FOR MALNUTRITION IN THE PEDIATRIC INTENSIVE CARE UNIT

One in every five children admitted to the PICU experiences acute or chronic malnutrition.[3,8,9] Because of the lack of systematic nutritional assessment at many centers, the true extent of malnutrition in the PICU population may not be appreciated. Pediatric malnutrition, also commonly known as protein-energy malnutrition (PEM), remains a significant health care problem in the developing world and the industrial world. The correlation between nutritional status and outcomes is complex and probably bidirectional.[12] On the one hand, underlying disease state and the duration of pre-PICU illness may influence the severity of malnourishment and predispose some children to critical illness. Malnutrition in children is associated with physiologic alterations; micronutrient imbalance; gastrointestinal dysfunction; and impairment of cell-mediated immunity, phagocytic function, and the complement system. On the other hand, up to 44% of hospitalized children in a variety of disease states develop malnutrition during acute or chronic illness.[13,14] The increased energy demands secondary to the metabolic stress response to critical illness, erratic prescription of nutrients, and failure to administer adequate nutrients are factors responsible for the subsequent worsening of nutritional status in children admitted to the PICU. Indeed, acute and chronic malnutrition has been shown to worsen at discharge from the PICU.[8]

Infants have a high basal metabolic rate and limited energy reserves, and they are particularly at risk for developing nutritional deficiencies during illness. Some groups of critically ill children may be at an increased risk for developing malnutrition. Children with congenital heart disease (CHD) have a high incidence of PEM, which contributes to the poor outcome in this cohort.[15] Common reasons for energy deficits in children with CHD include decreased intake, increased energy expenditure (attributable to cardiac failure or increased work of breathing), and malabsorption (attributable to increased right-sided heart pressure, lower cardiac output, or altered gastrointestinal function).[16–19] In a retrospective review of newborns with hypoplastic left heart syndrome who underwent the traditional Norwood procedure, the authors have reported a high incidence of PEM manifested by low weight-for-age z scores.[20] After initial ICU hospitalization in the first month of life, weight-for-age z scores and weight-for-length z scores decreased over time, and half of the infants were severely underweight when readmitted for subsequent major cardiac surgery. Longer length of hospital or ICU stay and frequency of readmission were significantly correlated with poor nutritional status in this cohort, and aggressive enteral nutrition (EN) and parenteral nutrition (PN) were associated with better nutritional status.

Another group of critically ill children at nutritional risk includes those with burn injuries. In these children, a hypermetabolic stress response and poor intake result in energy deficits, and the negative effects on nutritional status may persist for months after injury. Decrease in lean body mass was shown for up to a year after the burn injury, with delayed linear growth reported for up to 2 years after burn injury.[21,22] Duration of PICU stay is an important factor associated with the development of cumulative energy and protein deficits in critically ill children.[10] The development of deficits is most rapid during the first few days after admission. Duration of mechanical ventilation and need for surgical intervention are other factors associated with development of cumulative energy deficits, independent of PICU stay.[10]

Obesity is increasing in the pediatric population and places children at risk for a variety of health care issues.[23] Although caloric deficit is well recognized in hospitalized children, overfeeding is a largely underestimated problem in critically ill children. Provision of excessive calories during illness can result in deleterious consequences. Problems with estimation of energy requirement and strategies to prevent overfeeding are described elsewhere in this article.

CAUSES OF MALNUTRITION IN CRITICALLY ILL CHILDREN

The etiology of malnutrition developing during critical illness is multifactorial, and common factors contributing to the protein and energy deficits during the PICU course include (1) increased demands secondary to the metabolic stress response, (2) failure to estimate energy expenditure accurately, and (3) inadequate substrate delivery at the bedside.

The Metabolic Stress Response

The profound metabolic response to critical illness in children is not always predictable and varies in intensity and duration between individuals. The energy burden imposed by the metabolic response to injury, surgery, or inflammation may be proportional to the severity and duration of the stress but cannot always be accurately estimated. Importantly, nutritional support itself cannot reverse or prevent the metabolic stress response. Failure to provide optimal calories and protein during the acute stage of illness can result in an exaggeration of existing nutritional deficiencies or further exacerbate underlying nutritional status, however. Large energy imbalances attributable to underfeeding and overfeeding in critically ill children must be avoided.[24] This requires an individualized nutritional regimen that must be tailored for each child and reviewed regularly during the course of illness. A basic understanding of the metabolic events that accompany critical illness and surgery is essential for planning appropriate nutritional support in critically ill children.

The unique hormonal and cytokine profile manifested during critical illness is characterized by an elevation in serum levels of insulin, glucagon, cortisol, catecholamines, and proinflammatory cytokines.[25] Increased serum counterregulatory hormone concentrations induce insulin and growth hormone resistance, resulting in the catabolism of endogenous stores of protein, carbohydrate, and fat to provide essential substrate intermediates and energy necessary to support maintenance energy and micronutrient needs in addition to the ongoing metabolic stress response.[25]

Fig. 1 illustrates the basic pathways involved in the metabolic stress response.[26] In general, the net increase in muscle protein degradation, characteristic of the metabolic stress response, results in a large amount of free amino acids in the circulation. Free amino acids are used as the building blocks for the rapid synthesis of proteins that act as inflammatory response mediators and are used for tissue repair. Remaining amino acids not used in this way are channeled through the liver, wherein their carbon skeletons are used to create glucose through gluconeogenesis. Although the provision of optimal dietary protein does not eliminate the overall negative protein balance associated with the catabolic response to injury, it may slow the rate of net protein loss.[27] Carbohydrate turnover is simultaneously increased during the metabolic

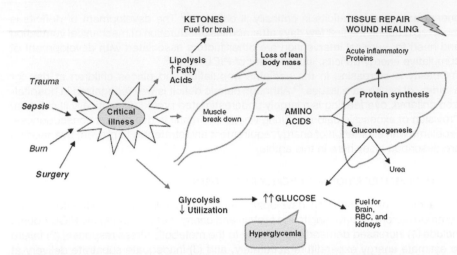

Fig. 1. Basic pathways of the metabolic stress response to injury. RBC, red blood cells. (*From* Mehta N, Jaksic T. The critically ill child. In: Duggan C, Watkins JB, Walker WA, editors. Nutrition in pediatrics. 4th edition. Hamilton, Ontario, Canada: BC Decker; 2008. p. 663–73; with permission.)

response, with a significant increase in glucose oxidation and gluconeogenesis.[28] The administration of exogenous glucose does not blunt the elevated rates of gluconeogenesis, however, and net protein catabolism continues unabated.[29] A combination of dietary glucose and protein may improve protein balance during critical illness, primarily by enhancing protein synthesis. The stress response is also characterized by increased rates of fatty acid oxidation.[30] As seen with the other catabolic changes associated with stress response, the provision of dietary glucose does not decrease fatty acid turnover in times of illness. The increased demand for lipid use in the setting of limited lipid stores puts the metabolically stressed neonate or previously malnourished child at high risk for the development of essential fatty acid deficiency.[31,32] Preterm infants are most at risk for developing essential fatty acid deficiency after a short period of a fat-free nutritional regimen.[33]

The metabolic alterations during critical illness may be dynamic during the course of illness. A wide range of metabolic states have been observed in mechanically ventilated children, with an average tendency toward hypermetabolism.[34] Children with severe burn injury demonstrate extreme hypermetabolism in the early stages of injury.[35] The standard equations used for estimating energy requirements may underestimate the resting energy expenditure (REE) and lead to underfeeding. Failure to provide adequate calories during this phase may lead to the loss of critical lean body mass and worsening of existing malnutrition. Stress or activity correction factors have traditionally been factored into basal energy requirement estimates to adjust for the nature of illness, its severity, and the activity level of hospitalized subjects.[36,37] These factors range from 1.2 to 2.0 times the estimated basal energy requirement. Low physical activity, decreased insensible fluid losses, and transient absence of growth during the acute illness may predispose some critically ill children to the risk for overfeeding, however.[38] The application of a uniform stress correction factor to the equation for estimated energy requirement in critically ill children may be too simplistic, likely to be inaccurate, and increase the risk for overfeeding. Overfeeding is associated with deleterious effects in the critically ill patient.[39,40] It increases ventilatory work by increasing carbon dioxide production and can potentially prolong the need for mechanical ventilation.[41] Overfeeding may also impair liver function by inducing steatosis and cholestasis and increase the risk for infection caused by hyperglycemia. To account for these dynamic alterations in energy metabolism secondary to an unpredictable stress response, measured REE values remain the only true guide for energy intake in critically ill children.

Estimation of Energy Requirement During Critical Illness

The energy requirements for critically ill children are often derived from commonly used equations based on patient demographics. These equations have been shown to be inaccurate in critical illness and may underestimate or overestimate the true energy requirements.[42–46] Thus, nutritional intake based on estimated requirements often results in underfeeding or overfeeding. The cumulative effect of inaccurate estimations and suboptimal delivery may result in significant caloric imbalances with potential for affecting outcomes.[24,47] Indirect calorimetry (IC), using a metabolic cart, can be performed at the bedside to measure the volume of oxygen consumed (VO_2) and the volume of carbon dioxide produced (VCO_2). The respiratory quotient (RQ), defined by the ratio of VCO_2 to VO_2, is partially determined by substrate use in the child. Underfeeding, which promotes use of endogenous fat stores, should cause decreases in the RQ, whereas overfeeding, which results in lipogenesis, should cause increases in the RQ.[48] The use of the RQ as a measure of substrate use in individual patients has a low specificity, however.[49] An RQ lower than 0.85 identified underfeeding with a low sensitivity (63%), high specificity (89%), and high negative predictive value (90%). An RQ higher than 1.0 indicated overfeeding with a poor sensitivity (21%) but a high specificity (97%) and a high positive predictive value (93%).[41] Food composition, notably high-carbohydrate intake, was responsible for an RQ exceeding 1.0 in the overfed group. An increasing value of the RQ in response to overfeeding has been associated with increased ventilatory demands and respiratory burden, and elevation of the measured RQ greater than 1.0 may be an indicator of reduced respiratory tolerance of the nutritional regimen (**Fig. 2**).[48]

To achieve optimal individualized nutritional support, energy goals should be identified regularly in critically ill children with the help of IC when feasible. With careful attention to its limitations and available expertise for interpretation, IC can be applied in a PICU and is indeed warranted in children at high risk for underfeeding and overfeeding.[24,47] Resource constraints and lack of available expertise restrict the regular use of IC in the PICU, however. In a multicenter study of nutritional practices in the

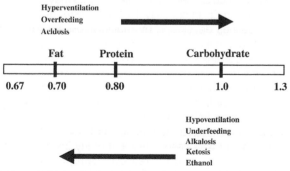

Fig. 2. Relation between RQ and substrate use. (*From* McClave SA, Lowen CC, Kleber MJ, et al. Clinical use of the respiratory quotient obtained from indirect calorimetry. JPEN J Parenter Enteral Nutr 2003;27(1):21–6; with permission.)

PICU, most European centers reported the use of estimated equations for energy expenditure when planning energy intake in critically ill children.[50] Targeted IC to obtain accurate measurement of REE may allow individualized nutritional therapy in high-risk children in the PICU and prevent cumulative caloric imbalances.[24]

Nutrient Intake at the Bedside: Prescription and Delivery

Barriers to nutritional intake in critically ill children have been described across centers all over the world.[51,52] After accurate estimation of energy needs, the actual delivery of requisite nutrients may be challenging and requires a multidisciplinary effort. In the first week of the PICU course, children received less than 60% of their prescribed calories.[53,54] Caloric deprivation in the PICU is prevalent, and its etiology is multifactorial.[52,55] In one study, less than half of the children in the PICU received nutrition on the first day of admission.[53] Delay in initiation of nutrition, suboptimal use of PN, and overall failure to prescribe adequate calories and protein were factors responsible for malnutrition during the PICU course of children in this study.

The PICU is a complex environment in which routine interventions and procedures are in constant conflict with bedside nutrient delivery. Early institution of EN is associated with beneficial outcomes in animal models and human studies,[56,57] and it has been increasingly implemented during critical illness, often using nutritional guidelines or protocols.[58,59] Despite its known benefits, EN is often delayed. Subsequent maintenance of enteral nutrient delivery remains elusive, because EN is frequently interrupted in the intensive care setting for a variety of reasons, some of which are avoidable.[52,60] Frequent interruptions in enteral nutrient delivery may affect clinical outcomes because of energy imbalance or overreliance on PN.[52] To realize the potential benefits of EN in the PICU, early initiation and maintenance of enteral feeds must be ensured. The authors reviewed bedside EN delivery in 112 children in their PICU using a multidisciplinary bedside audit tool. Despite early initiation of EN, feeds were interrupted in many critically ill children admitted to the authors' busy medical and surgical PICU.[61] Avoidable EN interruptions were associated with a more than threefold increase in the use of PN and a significant delay in reaching energy goals. Fasting for procedures and intolerance to EN were the most common reasons for prolonged EN interruptions. Interventions aimed at optimizing EN delivery must be designed after examining existing barriers to EN and directed at high-risk individuals who are most likely to benefit from these interventions. Infants, younger children, and those requiring mechanical ventilation were more likely to be fed by means of the postpyloric route and had a longer stay in the PICU. Educational intervention and practice changes targeted at these high-risk patients may decrease the incidence of avoidable interruptions to EN in critically ill children (**Fig. 3**).

Clinical practice guidelines developed by multidisciplinary expert consensus and based on existing evidence may help to improve nutritional support practices in the intensive care unit. The Canadian clinical practice guidelines for nutritional support in critically ill adults provide a model for evidence-based consensus-derived generation of practical recommendations, dissemination of recommendations, and then systematic evaluation of their impact on patient outcomes. Adherence to guidelines has been shown to increase EN intake and decrease hospital length of stay and was associated with a trend toward decreased mortality.[62-65] Implementation of an institutional feeding protocol was associated with early institution of EN, shortened time to reaching a caloric goal, and decreased interruptions to established EN in a study conducted in the PICU population.[66] There are no randomized trials examining the effect of such protocols for feeding in the PICU, and their application remains sporadic with mixed effects.[67,68] Guidelines for EN and PN for the critically ill child

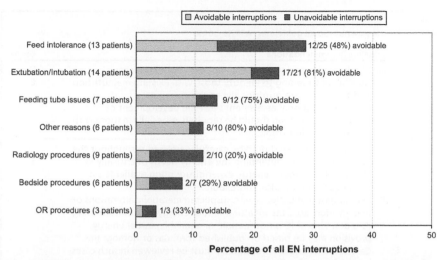

Fig. 3. Common reasons for EN interruption in a PICU. OR, operating room. (*From* Mehta NM, Hamilton S, McAleer D, et al. Challenges to enteral nutrient delivery in the critically ill child. JPEN J Parenter Enteral Nutr 2009, in press.)

were recently revised by the Guidelines Committee and Board of Directors of the American Society of Parenteral and Enteral Nutrition (ASPEN) (**Table 1**).[38]

NUTRITIONAL ASSESSMENT DURING CRITICAL ILLNESS

The nutritional assessment of critically ill children may be challenging from scientific and practical aspects. After admission, weights are infrequently obtained during the PICU course, and acute changes in nutritional status may be missed or detected late.[47] Failure to weigh children in the PICU is attributable to the perceived dangers of moving critically ill patients and the low priority among health care workers for nutritional assessment. In a review of hospitalized adults outside the intensive care unit, weights on admission were obtained in less than half of the patients.[11] The overall lack of enthusiasm for weighing critically ill children results in failure to estimate the true incidence of malnutrition in this cohort.

Anthropometric Assessment

Arm anthropometry (mid-upper arm circumference and triceps skinfold), body weights, body lengths, and body mass index are commonly used to assess the nutritional status of children. Hulst and colleagues[10] observed a correlation between energy deficits and deterioration in anthropometric parameters, such as midarm circumference and weight in a mixed population of critically ill children. The anthropometric abnormalities accrued during the PICU admission returned to normal by 6 months after discharge.[8] Using reproducible anthropometric measures, Leite and colleagues[7] reported a 65% prevalence of malnutrition on admission with increased mortality in this group compared with those without malnutrition. On follow-up, a significant portion of children with PEM had further deterioration in nutritional status.

Body Composition

Emerging literature supports the concept that body composition is a primary determinant of health and a predictor of morbidity and mortality in children. Preservation and

No.	Guideline Recommendations	Grade
Table 1		
Pediatric critical care nutritional guidelines: ASPEN, 2009		
1	(A) Children admitted with critical illnesses should undergo nutritional screening to identify those with existing malnutrition and those who are nutritionally at risk. (B) A formal nutritional assessment with the development of a nutritional care plan should be required, especially in those with preexisting malnutrition.	D E
2	(A) Energy expenditure should be carefully assessed throughout the course of illness to determine the energy needs of critically ill children. Estimates of energy expenditure using available standard equations are often unreliable. (B) In a subgroup of patients with suspected metabolic alterations or malnutrition, accurate measurement of energy expenditure using IC is desirable. If IC is not feasible or available, initial energy provision may be based on published formulas or nomograms. Caloric intake and anthropometry must be reviewed in such cases to avoid underfeeding or overfeeding.	D E
3	There are insufficient data to make evidence-based recommendations for macronutrient intake in critically ill children. After determination of energy needs for the critically ill child, the rational partitioning of the major substrates requires a basic understanding of protein metabolism and carbohydrate and lipid handling during critical illness.	E
4	(A) In children with a functioning gastrointestinal tract, EN is well tolerated. (B) A variety of barriers to EN exist in the PICU. Clinicians must identify and prevent avoidable interruptions to EN in critically ill children. (C) There are insufficient data to recommend the appropriate enteral access device site (gastric vs postpyloric/transpyloric) for enteral feeding in critically ill children. Postpyloric or transpyloric feeding may improve caloric intake when compared with administering nutrients into the stomach. Postpyloric feeding may be considered in children at high risk for aspiration or those who have failed a trial of gastric feeding.	C D C
5	Based on the available pediatric data, the routine use of immunonutrition, immune-enhancing diets/nutrients, or pharmaconutrients in critically ill children cannot be recommended.	D
6	A specialized NST in the PICU and aggressive feeding protocols may enhance the overall delivery of nutrition, with shorter time to goal nutrition, increased delivery of EN, and decreased use of PN. The impact of these strategies on patient outcomes has not been demonstrated.	E

Adapted from Mehta NM, Compher C. A.s.p.e.N. clinical guidelines: nutrition support of the critically ill child. JPEN J Parenter Enteral Nutr 2009;33(3):260–76; with permission.

accrual of lean body mass during illness have been shown to be important predictors of clinical outcomes in a variety of settings, including patients with sepsis, cystic fibrosis, and malnutrition.[69–71] Although bedside anthropometric methods are inexpensive, they are sporadically applied in hospitalized children, may be insensitive in the setting of critical illness, and are limited by significant interobserver variability.

Weight changes and other anthropometric measurements in critically ill children should be interpreted in the context of edema, fluid therapy, volume overload, and diuresis. In the presence of ascites or edema, ongoing loss of lean body mass may not be evident using weight monitoring. A variety of techniques of body composition measurement, including body densitometry by underwater weighing, neutron activation analysis, and total body potassium determination or dual-energy x-ray absorptiometry (DXA), have been described in the literature.[72-75] Most of these methods are not practical for application in the clinical management of a critically ill child. DXA is a radiographic technique that can determine the composition and density of different body compartments (fat, lean tissue, fat-free mass, and bone mineral content) and their distribution in the body. DXA has been used extensively in pediatric practice for determining fat-free mass, fat mass, and lean mass, and it is recognized as a reference method for body composition research.[76] Its results correlate well with direct chemical analyses, and there is good agreement between percentage body fat estimated by hydrodensitometry and DXA.[77] The application of DXA in the PICU is impractical, however. Bioelectric impedance analysis (BIA), in contrast, is a bedside technique that can be applied to pediatric patients without exposure to radiation and with ease. Electrical current is conducted by body water and is impeded by other body components. BIA estimates the volumes of body compartments, including extracellular water, and total body water (TBW). TBW measures can be used to estimate lean body mass by applying age-appropriate hydration factors.[77] BIA has not been validated in critically ill populations; hence, its use outside clinical studies is not recommended in the PICU. The search for an ideal bedside body composition measurement technique in critically ill patient continues, and some of these promising new methods require validation.

Biochemical Assessment

Nutritional status can also be assessed by measuring the visceral (or constitutive) protein pool, the acute-phase protein pool, nitrogen balance, and REE. Albumin, which has a large pool and much longer half-life (14–20 days), is not indicative of the immediate nutritional status and may be skewed by changes in fluid status. Serum albumin concentration may be affected by albumin infusion, dehydration, sepsis, trauma, and liver disease, and it is independent of nutritional status. Thus, its reliability as a marker of visceral protein status is questionable. Prealbumin, (also known as transthyretin or thyroxine-binding prealbumin) is a stable circulating glycoprotein synthesized in the liver. It binds with retinol-binding protein and is involved in the transport of thyroxine and retinol. Prealbumin, so named by its proximity to albumin on an electrophoretic strip, has a half-life of 24 to 48 hours and reflects more acute nutritional changes. Prealbumin concentration is diminished in liver disease. Prealbumin is readily measured in most hospitals and is a good marker for the visceral protein pool.[78,79] In children with burn injury, serum acute-phase protein levels increase within 12 to 24 hours of the stress because of hepatic reprioritization of protein synthesis in response to injury.[80] The increase is proportional to the severity of injury. Many hospitals are capable of measuring C-reactive protein (CRP) as an index of the acute-phase response. When measured serially, serum prealbumin and CRP are inversely related (ie, serum prealbumin levels decrease and CRP levels increase with the magnitude proportional to injury severity and then return to normal as the acute injury response resolves). In infants after surgery, decreases in serum CRP values to less than 2 mg/dL have been associated with the return of anabolic metabolism and are followed by increases in serum prealbumin levels.[81] Interleukin 6 (IL-6), a proinflammatory cytokine recognized as an early marker of the systemic inflammatory response syndrome (SIRS) in several disease models, might be used to determine whether the inflammatory response is intact. Serum concentrations of IL-6 may be useful in identifying patients at risk for nutritional deterioration.

MICRONUTRIENT DEFICIENCY IN CRITICALLY ILL CHILDREN

The antioxidant properties of certain micronutrients have renewed interest in their role during critical illness. Vitamins C and E have important antioxidant properties. Selenium has also been shown to be a critical micronutrient with antioxidant functions in patients with thermal injury and trauma.[82] A complex system of special enzymes, their cofactors (selenium, zinc, iron, and manganese), sulfhydryl group donors (glutathione), and vitamins (E and C) form a defense system to counter the oxidant stress seen in the acute phase of injury or illness. Critically ill patients may have variable deficiencies of micronutrients in the early phase of illness. Vitamins and trace elements are redistributed from central circulation to tissues and organs during SIRS.[83,84] Levels of trace elements, such as iron, selenium, and zinc, and water-soluble vitamins are decreased, whereas copper and manganese levels may be increased.[84,85] In addition, trauma and thermal injuries are characterized by extensive losses of biologic fluids through wound exudates, drains, and hemorrhage, which cause negative micronutrient balances. The reduced stores of these enzyme cofactors, vitamins, and trace elements decrease rapidly after injury and remain at subnormal levels for weeks. Low endogenous stores of antioxidants are associated with an increase in free radical generation, augmented systemic inflammatory response, cell injury, and increased morbidity and mortality in the critically ill.[86,87] Recently, there has been increased interest in the role of vitamin D as an antioxidant. Serum levels of vitamin D are decreased in children with severe burns.[88] Vitamin D status may be compromised for months after burn injury. The concept of early micronutrient supplementation to prevent the development of acute deficiency, to rectify the oxidant-antioxidant balance, and to reduce oxidative-mediated injuries to organs has driven recent trials in critically ill patients.[89]

Antioxidant research in the critically ill has focused on copper, selenium, zinc, vitamins C and E, and the vitamin B group.[89] Most of these studies were performed in relatively small patient populations presenting with heterogeneous diseases, such as trauma, burns, sepsis, or acute respiratory distress syndrome, however, and thus are underpowered to detect a treatment effect on clinically important outcomes. Heyland and colleagues[82] performed a systematic review of trials supplementing critically ill patients with antioxidants, trace elements, and vitamins with an aim to improve survival. These researchers concluded that trace elements and vitamins that support antioxidant function, particularly high-dose parenteral selenium alone or in combination with other antioxidants, are reportedly safe and may be associated with a reduction in mortality in critically ill patients.

Electrolyte management in critically ill children can be complicated because of existing deficiencies, fluid shifts, increased insensible losses, drainage of bodily secretions, and renal failure. Intravenous fluids or PN prescriptions need to be reviewed daily in light of the basic electrolytes (Na^+, K^+, Cl^-, HCO_3^-, and Ca^{2+}) and blood sugar levels. In children with significant gastrointestinal fluid loss (gastric, pancreatic, small intestinal, or bile), the actual measurement of electrolytes from the drained fluid may assist in prescribing replacement fluids. Acute changes in serum electrolytes that require urgent electrolyte replacement must not be managed by changes in the PN infusion rate or composition, because this method may be imprecise and potentially dangerous. Phosphate and magnesium levels are often abnormal in critically ill children, especially in those with existing nutritional deficiencies, sepsis, or ongoing deprivation of EN. Hypophosphatemia may be associated with hemolytic anemia, respiratory muscle dysfunction, and cardiac failure. A significant decrease in serum phosphate also may be seen with the refeeding syndrome. In contrast, children with renal insufficiency may present with increased serum levels of phosphate and potassium. Deficiency of magnesium can cause fatal cardiac arrhythmia in children and adults alike. Abnormalities of acid-base physiology also can influence the nutritional regimen of the hospitalized child. If metabolic alkalosis from active diuresis or gastric suction occurs, chloride (Cl⁻) administration should be used to correct the alkalosis. Severe, untreated alkalemia may inhibit the patient's respiratory drive, shift potassium intracellularly, decrease ionized calcium concentrations by increasing the affinity of albumin for calcium, and promote refractory cardiac arrhythmias. Metabolic acidosis is often seen in critically ill children and may be associated with hypotension, ischemia, or renal failure. In this case, the provision of supplemental acetate in the PN regimen may be of use.[90]

PREVENTION OF NUTRITIONAL DETERIORATION DURING CRITICAL ILLNESS

The first step in improving the nutritional status of critically ill children is to acknowledge the magnitude of the problem. Description of the epidemiology of malnutrition requires accurate and regular monitoring of nutritional parameters in hospitalized children. Despite the association between malnutrition in hospitalized patients and poorer outcomes, less than half of the patients actually have their nutritional assessment recorded in their notes and fewer are referred for specialized nutritional consultation.[91] In many of these cases, simple interventions may halt or reverse nutritional deterioration. The recently revised ASPEN guidelines recommend nutritional screening of all children admitted to the PICU to identify those with existing nutritional deficiencies and those who are at risk for further deterioration (see **Table 1**).[92]

The Joint Commission for Accreditation of Healthcare Organizations (JCAHO) guidelines describe the importance of nutritional screening in children admitted to the hospital to identify those at high risk for nutritional deterioration.[93] Nutritional screening procedures must be established and implemented in all PICUs. Objective data, such as height, weight, change in weight, and estimation of nutritional requirements, must be recorded in patients within 24 hours of admission to the PICU. A single nutritional assessment may fail to detect dynamic changes during the course of acute illness.[94] Serial nutritional assessments may allow early detection of nutritional deficiencies and ensure the adequacy of nutritional therapy in critically ill children. With dedicated staff and newer technology, basic anthropometry can be safely recorded in critically ill children. A dedicated NST has become an integral part of the multidisciplinary critical care team at many centers. The availability of such a team may be of great assistance in the nutritional screening, assessment, and follow-up of children admitted to the PICU. Dedicated nutritionists or dieticians may perform the comprehensive nutritional assessment after PICU admission, identify high-risk children, plan nutrient intake based on accurate estimation or measurement of energy expenditure, and plan the method of nutrient delivery along with the health care team. The implementation of a dedicated NST has been associated with increased use of EN, decreased reliance on PN, and improved patient outcomes in the PICU.[66] In the absence of evidence for many feeding practices in the PICU, feeding protocols and guidelines based on consensus and adult literature have been implemented in many centers. Protocolized and aggressive feeding strategies have yet to be shown to improve outcomes in critically ill children. In a recent cluster randomized controlled trial in the adult critical care population, evidence-based feeding guidelines were successfully incorporated, including specific nutritional support strategies, using educational interventions.[95] Intensive care units in the intervention group, adhering to the guidelines, achieved early EN (0.75 days vs 1.37 days from admission) compared with the control group, with a marginal increase in caloric adequacy. There were no statistical differences between the groups for clinical outcomes, such as mortality, or hospital and intensive care unit length of stay.

Variable energy requirements and the inaccuracies of commonly used equations for estimating energy expenditure are factors that predispose critically ill children to the risk for underfeeding or overfeeding.[43,96] IC allows accurate measurement of energy expenditure under steady-state conditions and can be used for nutritional assessment in critically ill children.[97,98] **Fig. 4** illustrates IC results during two time periods in a child with hypoxic brain injury who experienced severe unexplained weight loss in the PICU.[47] Steady-state data from time point 1 (first shaded box) show severe hypermetabolism with energy demands far in excess for energy provision.

With the help of a dedicated NST, the authors have successfully used IC in selected patients in the PICU, in whom it has allowed early detection of underfeeding and overfeeding.[24,47] Nutritional intake based on the results of IC in such patients may prevent cumulative caloric imbalances. Cumulative caloric and protein imbalances accumulate over the course of critical illness and are associated with poor anthropometric and clinical outcomes in pediatric and adult populations.[10,99] Currently, the use of IC is sporadic, and its cost-effectiveness and impact on patient outcomes need to be described.[50]

Finally, individualized nutritional regimens aimed at minimizing protein accretion and to meet the energy requirement remain the ultimate goal of nutritional therapy for children in the PICU. Using a multidisciplinary nutrition team comprising a dietician and a pharmacist, judicious use of institutional feeding guidelines, based on consensus and evidence, should allow safe nutrient delivery in the critically ill child. Electrolyte and micronutrient deficiencies must be identified and corrected using an institutional care plan for monitoring.[38] Individual centers must audit their nutritional practices and evaluate the ability to reach nutritional goals, examine local deficiencies in practice, and implement practice change when required.

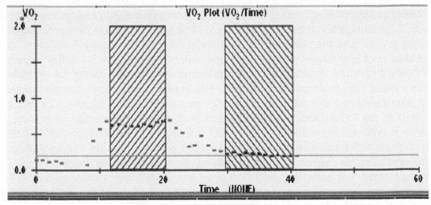

Fig. 4. Graphic plot of VO_2 in liters per minute over time. Steady-state periods are shown as shaded boxes. (*Adapted from* Mehta NM, Bechard LJ, Leavitt K, et al. Severe weight loss and hypermetabolic paroxysmal dysautonomia following hypoxic ischemic brain injury: the role of indirect calorimetry in the intensive care unit. JPEN J Parenter Enteral Nutr 2008;32(3):281–4; with permission.)

SUMMARY

Malnutrition is prevalent in children admitted to the PICU, and their nutritional status may further deteriorate during the course of critical illness. Assessment of nutritional status on admission to the PICU allows identification of those children at high risk for further nutritional deterioration. A basic understanding of the metabolic stress response and accurate assessment of energy expenditure are essential for designing individually tailored nutritional prescriptions for critically ill children. Individualized nutritional regimens may prevent underfeeding and overfeeding in the PICU and have a positive impact on outcomes from critical illness. Hospital-acquired malnutrition may be avoidable in some cases, and individual institutions need to address it by means of multidisciplinary efforts. Accurate measurement of energy expenditure, availability of an NST, use of nutritional therapy guidelines, and protocolized assessment of nutritional parameters at admission and regularly during the PICU course are some steps to improve the nutritional state of children admitted to the PICU.

REFERENCES

1. Butterworth CE Jr. Malnutrition in the hospital [editorial]. JAMA 1974;230(6):879.
2. Bistrian BR, Blackburn GL, Vitale J, et al. Prevalence of malnutrition in general medical patients. JAMA 1976;235(15):1567–70.
3. Merritt RJ, Suskind RM. Nutritional survey of hospitalized pediatric patients. Am J Clin Nutr 1979;32(6):1320–5.
4. Chima CS, Barco K, Dewitt ML, et al. Relationship of nutritional status to length of stay, hospital costs, and discharge status of patients hospitalized in the medicine service. J Am Diet Assoc 1997;97(9):975–8 [quiz: 979–80].
5. Correia MI, Waitzberg DL. The impact of malnutrition on morbidity, mortality, length of hospital stay and costs evaluated through a multivariate model analysis. Clin Nutr 2003;22(3):235–9.
6. Pollack MM, Ruttimann UE, Wiley JS. Nutritional depletions in critically ill children: associations with physiologic instability and increased quantity of care. JPEN J Parenter Enteral Nutr 1985;9(3):309–13.
7. Leite HP, Isatugo MK, Sawaki L, et al. Anthropometric nutritional assessment of critically ill hospitalized children. Rev Paul Med 1993;111(1):309–13.
8. Hulst J, Joosten K, Zimmermann L, et al. Malnutrition in critically ill children: from admission to 6 months after discharge. Clin Nutr 2004;23(2):223–32.
9. Pollack MM, Wiley JS, Kanter R, et al. Malnutrition in critically ill infants and children. JPEN J Parenter Enteral Nutr 1982;6(1):20–4.
10. Hulst JM, van Goudoever JB, Zimmermann LJ, et al. The effect of cumulative energy and protein deficiency on anthropometric parameters in a pediatric ICU population. Clin Nutr 2004;23(6):1381–9.
11. McWhirter JP, Pennington CR. Incidence and recognition of malnutrition in hospital. BMJ 1994;308(6934):945–8.
12. Jeejeebhoy KN. Nutritional assessment. Nutrition 2000;16(7-8):585–90.
13. Hendricks KM, Duggan C, Gallagher L, et al. Malnutrition in hospitalized pediatric patients. Current prevalence. Arch Pediatr Adolesc Med 1995;149(10):1118–22.
14. Reilly JJ, Weir J, McColl JH, et al. Prevalence of protein-energy malnutrition at diagnosis in children with acute lymphoblastic leukemia. J Pediatr Gastroenterol Nutr 1999;29(2):194–7.
15. Cameron JW, Rosenthal A, Olson AD. Malnutrition in hospitalized children with congenital heart disease. Arch Pediatr Adolesc Med 1995;149(10):1098–102.

16. Barton JS, Hindmarsh PC, Scrimgeour CM, et al. Energy expenditure in congenital heart disease. Arch Dis Child 1994;70(1):5–9.

17. Forchielli ML, McColl R, Walker WA, et al. Children with congenital heart disease: a nutrition challenge. Nutr Rev 1994;52(10):348–53.

18. Norris MK, Hill CS. Nutritional issues in infants and children with congenital heart disease. Crit Care Nurs Clin North Am 1994;6(1):153–63.

19. Schwarz SM, Gewitz MH, See CC, et al. Enteral nutrition in infants with congenital heart disease and growth failure. Pediatrics 1990;86(3):368–73.

20. Kelleher DK, Laussen P, Teixeira-Pinto A, et al. Growth and correlates of nutritional status among infants with hypoplastic left heart syndrome (HLHS) after stage 1 Norwood procedure. Nutrition 2006;22(3):237–44.

21. Hart DW, Wolf SE, Mlcak R, et al. Persistence of muscle catabolism after severe burn. Surgery 2000;128(2):312–9.

22. Rutan RL, Herndon DN. Growth delay in postburn pediatric patients. Arch Surg 1990;125(3):392–5.

23. Flegal KM, Troiano RP. Changes in the distribution of body mass index of adults and children in the US population. Int J Obes Relat Metab Disord 2000;24(7): 807–18.

24. Mehta NM, Bechard LJ, Leavitt K, et al. Cumulative energy imbalance in the pediatric intensive care unit: role of targeted indirect calorimetry. JPEN J Parenter Enteral Nutr 2009;33(3):336–44.

25. de Groof F, Joosten KF, Janssen JA, et al. Acute stress response in children with meningococcal sepsis: important differences in the growth hormone/insulin-like growth factor I axis between nonsurvivors and survivors. J Clin Endocrinol Metab 2002;87(7):3118–24.

26. Mehta N, Jaksic T. The critically ill child. In: Duggan C, Watkins JB, Walker WA, editors. Nutrition in pediatrics. 4th edition. Hamilton (ON): BC Decker Inc; 2008. p. 663–73.

27. Munro HN. Nutrition and muscle protein metabolism: introduction. Fed Proc 1978; 37(9):2281–2.

28. Whyte RK, Haslam R, Vlainic C, et al. Energy balance and nitrogen balance in growing low birthweight infants fed human milk or formula. Pediatr Res 1983; 17(11):891–8.

29. Long CL, Kinney JM, Geiger JW. Nonsuppressability of gluconeogenesis by glucose in septic patients. Metabolism 1976;25(2):193–201.

30. Coss-Bu JA, Klish WJ, Walding D, et al. Energy metabolism, nitrogen balance, and substrate utilization in critically ill children. Am J Clin Nutr 2001;74(5): 664–9.

31. Friedman Z, Danon A, Stahlman MT, et al. Rapid onset of essential fatty acid deficiency in the newborn. Pediatrics 1976;58(5):640–9.

32. Paulsrud JR, Pensler L, Whitten CF, et al. Essential fatty acid deficiency in infants induced by fat-free intravenous feeding. Am J Clin Nutr 1972;25(9):897–904.

33. Giovannini M, Riva E, Agostoni C. Fatty acids in pediatric nutrition. Pediatr Clin North Am 1995;42(4):861–77.

34. Coss-Bu JA, Jefferson LS, Walding D, et al. Resting energy expenditure and nitrogen balance in critically ill pediatric patients on mechanical ventilation. Nutrition 1998;14(9):649–52.

35. Suman OE, Mlcak RP, Chinkes DL, et al. Resting energy expenditure in severely burned children: analysis of agreement between indirect calorimetry and prediction equations using the Bland-Altman method. Burns 2006;32(3):335–42.

36. Briassoulis G, Filippou O, Hatzi E, et al. Early enteral administration of immunonutrition in critically ill children: results of a blinded randomized controlled clinical trial. Nutrition 2005;21(7–8):799–807.
37. Goran MI, Kaskoun M, Johnson R. Determinants of resting energy expenditure in young children. J Pediatr 1994;125(3):362–7.
38. Guidelines for the use of parenteral and enteral nutrition in adult and pediatric patients. JPEN J Parenter Enteral Nutr 2002;26(Suppl 1):1SA–138SA.
39. Askanazi J, Rosenbaum SH, Hyman AI, et al. Respiratory changes induced by the large glucose loads of total parenteral nutrition. JAMA 1980;243(14):1444–7.
40. Grohskopf LA, Sinkowitz-Cochran RL, Garrett DO, et al. A national point-prevalence survey of pediatric intensive care unit-acquired infections in the United States. J Pediatr 2002;140(4):432–8.
41. MacIntyre NR, Cook DJ, Ely EW Jr, et al. Evidence-based guidelines for weaning and discontinuing ventilatory support: a collective task force facilitated by the American College of Chest Physicians; the American Association for Respiratory Care; and the American College of Critical Care Medicine. Chest 2001;120 (Suppl 6):375S–95S.
42. Framson CM, LeLeiko NS, Dallal GE, et al. Energy expenditure in critically ill children. Pediatr Crit Care Med 2007;8(3):264–7.
43. Hardy CM, Dwyer J, Snelling LK, et al. Pitfalls in predicting resting energy requirements in critically ill children: a comparison of predictive methods to indirect calorimetry. Nutr Clin Pract 2002;17(3):182–9.
44. Derumeaux-Burel H, Meyer M, Morin L, et al. Prediction of resting energy expenditure in a large population of obese children. Am J Clin Nutr 2004;80(6):1544–5.
45. White MS, Shepherd RW, McEniery JA. Energy expenditure in 100 ventilated, critically ill children: improving the accuracy of predictive equations. Crit Care Med 2000;28(7):2307–12.
46. Vazquez Martinez JL, Martinez-Romillo PD, Diez Sebastian J, et al. Predicted versus measured energy expenditure by continuous, online indirect calorimetry in ventilated, critically ill children during the early postinjury period. Pediatr Crit Care Med 2004;5(1):19–27.
47. Mehta NM, Bechard LJ, Leavitt K, et al. Severe weight loss and hypermetabolic paroxysmal dysautonomia following hypoxic ischemic brain injury: the role of indirect calorimetry in the intensive care unit. JPEN J Parenter Enteral Nutr 2008;32(3):281–4.
48. McClave SA, Lowen CC, Kleber MJ, et al. Clinical use of the respiratory quotient obtained from indirect calorimetry. JPEN J Parenter Enteral Nutr 2003;27(1):21–6.
49. Guenst JM, Nelson LD. Predictors of total parenteral nutrition-induced lipogenesis. Chest 1994;105(2):553–9.
50. Van der Kuip M, Oosterveld MJ, van Bokhorst-de van der Schueren MA, et al. Nutritional support in 111 pediatric intensive care units: a European survey. Intensive Care Med 2004;30(9):1807–13.
51. Adam SK, Webb AR. Attitudes to the delivery of enteral nutritional support to patients in British intensive care units. Clin Intensive Care 1990;1(4):150–6.
52. Rogers EJ, Gilbertson HR, Heine RG, et al. Barriers to adequate nutrition in critically ill children. Nutrition 2003;19(10):865–8.
53. de Neef M, Geukers VG, Dral A, et al. Nutritional goals, prescription and delivery in a pediatric intensive care unit. Clin Nutr 2008;27(1):65–71.

54. Taylor RM, Preedy VR, Baker AJ, et al. Nutritional support in critically ill children. Clin Nutr 2003;22(4):365–9.
55. Hulst JM, Joosten KF, Tibboel D, et al. Causes and consequences of inadequate substrate supply to pediatric ICU patients. Curr Opin Clin Nutr Metab Care 2006; 9(3):297–303.
56. Moore FA, Moore EE, Haenel JB. Clinical benefits of early post-injury enteral feeding. Clin Intensive Care 1995;6(1):21–7.
57. Hamaoui E, Lefkowitz R, Olender L, et al. Enteral nutrition in the early postoperative period: a new semi-elemental formula versus total parenteral nutrition. JPEN J Parenter Enteral Nutr 1990;14(5):501–7.
58. Moore FA, Feliciano DV, Andrassy RJ, et al. Early enteral feeding, compared with parenteral, reduces postoperative septic complications. The results of a meta-analysis. Ann Surg 1992;216(2):172–83.
59. Chellis MJ, Sanders SV, Webster H, et al. Early enteral feeding in the pediatric intensive care unit. JPEN J Parenter Enteral Nutr 1996;20(1):71–3.
60. Adam S, Batson S. A study of problems associated with the delivery of enteral feed in critically ill patients in five ICUs in the UK. Intensive Care Med 1997; 23(3):261–6.
61. Mehta NM, Hamilton S, McAleer D, et al. Challenges to enteral nutrient delivery in the critically ill child. JPEN J Parenter Enteral Nutr 2009, in press.
62. Heyland DK, Dhaliwal R, Day A, et al. Validation of the Canadian clinical practice guidelines for nutrition support in mechanically ventilated, critically ill adult patients: results of a prospective observational study. Crit Care Med 2004; 32(11):2260–6.
63. Heyland DK, Dhaliwal R, Drover JW, et al. Canadian clinical practice guidelines for nutrition support in mechanically ventilated, critically ill adult patients. JPEN J Parenter Enteral Nutr 2003;27(5):355–73.
64. Jain MK, Heyland D, Dhaliwal R, et al. Dissemination of the Canadian clinical practice guidelines for nutrition support: results of a cluster randomized controlled trial. Crit Care Med 2006;34(9):2362–9.
65. Martin CM, Doig GS, Heyland DK, et al. Multicentre, cluster-randomized clinical trial of algorithms for critical-care enteral and parenteral therapy (ACCEPT). CMAJ 2004;170(2):197–204.
66. Gurgueira GL, Leite HP, Taddei JA, et al. Outcomes in a pediatric intensive care unit before and after the implementation of a nutrition support team. JPEN J Parenter Enteral Nutr 2005;29(3):176–85.
67. Lambe C, Hubert P, Jouvet P, et al. A nutritional support team in the pediatric intensive care unit: changes and factors impeding appropriate nutrition. Clin Nutr 2007;26(3):355–63.
68. Petrillo-Albarano T, Pettignano R, Asfaw M, et al. Use of a feeding protocol to improve nutritional support through early, aggressive, enteral nutrition in the pediatric intensive care unit. Pediatr Crit Care Med 2006;7(4):340–4.
69. Brambilla P, Rolland-Cachera MF, Testolin C, et al. Lean mass of children in various nutritional states. Comparison between dual-energy X-ray absorptiometry and anthropometry. Ann N Y Acad Sci 2000;904:433–6.
70. Sood M, Adams JE, Mughal MZ. Lean body mass in children with cystic fibrosis [letter]. Arch Dis Child 2003;88(9):836.
71. Streat SJ, Beddoe AH, Hill GL. Aggressive nutritional support does not prevent protein loss despite fat gain in septic intensive care patients. J Trauma 1987; 27(3):262–6.

72. Cohn SH, Ellis KJ, Wallach S. In vivo neutron activation analysis. Clinical potential in body composition studies. Am J Med 1974;57(5):683–6.
73. Johnson J, Dawson-Hughes B. Precision and stability of dual-energy X-ray absorptiometry measurements. Calcif Tissue Int 1991;49(3):174–8.
74. Krzywicki HJ, Ward GM, Rahman DP, et al. A comparison of methods for estimating human body composition. Am J Clin Nutr 1974;27(12):1380–5.
75. Talso PJ, Miller CE, Carballo AJ, et al. Exchangeable potassium as a parameter of body composition. Metabolism 1960;9:456–71.
76. Elberg J, McDuffie JR, Sebring NG, et al. Comparison of methods to assess change in children's body composition. Am J Clin Nutr 2004;80(1):64–9.
77. Prior BM, Cureton KJ, Modlesky CM, et al. In vivo validation of whole body composition estimates from dual-energy X-ray absorptiometry. J Appl Physiol 1997;83(2):623–30.
78. Robinson MK, Trujillo EB, Mogensen KM, et al. Improving nutritional screening of hospitalized patients: the role of prealbumin. JPEN J Parenter Enteral Nutr 2003; 27(6):389–95 [quiz: 439].
79. Measurement of visceral protein status in assessing protein and energy malnutrition: standard of care. Prealbumin in Nutritional Care Consensus Group. Nutrition 1995;11(2):169–71.
80. Dickson PW, Bannister D, Schreiber G. Minor burns lead to major changes in synthesis rates of plasma proteins in the liver. J Trauma 1987;27(3):283–6.
81. Letton RW, Chwals WJ, Jamie A, et al. Early postoperative alterations in infant energy use increase the risk of overfeeding. J Pediatr Surg 1995;30(7):988–92 [discussion: 992–3].
82. Heyland DK, Dhaliwal R, Suchner U, et al. Antioxidant nutrients: a systematic review of trace elements and vitamins in the critically ill patient. Intensive Care Med 2005;31(3):327–37.
83. Galloway P, McMillan DC, Sattar N. Effect of the inflammatory response on trace element and vitamin status. Ann Clin Biochem 2000;37(Pt 3):289–97.
84. Maehira F, Luyo GA, Miyagi I, et al. Alterations of serum selenium concentrations in the acute phase of pathological conditions. Clin Chim Acta 2002;316(1–2): 137–46.
85. Gaetke LM, McClain CJ, Talwalkar RT, et al. Effects of endotoxin on zinc metabolism in human volunteers. Am J Physiol Endocrinol Metab 1997;272:E952–6.
86. Goode HF, Cowley HC, Walker BE, et al. Decreased antioxidant status and increased lipid peroxidation in patients with septic shock and secondary organ dysfunction. Crit Care Med 1995;23(4):646–51.
87. Metnitz PG, Bartens C, Fischer M, et al. Antioxidant status in patients with acute respiratory distress syndrome. Intensive Care Med 1999;25(2):180–5.
88. Gottschlich MM, Mayes T, Khoury J, et al. Hypovitaminosis D in acutely injured pediatric burn patients. J Am Diet Assoc 2004;104(6):931–41 [quiz: 1031].
89. Berger MM. Antioxidant micronutrients in major trauma and burns: evidence and practice. Nutr Clin Pract 2006;21(5):438–49.
90. Peters O, Ryan S, Matthew L, et al. Randomised controlled trial of acetate in preterm neonates receiving parenteral nutrition. Arch Dis Child Fetal Neonatal Ed 1997;77(1):F12–5.
91. McWhirter JP, Hill K, Richards J, et al. The use, efficacy and monitoring of artificial nutritional support in a teaching hospital. Scott Med J 1995;40(6):179–83.
92. Mehta NM, Compher C. A.s.p.e.N. clinical guidelines: nutrition support of the critically ill child. JPEN J Parenter Enteral Nutr 2009;33(3):260–76.

93. Joint Commission for Accreditation of Healthcare Organizations: comprehensive accreditation manual for hospitals. Oakbrook Terrace (IL) 2000. Available at: http://www.jcrinc.com/Accreditation-Manuals/2009-CAMH-OFFICIAL-HANDBOOK/ 1377/.
94. Baxter JP. Problems of nutritional assessment in the acute setting. Proc Nutr Soc 1999;58(1):39–46.
95. Doig GS, Simpson F, Finfer S, et al. Effect of evidence-based feeding guidelines on mortality of critically ill adults: a cluster randomized controlled trial. JAMA 2008;300(23):2731–41.
96. Reid CL. Nutritional requirements of surgical and critically-ill patients: do we really know what they need? Proc Nutr Soc 2004;63(3):467–72.
97. Lafeber HN. The art of using indirect calorimetry for nutritional assessment of sick infants and children. Nutrition 2005;21(2):280–1.
98. van der Kuip M, de Meer K, Oosterveld MJ, et al. Simple and accurate assessment of energy expenditure in ventilated paediatric intensive care patients. Clin Nutr 2004;23(4):657–63.
99. Bartlett RH, Dechert RE, Mault JR, et al. Measurement of metabolism in multiple organ failure. Surgery 1982;92(4):771–9.

Optimizing Nutritional Management in Children with Chronic Liver Disease

Scott Nightingale, BMed (Hons), FRACP[a,b], Vicky Lee Ng, MD, FRCP[a,b,c],*

KEYWORDS

- Malnutrition • Chronic liver disease • Biliary atresia
- Cirrhosis • Growth failure

The liver plays a central role in energy and nutrient metabolism. Liver disease results in complex pathophysiologic disturbances affecting nutrient digestion, absorption, distribution, storage, and use. In children, chronic liver disease (CLD) is most commonly cholestatic in nature and include such conditions as biliary atresia, α_1-antitrypsin deficiency, Alagille syndrome, and progressive familial intrahepatic cholestasis (**Box 1**). Malnutrition in children with CLD is often underrecognized, because the clinical assessment of nutritional status with such parameters as weight-for-age, height-for-age, and weight-for-height percentiles frequently overestimates nutritional adequacy. High energy and growth requirements make infants and children with CLD particularly vulnerable to the debilitating effects of malnutrition. For those patients with end-stage liver disease awaiting liver transplantation (LT), malnutrition is associated with poorer outcomes, including increased risks for pre- and post-LT morbidity and mortality,[1–3] poorer neurocognitive development,[4,5] and growth even after LT.[6]

This article reviews the pathophysiology of malnutrition in pediatric CLD and provides an approach to the assessment, diagnosis, and treatment of the most commonly seen nutritional deficiencies in children with CLD.

This work was supported by a grant from the Eric Burnard Trust, Royal Australasian College of Physicians.

[a] SickKids Transplant Center, Hospital for Sick Children, 555 University Avenue, Toronto, Ontario, Canada M5G 1X8

[b] Division of Gastroenterology, Hepatology, and Nutrition, Hospital for Sick Children, 555 University Avenue, Toronto, Ontario, Canada M5G 1X8

[c] Department of Pediatrics, 555 University Avenue, Toronto, Ontario, Canada M5G 1H4

* Corresponding author. Division of Gastroenterology, Hepatology, and Nutrition, Hospital for Sick Children, 555 University Avenue, Toronto, Ontario, Canada M5G 1X8.

E-mail address: vicky.ng@sickkids.ca (V.L. Ng).

Box 1
More common causes of chronic childhood cholestasis

Obstruction to normal biliary flow

Extrahepatic

  Biliary atresia

  Autoimmune sclerosing cholangitis

  Choledochal cyst

Intrahepatic

  Alagille syndrome

  Cystic fibrosis

  Congenital hepatic fibrosis, Caroli disease

Bile formation and transport

PFIC types 1, 2, and 3

BRIC

Bile acid synthetic defects

Hepatocellular cholestasis

Metabolic conditions

  α_1-Antitrypsin deficiency

  Mitochondrial disorders

  Amino acid metabolism: tyrosinemia

  Carbohydrate metabolism: galactosemia, fructosemia, GSD IV

  Lipid metabolism: Wolman, Niemann-Pick, and Gaucher diseases

Endocrinopathies

  Hypopituitarism

  Hypothyroidism

Acquired

  Infective: TORCH, echovirus, parvovirus B19

  Parenteral nutrition-associated liver disease

  Drugs

Idiopathic

Idiopathic neonatal hepatitis

Abbreviations: BRIC, benign recurrent intrahepatic cholestasis; GSD, glycogen storage disease; PFIC, progressive familial intrahepatic cholestasis; TORCH, toxoplasmosis, other (syphilis), rubella, cytomegalovirus, herpes simplex virus.

PATHOPHYSIOLOGY OF MALNUTRITION IN CHILDHOOD LIVER DISEASE

The development of malnutrition in children with CLD is complex and involves multiple mechanisms, including decreased dietary intake, malabsorption, increased energy expenditure, and disordered substrate use (**Box 2**).

Etiology of Malnutrition in Childhood Chronic Liver Disease

Decreased dietary intake

Children with CLD on ad libitum diets ingest less than the recommended daily energy requirements.[7] Anorexia, altered taste perception, early satiety, nausea, and vomiting

---

Box 2
Mechanisms of malnutrition in childhood liver disease

Decreased dietary intake

- Anorexia
- Altered taste perception, unpalatability of diet
- Early satiety from tense ascites, organomegaly
- Nausea and vomiting due to inflammatory cytokines or medications

Impaired nutrient digestion and absorption

- Reduced luminal bile concentration
- Pancreatic insufficiency as seen in Alagille syndrome or Byler disease
- Congestive enteropathy from portal hypertension
- Small bowel bacterial overgrowth

Increased energy requirements

- Underlying disease process, such as inflammation
- Recovery from major insults, such as variceal hemorrhage, infection, or surgery
- Increased respiratory effort from ascites and organomegaly

Disordered substrate use

- Decreased glycogen stores
- Impaired carbohydrate use and insulin resistance
- Negative protein balance
- Increased fat oxidation

---

are all common symptoms in children with CLD and contribute to insufficient protein and calorie intake. Anorexia is related to altered amino acid metabolism causing elevated plasma tryptophan levels and resultant increased brain serotonergic activity.[8] Zinc or magnesium deficiency may contribute to altered taste perception, which, in addition to the prescription of unpalatable diets, may further exacerbate anorexia and already reduced energy intake. Early satiety results from the mechanical effect of abdominal distention secondary to organomegaly or ascites.[9] Nausea and vomiting may be related to elevated proinflammatory cytokines, in addition to adverse effects of concurrent medications.[10] Intercurrent illness episodes, in addition to iatrogenic fasting, such as for investigations or procedures, also influence a child's ability to ingest adequate calories and nutrients.

Impaired nutrient digestion and absorption

Impaired digestion and absorption of fat in cholestatic CLD results from reduced delivery of bile to the small bowel.[11] Because infants derive a large proportion of total energy from fat sources, the implications of fat malabsorption are particularly significant for those with CLD. Vascular congestion in the gut secondary to portal hypertension can result in an enteropathy that may contribute to nutrient malabsorption.[12] Bacterial overgrowth from a blind loop of gut (eg, Roux-en-Y loop in infants who have biliary atresia and have undergone a Kasai portoenterostomy) can result in bile salt deconjugation,[13] further contributing to fat malabsorption. Fat-soluble vitamin malabsorption is discussed in elsewhere in this article.

Increased energy requirements

In adults with CLD, resting energy expenditure (REE) is increased, even when corrected for lean mass.[14] In children with CLD mainly attributable to biliary atresia, REE was reported to be around 30% higher than normal.[15,16] This increased energy expenditure may be related to disordered metabolism leading to inefficient energy use; disease-specific variables, such as inflammation; and complications of the disease, including episodes of recurrent ascending cholangitis or variceal hemorrhage. REE is also increased by the presence of ascites as a result of increased respiratory effort and "third space" loss of protein.[17]

Disordered substrate use

Interrelated abnormalities of carbohydrate, protein, and fat metabolism occur with CLD, including decreased glycogen stores, negative nitrogen balance, and increased fat oxidation. These factors result in inefficient use of available substrates and depletion of body stores.

Specific Macro- and Micronutrient Abnormalities

Carbohydrates

Children with CLD are at increased risk for fasting hypoglycemia, because the capacity for glycogen storage and gluconeogenesis is reduced as a result of abnormal hepatocyte function and loss of hepatocyte mass.[18] Infants and smaller children are particularly at risk because of lower nutritional reserve. The development of postprandial hyperglycemia and reduced glucose use, despite elevated insulin levels, in cirrhotic patients is postulated to relate to reduced catabolism of insulin by the liver or to portosystemic shunting.[19,20]

Proteins

Disordered carbohydrate metabolism results in increased use of amino acids for gluconeogenesis.[21] The negative nitrogen balance seen in adults with cirrhosis[14] has also been observed in children with biliary atresia.[15] The liver's capacity for plasma protein synthesis is impaired by reduced substrate availability, impaired hepatocyte function, and increased catabolism. This results in hypoalbuminemia, leading to peripheral edema and contributing to ascites. Reduced synthesis of insulin-like growth factor (IGF)-1 and its binding protein IGF-BP3 by the chronically diseased liver results in growth hormone resistance[22,23] and may contribute to the poor growth observed in these children.

Protein catabolism results in an increased load of nitrogenous wastes, chiefly ammonia, which must be converted to urea in the liver for excretion. Dietary protein restriction is often recommended for patients with advanced liver disease in an attempt to prevent the development of clinical hepatic encephalopathy. In children, this empiric recommendation is less appropriate given the increased protein demands for growth. Protein intake of up to 4 g/kg of body weight per day has been shown not to precipitate encephalopathy in children with severe CLD mostly caused by biliary atresia.[24]

The role of branched-chain amino acids (BCAAs) is of particular interest in understanding protein metabolism in CLD. BCAAs comprise three essential amino acids (leucine, isoleucine, and valine) whose metabolism differs from the seven aromatic amino acids (AAAs). BCAAs are predominantly metabolized in skeletal muscle, wherein they are taken up by means of an insulin-dependent mechanism. In contrast, AAAs are metabolized by the liver. Serum BCAA levels have been found to be depressed relative to AAA levels in adults with cirrhosis[25] and children with CLD secondary to biliary atresia.[26] An abnormal AAA/BCAA ratio has been implicated in the etiopathogenesis of hepatic encephalopathy, through promotion of cerebral uptake of AAAs resulting in formation of false neurotransmitters and neurologic dysfunction.[27] Dietary and parenteral BCAA supplementation to treat or prevent hepatic encephalopathy in adults had mixed results.[28] BCAA supplementation can also increase protein synthesis in the liver.[29] A large, double-blind, randomized controlled trial in cirrhotic adults showed an advantage of oral BCAA supplementation in decreasing mortality, progression of liver disease, and hospital admissions, in addition to improving quality of life, although the poor palatability of the BCAA supplement caused a high dropout rate.[30] A meta-analysis (which did not include this study) found no benefits of BCAA supplements in treatment of encephalopathy or in survival when studies with serious methodologic flaws were excluded.[31] A small, crossover, randomized controlled trial (using a BCAA-fortified formula compared with a semielemental formula with the same caloric density) showed improved short-term growth, nutritional state, and nitrogen balance in children with CLD awaiting transplantation.[32]

Fats

There is increased fat oxidation in children with end-stage liver disease in the fed and fasting states compared with controls,[16] which is probably related to reduced carbohydrate availability. The increased lipolysis results in a decrease in fat stores, which may not be easily replenished in the setting of the fat malabsorption that accompanies cholestasis.

Reduced bile delivery to the gut results in impaired fat emulsification, and hence digestion. The products of fat digestion are also poorly absorbed, because bile is also required for micelle formation. In various liver diseases, there may be reduced bile production by inadequately functioning hepatocytes, reduced hepatocyte excretion into the bile canaliculus (as in PFIC), or obstruction to biliary flow (as occurs in biliary atresia). The circulating bile salt pool may be depleted secondary to treatment with binding agents, such as cholestyramine, which is often prescribed for pruritus in cholestatic patients. Pancreatic insufficiency may further exacerbate fat malabsorption in certain cholestatic liver diseases, such as PFIC type I (Byler's disease)[33] and Alagille syndrome.[34]

In the setting of cholestasis, impaired digestion and absorption of long-chain triglycerides (LCTs) are affected more than digestion and absorption of medium-chain triglycerides (MCT), which are more water soluble and are readily absorbed by enterocytes in the absence of micelles.[35] Micelle formation is also important for absorption of essential fatty acids and fat-soluble vitamins (A, D, E, and K). Essential fatty acids (ie, linoleic, linolenic acids), which, by definition, cannot be synthesized by the body and must be sourced from the diet, are most abundant in vegetable oils. The liver uses these essential fatty acids to form long-chain polyunsaturated fatty acids (LCPUFAs). Two important LCPUFAs are arachidonic acid and docosahexanoic acid, which are important for eicosanoid formation, neurologic development, and growth in children.[36–38]

Vitamin A

Vitamin A comprises a group of fat-soluble substances that have the activity of all-trans retinol. These are sourced from the diet as retinyl palmitate found in animal sources (eg, fish oils, liver, dairy products, eggs) or as carotenoids from plants (eg, green leafy vegetables, orange-colored fruit, and vegetables). Vitamin A deficiency occurs in cholestatic CLD, because reduced intraluminal bile limits the hydrolysis of retinyl esters to retinol and the formation of micelles, which assist absorption. Utilization may also be impaired in liver disease, because the liver synthesizes retinol-binding protein (RBP), which transports the vitamin to peripheral tissues. Retinol is required for (1) formation of rhodopsin, a pigment that is essential for normal functioning of rod cells in the retina and dark adaptation, and (2) normal cell differentiation. Chronic vitamin A deficiency may result in night blindness and irreversible damage to the cornea in the form of xerophthalmia and keratomalacia. Its role in immune function has been suggested by the decreased morbidity and mortality in certain forms of diarrheal illness, measles, HIV infection, and malaria observed with vitamin A supplementation in malnourished children.[39] Cirrhotic adults with vitamin A deficiency have been found to have increased circulating endotoxin levels; however, a role for vitamin A in prevention of infections in the setting of CLD is yet to be evaluated.[40] Vitamin A deficiency was present in 69% of children with end-stage liver disease.[7]

Vitamin D

Vitamin D refers to a group of fat-soluble prohormones and their metabolites, the two major forms of which are vitamin D_2 (ergocalciferol) and vitamin D_3 (cholecalciferol). These prohormones must be activated by two stages of hydroxylation: in the liver first (to form 25-hydroxy vitamin D [25-OH D]) and then in the kidney (to form $1\alpha,25$-dihydroxy vitamin D or 24,25-dihydroxy vitamin D). Foods rich in vitamin D include fish oils and fortified dairy products, although adequate amounts can be synthesized in the skin when cholesterol is exposed to sufficient ultraviolet B light. In CLD, vitamin D deficiency can result from decreased ingestion, malabsorption (if cholestatic), impaired hepatic hydroxylation, and decreased sunlight exposure. The vitamin plays an important role in the regulation of calcium and phosphorus, and hence in bone homeostasis. Vitamin D deficiency results in defective bone mineralization, causing rickets in children. Around 25% of children with CLD have low serum 25-OH D levels, 17% have radiologic evidence of rickets, and 11% experience fractures, and bone mineral densitometry is often more than 3 SDs less than the mean.[7,41,42] Infants with chronic cholestasis are particularly affected, with bone mineral content deteriorating markedly over the first 2 years of life.[43] Because human milk has low levels of vitamin D,[44] breastfed infants with liver disease have additional risk for deficiency.

Vitamin E

Vitamin E is the collective name for a group of tocopherols or corresponding tocotrienols that are fat soluble and have important antioxidant properties. Of these, α-tocopherol has been most studied because it has the highest bioavailability. Foods with particularly high levels of vitamin E include nuts, green leafy vegetables, and vegetable oils. Vitamin E deficiency causes neurologic problems because of poor nerve conduction. These include peripheral neuropathy, myopathy, and spinocerebellar dysfunction. Vitamin E deficiency can also result in hemolytic anemia because of oxidative damage to red blood cells. Decreased intraluminal bile concentration results in malabsorption of vitamin E.[45] Between 62% and 75% of children with cholestatic CLD are deficient in vitamin E.[7,46] In the setting of hyperlipidemia, such as may accompany chronic cholestasis, vitamin E may move out of cellular membranes and into circulating lipids, thereby preserving serum levels even when total body levels are low.

Vitamin K

Vitamin K_1 (phylloquinone) is the main dietary source of vitamin K in humans and is found in high concentrations in green leafy vegetables, dairy products, and liver. Small amounts of vitamin K_2 (the menaquinones) are derived from bacterial metabolism within the gut but are not believed to be sufficient in the absence of dietary vitamin K_1. Vitamin K is required for posttranslational carboxylation of glutamic acid residues on coagulation factors II, VII, IX, and X, in addition to proteins C and S within the liver.

Without vitamin K activity, the proteins formed are collectively referred to as PIVKA (proteins induced in vitamin K absence)-II. The abnormal coagulation function manifests as easy bruising or a bleeding diathesis. Other proteins requiring vitamin K-dependent carboxylation include osteocalcin, suggesting a possible link between vitamin K deficiency and bone disease.[47] The body has limited storage capacity for this vitamin; hence, it is one of the earliest to manifest in fat-soluble vitamin deficiency.[48] Around 23% of children with CLD have a coagulopathy caused by vitamin K deficiency.[49]

Water-soluble vitamins
Water-soluble vitamins include a group of B-complex vitamins and vitamin C, which are stored within the body but eliminated in the urine. Because storage is limited, these vitamins must be supplied in the diet regularly. The B-complex group includes thiamine, riboflavin, niacin, pyridoxine, and biotin, which function as cofactors in enzymatic reactions that use energy substrates. Folate (also a B-complex vitamin) is required for nucleotide synthesis, and vitamin B_{12} (cobalamin) assists in folate recycling. Vitamin C (ascorbic acid) is important for wound healing and immune function and assists in iron absorption from the gut. Deficiencies in multiple water-soluble vitamins are well described in studies of adults with mainly alcoholic cirrhosis.[50,51] Although decreased intake and malabsorption secondary to enteropathy may be risk factors for deficiency in children with CLD, the prevalence of deficiencies of these vitamins is not currently known.

Trace elements
Trace elements are minerals and metals required in small quantities to enable the normal functioning of many enzymes within the body. In healthy children eating normal diets, deficiency is rare except for situations of environmental deficiency, such as that found with endemic goitre (iodine) or Keshan disease (selenium). In children with reduced oral intake or abnormal gut function or structure, such as with fat malabsorption, portal hypertension, or atrophic changes associated with protein-calorie malnutrition, potential for deficiency exists. Little is described about trace element deficiency in childhood liver disease.

Calcium and magnesium metabolism is closely related to vitamin D status. Depletion of both occurs in CLD because of reduced vitamin D-stimulated intestinal absorption. Both also become bound to unabsorbed fatty acids (saponification) in the gut, further reducing absorption.

In addition to its requirement for synthesis of hemoglobin, iron seems to have an important role in neurologic development of children.[52] Approximately one third of children with CLD are iron deficient.[7] Iron deficiency occurs because of reduced intake or increased losses from overt or occult gastrointestinal hemorrhage, such as occurs with portal hypertension. Zinc has a wide variety of functions, including assistance with wound healing, immune functions, and growth. Approximately 40% of children with CLD are zinc deficient, which is likely attributable to malabsorption and to increased urinary loss, given that zinc is normally albumin bound.[53] Selenium is required for the function of the enzyme glutathione peroxidase, which is important in protecting cells from oxidative damage. It is found in seafood, liver, and meat products and also in grains from areas with adequate selenium concentrations in the soil. Selenium deficiency can manifest as cardiomyopathy. Low plasma selenium levels have been described in cirrhotic adults[54] and children with end-stage liver disease;[7] however, glutathione peroxidase activity was not measured in these studies. Elevated levels of copper and manganese may occur in cholestatic patients, because these metals are primarily excreted in bile.[55,56] Cholestatic patients receiving total parenteral nutrition are particularly at risk for manganese toxicity, which can cause symptomatic disease from manganese deposition in the basal ganglia.[57,58]

APPROACH TO THE ASSESSMENT OF NUTRITIONAL STATUS IN CHILDREN WITH LIVER DISEASE

Routine nutritional assessment of an infant or child with CLD is a cornerstone of management and should be undertaken at every visit. An approach encompassing a comprehensive history and physical examination, including anthropometry when possible, followed by laboratory testing and specialized investigations as necessary is enhanced by the involvement of a multidisciplinary team (**Table 1**).

History

A thorough clinical history must include a detailed feeding history. For those infants and children taking formula, specific volumes of feed and the type of feed and its concentration (if applicable) are crucial in determining caloric intake. Breast milk, in addition to most standard infant formulas, has a caloric density of 0.67 kcal/mL. Thus, the clinician can readily calculate the caloric contribution of feeds that an infant is receiving. Of course, this becomes more complicated for those taking concentrated or fortified feeds. Nonetheless, a careful feeding history is valuable in identifying deficiencies that can be addressed in management. The clinician should also enquire about the variety of foods ingested by older infants and children, which may identify potential risks for micronutrient deficiency. Parents can usually provide a good history of the child's intake, and a food diary may be of assistance. Maternal dietary restriction (eg, veganism) places the infant at risk for vitamin B_{12} deficiency, and maternal sunlight avoidance (eg, for cultural or religious reasons) may predispose to vitamin D deficiency. Breastfed cholestatic infants, as mentioned previously, are at increased risk for vitamin D and K deficiency. A pediatric dietitian is a valuable resource who can provide a detailed assessment of current intake.

Symptoms of liver disease relevant to nutritional assessment should also be enquired about. These include frequency and approximate volume of vomiting, stool frequency, and steatorrhea. Increasing stool pallor or pruritus suggests worsening cholestasis. The parent or caregiver should also be asked about his or her perception of the child's neurocognitive developmental progress, because a history of increased clumsiness or loss of motor milestones may signify vitamin E or B_{12} deficiency. A history of bruising with minimal trauma or of recurrent or prolonged epistaxis suggests vitamin K deficiency. An older child may describe the night blindness associated with vitamin A deficiency.

A psychosocial history provides useful insights into how the child and family are coping with the child's illness and factors that may be having an impact on compliance with nutritional and other management. Specifically, the family structure, ability to afford medications and specialized formulae or supplements, attitudes toward feeding, child behavioral problems, maternal depression, and current psychosocial stressors within the household are key aspects. Opportunities for assistance or support by various professionals, such as social workers and psychologists, can then be identified.

Physical Examination

A thorough physical examination is indicated not only to monitor for progression of the primary liver disease and the development of complications but to provide possible clues to nutritional deficiencies.

The child's weight, height, and head circumference (if younger than 3 years of age) should be measured and plotted on gender-specific percentile charts at each encounter using standardized techniques. Body weight for age can be misleading in CLD, because organomegaly, ascites, and edema can mask underlying weight loss. Measurement of height for age provides a more reliable indicator of nutritional adequacy over the long term but is not sensitive to short-term changes. On general inspection, the clinician should pay particular attention to muscle bulk (most evident in the gluteal, temporalis, and interosseus muscles) and fat deposits (thigh creases, cheeks, and chest and abdominal wall), which provide a gross impression of protein and fat status. Bowed lower limbs, rachitic rosary, or a persistently open anterior fontanelle signifies vitamin D deficiency. Examination of the skin may reveal signs suggestive of zinc deficiency (periorificial desquamating rash) or essential fatty acid deficiency (generalized dry and desquamating skin). Excessive bruising suggests vitamin K deficiency. The hair may be dull or even falling out with severe protein-energy malnutrition and zinc or essential fatty acid deficiency. Conjunctival and palmar crease pallor suggests anemia, and nail changes, such as koilonychia, suggest iron deficiency. The mouth and oropharynx should be examined for stomatitis or cheilitis (iron, folate, or riboflavin deficiency), for glossitis (vitamin B_{12}, folate, riboflavin, or niacin deficiency), and for dental status (vitamin D or calcium deficiency). The neurologic manifestations of vitamin E deficiency tend to occur in a stepwise fashion: initially, there is a loss of deep tendon reflexes and lower limb weakness, followed by gait ataxia, posterior column dysfunction, and even progression to retinopathy.[59] Thus, assessment of lower limb reflexes should be part of the routine clinical examination.

Anthropometry

As mentioned previously, weight-for-age and weight-for-height measurements in children with CLD can be inaccurate, and these may overestimate nutritional status. Serial height-for-age plots may be less accurate in certain genetic pediatric chronic liver conditions, such as Alagille syndrome, in which short stature is a feature. Despite these limitations, approximately 60% of infants with biliary atresia awaiting LT have height or weight z scores of 2 or less (ie, more than 2 SDs less than the mean).[60] In children with CLD, height z scores are lower than weight z scores.[2] Weight-for-height z scores are often normal.[61]

Serial triceps skinfold thickness and midarm circumference measurements compared with age- and height-matched normal values are used to estimate body fat and muscle bulk, respectively. With malnutrition, these measurements decline before changes in weight or height are apparent.[62] These upper limb measurements are less likely to be influenced by edema than measurements on the trunk or lower limbs. Such anthropometric measurements require experienced personnel (typically, a pediatric dietitian) to achieve reliable results, and may thus not be readily available. In children with CLD, triceps skinfold thickness has been shown to be more sensitive to malnutrition than weight-for-height z scores.[61] Infants with liver disease are more likely than older children to have severe malnutrition, as assessed by several anthropometric indices.[63]

Laboratory and Radiologic Investigations

Directed laboratory investigation can screen for or confirm nutritional deficiencies before they manifest clinically, allowing the clinician to intervene. Laboratory assessment of micronutrient status is particularly important in these children because their micronutrient status does not correlate with overall clinical appearance or with

Table 1
Approach to the assessment of nutritional deficiencies in children with liver disease

Element	Important Aspects	Significance
History	Feeding history	Are adequate calories being ingested?
		Are there any important dietary restrictions?
	Diarrhea, vomiting	Loss of ingested calories or nutrients
	Stool pallor, steatorrhea, pruritus	Worsening cholestasis, fat malabsorption
	Neurodevelopment	Vitamin E, vitamin B_{12} deficiency
	Epistaxis, easy bruising	Vitamin K deficiency
	Night blindness	Vitamin A deficiency
	Bone fractures	Vitamin D deficiency
Examination	Basic measurements: height, weight, HC	Abrupt weight increase may indicate edema or ascites, height and HC for age indicate overall nutritional status
	Reduced muscle bulk	Protein catabolism
	Reduced fat stores	Increased lipolysis, fat malabsorption
	Bowed legs, rachitic rosary, craniotabes, delayed fontanelle closure	Vitamin D deficiency
	Excessive bruising	Vitamin K deficiency
	Skin dryness, peeling	Essential fatty acid, zinc, niacin deficiency
	Alopecia	Protein-energy malnutrition, essential fatty acid or zinc deficiency
	Pallor	Iron, vitamin B_{12}, or folate deficiency; occult gastrointestinal bleeding
	Koilonychia (spooning of nails)	Iron deficiency
	Stomatitis, cheilitis	Iron, folate, riboflavin deficiency
	Glossitis	Vitamin B_{12}, folate, riboflavin, niacin deficiency
	Poor dentition	Vitamin D, calcium deficiency
	Depressed or absent lower limb tendon reflexes	Vitamin E deficiency

Anthropometry	Triceps or subscapular skinfold thickness	Estimates body fat stores
	Middle upper arm circumference	Estimates body protein stores
Laboratory investigations[a]	Glucose	Fasting hypoglycemia, postprandial hyperglycemia
	Albumin, prealbumin	Low levels can signify protein malnutrition
	Serum retinol, RDR	Vitamin A deficiency
	Triene/tetraene ratio	Essential fatty acid deficiency
	Serum 25-OH D, calcium, phosphorus, plain radiographs, bone densitometry (older children)	Vitamin D deficiency and its complications
	Plasma tocopherol and tocopherol/cholesterol ratio	Vitamin E deficiency
	PT, INR	Vitamin K deficiency, if elevated and corrects with parenteral vitamin K administration
	Serum iron, ferritin, transferring saturation	Iron deficiency
	Serum zinc	Zinc deficiency
Specialized testing[b]	DEXA, TBK	Provides accurate body composition analysis
	Indirect calorimetry	Measures REE and provides energy requirements

Abbreviations: HC, head circumference; INR, international normalized ratio; 25-OH D, 25-hydroxy vitamin D; PT, prothrombin time; RDR, retinal dose response.
[a] Many of these need to be interpreted with care in children who have CLD (see text).
[b] Usually restricted to research settings.

anthropometry.[7] Testing should also be used to monitor response to therapy, particularly with fat-soluble vitamins, from which toxicity caused by oversupplementation can occur.

Assessing overall protein-energy nutritional status

Monitoring blood glucose levels is important for detecting hypoglycemia, particularly in small infants and children who are fasting. Serum levels of protein markers synthesized by the liver, such as albumin, prealbumin, and transferrin, are of little value in assessing nutrition in CLD and should not be relied on in isolation. Hypoalbuminemia can also result from hepatic synthetic dysfunction, inflammation, or acute physiologic stress.[64] Serum albumin levels may be artificially elevated if the patient has recently received an albumin transfusion. Depressed serum levels of prealbumin (also known as transthyretin because it binds thyroid hormone, retinol, and RBP) are believed to be a more sensitive marker of early malnutrition, because prealbumin has a much shorter half-life than albumin (around 2 days versus 18–20 days); however, current assays may be imprecise, and normal levels can be found with chronic malnutrition.[65] Because depressed levels also occur with inflammation, C-reactive protein levels are often used to assist in interpretation of prealbumin levels. Transferrin has also been examined as a serum marker for protein malnutrition; however, because it is an acute-phase reactant, it is less reliable. Overall, these drawbacks limit the usefulness of plasma proteins as markers of nutritional status, and they are not recommended.[66]

Essential fatty acid deficiency can be demonstrated by an increased serum triene/tetraene ratio (>0.4). Deficiency is common in adults with end-stage liver disease[67] and was found in one third of children with end-stage liver disease awaiting LT.[7] Thrombocytopenia can occur with essential fatty acid deficiency, although it is more commonly attributable to splenic sequestration secondary to portal hypertension in patients with CLD.

Fat-soluble vitamins

Vitamin A There is no "gold standard" test for vitamin A status. Investigations may include serum retinol, the serum retinol/RBP ratio, the retinol dose response (RDR) test, the liver retinol level, and various ophthalmologic tests (eg, conjunctival impression cytology, tear film break-up time, Schirmer's test, dark field adaptation). Serum retinol level is the most convenient and practical test, although the RDR is believed to be the most reliable.[68,69] The RDR is based on the observation that serum retinol levels increase sharply after an oral or parenteral dose of vitamin A in patients who are deficient in vitamin A. Many of the other tests have not been well studied in children.

Vitamin D Serum levels of 25-OH D are commonly measured, because 25-OH D is the most abundant vitamin D metabolite in the body. Low serum levels of 25-OH D are associated with reduced bone mineral density in children with CLD, but there does not seem to be a linear correlation.[43] Plain radiographs may demonstrate osteopenia or even pathologic fractures. Bone mineral densitometry can quantify osteopenia, although interpretation of results is difficult in young children.[70] Serum calcium and phosphorus levels may be low.

Vitamin E Serum tocopherol levels are widely used as a measure of vitamin E status. A tocopherol/total lipids ratio is more specific, particularly in cholestatic patients, in whom normal serum tocopherol levels may be found, even with clinical evidence of vitamin E deficiency.[71] This is probably because elevated serum lipids draw vitamin E out from cellular membranes in the setting of cholestasis. The tocopherol/

cholesterol ratio (< 2.22 μmol/mmol in deficiency) performs well as a practical alternative, because cholesterol levels are more readily obtainable in most laboratories than total lipid levels.[72]

Vitamin K Vitamin K deficiency can be diagnosed by the improvement in elevated prothrombin time (PT) or international normalized ratio (INR) after a parenteral dose. Vitamin K_1 levels in the serum reflect recent intake and are not indicative of functional deficiency. The PIVKA-II assay is much more sensitive to milder vitamin K deficiency than changes in coagulation studies, although it is not as widely available.[73,74]

Water-soluble vitamins

Measuring plasma levels of water-soluble vitamins has limited value unless a particular deficiency is suspected clinically. The incidence of such deficiencies is low in practice, probably because many infant and supplemental feeds are fortified with these vitamins and also because multivitamin supplements are widely used. The more commonly measured vitamins are vitamin C, folate (measured as red cell folate), and vitamin B_{12}. Vitamin B_{12} levels are indicated for children on long-term proton pump inhibitors and for infants of vegan mothers.

Trace elements

Commonly measured trace elements include serum iron, calcium, magnesium, phosphorus, and zinc. Other elements, such as selenium, copper, manganese, and aluminium, need only be measured when severe dietary restriction is occurring or for those on long-term parenteral nutrition in whom toxicity is suspected.

Other Investigations

Indirect calorimetry, which measures a subject's oxygen consumption, can be used to estimate REE. Individuals with increased REE are consuming caloric reserves rapidly and quickly become protein-energy depleted if they are not maintaining increased energy intake. Indirect calorimetry may be a technically difficult procedure to complete in unwell or uncooperative children and may not be easily available.

Body composition can be predicted to some extent by equations using skinfold thickness measurements, or it can be measured using a variety of specialized methods, such as dual-energy x-ray absorptiometry (DEXA), total body potassium (TBK) measurement, neutron activation analysis, hydrometry, and bioelectric impedance.[75,76] Because DEXA and TBK measurement results are not distorted by edema or ascites and they involve minimal or no radiation, they are more appropriate for use in children with CLD. DEXA is based on the principle that different tissues absorb photons to differing extents. TBK measurement is estimated by detection of the naturally occurring isotope ^{40}K, which translates to body cell mass, because potassium is predominantly found within all body cells except adipocytes. These studies provide detailed information on the relative proportions of various body compartments (eg, fat mass, fat-free mass, body cell mass) and can be used to detect changes associated with early malnutrition, although they are normally used in the realm of research rather than in clinical practice.

NUTRITIONAL MANAGEMENT IN CHILDREN WITH LIVER DISEASE
General Management Issues

Nutritional management must be tailored to the nature and degree of malnutrition of the infant or child with CLD. The goal of early intervention is to prevent or correct deficiencies, improve growth, and, ultimately, reduce morbidity and mortality. Nutritional intervention must attempt to compensate for anorexia, increased energy requirements, malabsorption, and abnormal substrate use.

Current caloric intake needs to be regularly reviewed and compared with the child's needs. Based on weight, estimates of the basal metabolic rate for children can be derived from validated equations or tables,[77,78] which are then modified depending on the activity of the child and any fever, illness, or injuries present. It is important that ideal body weight be used in these calculations (ie, the 50th percentile weight for the child's height). Because of the increased energy expenditure outlined previously, children with CLD require at least 130% of the calories that healthy children do,[15,16] and often much more. It should be emphasized that such calculations are an initial guide only and that re-evaluation of growth parameters is a better guide to the adequacy of energy intake.

A prescribed feeding plan providing specific goal quantities can be devised with the assistance of a dietician. Assistance from a psychologist or social worker may help with behavioral aspects of feeding problems. An infant's formula can be concentrated or fortified with extra carbohydrates or fat. Concentrating formulae (by adding less water) and adding carbohydrates (usually in the form of glucose polymer) increase the osmolality of the feed and may result in diarrhea if not carefully introduced. Added fat should ideally be in the form of MCTs for cholestatic infants, although a mix of LCTs and MCTs may be required to improve palatability. With these measures, the caloric density of infant formula can be increased from 0.67 kcal/mL to more than 1 kcal/mL if required. Specialized MCT-enriched formulae are available, which can also be concentrated or fortified as necessary. For breastfed infants, options include fortifying expressed breast milk as described previously or administering oral MCT oil doses during feeds. Older children can be prescribed calorie-dense nutritional supplements to be taken in addition to their usual diet. These children should be encouraged to consume high-calorie diets and to avoid low-fat varieties unless significant steatorrhea is affecting their quality of life.

The child's inability to ingest the required calories or poor growth warrants insertion of a feeding tube for supplementation with bolus feeds, continuous pump feeds, or both. In the setting of portal hypertension, gastrostomy tubes are best avoided because of the risk for portosystemic varices developing at the site. There is often anxiety among clinicians about inserting nasogastric or nasoenteric feeding tubes in patients with gastroesophageal varices, though available evidence from the literature does not suggest that they increase variceal bleeding,[24,79–81] except, possibly, for those patients who have bled in the preceding days.[82] The European Society for Parenteral and Enteral Nutrition (ESPEN) guidelines explicitly support the use of feeding tubes when necessary in these patients.[83] Particularly when using fine-bore soft tubes, the authors would argue that the risk for harm is greater in allowing the patient to become more malnourished. Nocturnal feeds by means of a pump are often well tolerated, are convenient if the child is managing reasonable intake or can tolerate bolus top-ups during the day, and have been shown to improve nutritional status in children with CLD.[84] For infants and children with severe liver disease whose oral intake is poor and who may not tolerate bolus tube feeds, continuous feeds throughout most of the day improve nutritional status.[24] A continuous source of carbohydrate can also prevent hypoglycemia in end-stage liver disease. Concentrating or increasing the volume of enteral feeds should be done gradually to ensure that the changes are tolerated by a gut that may already be poorly functioning secondary to portal hypertension. It is important to encourage some ongoing oral intake, particularly in infants, to avoid later feeding problems related to poor oromotor skills or oral aversion. Early involvement of a speech or occupational therapist may be warranted.

Some patients with severe liver disease are unable to tolerate sufficient enteral feeds to maintain an adequate nutritional state. In this situation, parenteral nutrition is the only option until LT, if indicated, can occur. The risks for catheter-associated infections and potential for accelerating liver dysfunction[85] are then assumed.

There is evidence that providing tube feeds to malnourished adults with cirrhosis improves clinical status and short-term mortality.[79] Supplemental nocturnal tube feeds have improved anthropometric indices in small trials in children with chronic cholestatic liver disease,[84] without precipitating encephalopathy.[24] The only randomized trial in children was a small trial (n = 19) that showed weight gain in children with end-stage liver disease awaiting LT with supplemental nasogastric feeds of BCAA-containing formula but not a standard formula.[86]

Early referral to a transplant center is important for the appropriate assessment and long-term management of infants and children with CLD. Children are also able to access specialized dietitian services that may not be available at smaller centers.

Management Related to Specific Macronutrients

Carbohydrates
Infants and small children with CLD are at high risk for hypoglycemia, particularly when fasting (eg, for procedures or investigations) or during intercurrent illnesses. In these situations, close blood glucose monitoring should be instituted. Intravenous access may be prudent to allow rapid treatment of serious hypoglycemia in some situations. Given the risk for permanent neurologic sequelae, prevention of severe hypoglycemia is critical in pediatric patients.

Proteins
Children with CLD should not be protein restricted unless encephalopathic. Protein supplementation up to 4 g/kg/d is generally safe and probably necessary given their growth demands and tendency to catabolism. There is insufficient evidence at present to recommend routine dietary BCAA supplementation for children with CLD. BCAA supplementation may be helpful in cases of refractory encephalopathy. Exogenous growth hormone therapy is not beneficial to children with CLD.

Fats
As the most calorie-dense macronutrient, fat is particularly important for children with reduced enteral intake. Although MCT supplementation is central in the nutritional management of children with cholestatic CLD, it is important not to eliminate LCTs from the diet because they provide essential fatty acids and assist in fat-soluble vitamin absorption. Around 30% to 50% of total fat should be provided as MCTs, although compliance can be problematic because of its poor palatability.

Management Related to Specific Micronutrients

Clinical and laboratory assessment of fat-soluble vitamin levels should be undertaken periodically to detect deficiency and to monitor response to any supplementation, because the potential for toxicity of fat-soluble vitamin exists. Toxicity in cholestatic patients is rare using standard doses (**Table 2**), and the doses usually need to be increased. In situations in which oral supplementation at high doses is insufficient, parenteral supplementation is required.

Vitamin A
Monitoring serum levels is most practical, because RDR testing is not widely available. It is particularly important to monitor levels with supplementation, because hypervitaminosis A leads to hepatotoxicity and can potentially be fatal. One should be

Table 2
Nutritional management strategies in childhood liver disease

	Focus	Specific Recommendations
General principles	Regular assessment of nutritional status	Feeding history, examination, growth parameters at each visit; anthropometry when available
	Multidisciplinary involvement	Dietitian for dietary assessment, practical advice for family, and anthropometry
		Social worker or psychologist for assistance with psychosocial aspects or behavioral problems
		Speech therapist, occupational therapist to help manage feeding problems and oral aversion
	Long-term prognosis	Timely referral to a liver transplant center
Macronutrient considerations	Caloric intake	At least 130% of standard requirements initially based on ideal weight, and much more is probably required[15,16]
		May require feed fortification/concentration or supplements for older children
		Early introduction of tube feeding if unable to ingest necessary quantities
		Parenteral nutrition if unable to tolerate required enteral volumes
	Carbohydrate	Monitor for hypoglycemia during fasting, illness, or reduced intake
	Protein	Do not restrict unless encephalopathic; give 2–4 g/kg/d
	Fat	Give 30%–50% of total fat as MCTs in cholestatic patients
Micronutrient supplementation[a]	Vitamin A	5000–25,000 U/d
		Coadminister with TPGS to improve absorption
	Vitamin D	400 IU/d, preferably in 25-OH D$_3$ form
		Monitor calcium, phosphorus, and 25-OH D levels
		Coadminister with TPGS to improve absorption
	Vitamin E	15–25 IU/kg/d, preferably as TPGS
	Vitamin K	2.5–5 mg/d
	Water-soluble vitamins	Multivitamin preparation providing at least 100% of the recommended dietary allowance
	Trace elements	Iron: 6 mg/kg/d in the form of elemental iron, reassess after a month
		Zinc: 1 mg/kg/d

Abbreviations: 25-OH D$_3$, 25-hydroxy vitamin D$_3$.
[a] Fat-soluble vitamin doses provided are for the oral route or administered by means of a feeding tube, as derived from other sources;[87–90] levels of fat-soluble vitamins and trace elements should be used for monitoring response.

especially cautious in pregnant patients or in those who may become pregnant, because oversupplementation has been shown to be teratogenic.

Vitamin D

There is controversy in the adult literature about whether vitamin D supplementation in patients with CLD and osteopenia is beneficial in terms of stopping progression of osteoporosis or reducing fractures.[91] Until more is known, supplementation in children with low 25-OH D levels, known osteopenia, or pathologic fractures seems prudent. An important difference between children and adults is that children are actively trying to accrete bone mass, whereas bone mass normally declines in adults. Optimizing vitamin D, and possibly bone status, before LT is important, because subsequent insults to bone health are likely (eg, corticosteroid use) and recovery of bone status is less likely if the pretransplant condition was poorer or the transplant becomes complicated.[92] Cosupplementation with a micellar vitamin E formulation has been shown to improve vitamin D absorption in children with cholestatic liver disease[93] but did not translate to improved bone mineral density. 25-OH D_3 is more water soluble and better absorbed in cholestatic children than vitamin D_2.[94] Serum levels of 25-hydroxy vitamin D should be monitored in all children with CLD of any etiology, as should response to any therapy. Calcium and phosphorus levels should also be monitored, because elevations may be a sign of overdosing of vitamin D. The clinician should have a high index of suspicion for fractures in cholestatic infants who have unexplained irritability. This should be pursued with radiographs and bone scintigraphy as required.

Vitamin E

The clinician should monitor vitamin E status in children with CLD, particularly those with cholestasis, with a directed neurologic history and examination. Plasma tocopherol or the tocopherol/cholesterol ratio should be used to screen for deficiency in these children and to monitor response to therapy. Absorption of oral vitamin E in cholestatic patients can be improved by using the form d-α-tocopheryl polyethylene glycol 1000 succinate (TPGS), which is amphipathic in structure, and thus can form micelles without the need for bile salts. This has allowed rapid correction of serum vitamin E levels and reversal of neurologic complications.[95] Correction of vitamin E status may not reverse severe spinocerebellar degeneration.[96]

Vitamin K

All cholestatic children should have their vitamin K status monitored, with particular attention to breastfed infants, in whom deficiency can present with catastrophic hemorrhage.[97] When the PIVKA-II assay is unavailable, vitamin K status can be most easily achieved by monitoring coagulation indices, such as PT or INR, and their response to parenteral vitamin K (0.3 mg/kg given intramuscularly or intravenously) if elevated. Oral supplementation can be used; however, absorption is poor. Even a mixed micellar form of phylloquinone (K_1) has been found to be poorly absorbed by cholestatic infants[98]; thus, intermittent parenteral supplementation may be necessary. Other medications may potentially exacerbate vitamin K deficiency; for example, lactulose and neomycin prescribed for encephalopathy may reduce intestinal luminal bacterial production of vitamin K.

Water-soluble vitamins

It is prudent to provide all infants and children who have CLD with a multivitamin preparation to ensure adequate intake of water-soluble vitamins. Although it is not evidence based, the authors recommend that at least the recommended dietary allowance[99] be supplemented initially. The clinician needs to be aware that many available preparations also contain quantities of fat-soluble vitamins.

Trace elements

Iron deficiency should be identified and treated. Given the role in immune function and tissue repair, zinc repletion may also be important for children with CLD, particularly for those requiring imminent LT. Supplementation of low magnesium levels may improve bone status in children with cholestatic CLD.[100]

SUMMARY

Malnutrition is common in children with CLD and may easily be underestimated by clinical appearance alone. Infants with CLD are more at risk than older children for severe malnutrition and have lower reserves. The cause of malnutrition in CLD is multifactorial, although insufficient dietary intake is probably the most important cause and is correctable. Fat malabsorption occurs in cholestatic disorders, and one must also consider any accompanying fat-soluble vitamin and essential fatty acid deficiencies. Breastfed infants with CLD are at high risk for vitamin D and K deficiencies. The clinician should proactively evaluate, treat, and re-evaluate response to treatment of nutritional deficiencies. Because a better nutritional state is associated with better survival before and after LT, aggressive nutritional management is an important part of the care of these children.

REFERENCES

1. Chin SE, Shepherd RW, Cleghorn GJ, et al. Survival, growth and quality of life in children after orthotopic liver transplantation: a 5 year experience. J Paediatr Child Health 1991;27(6):380–5.
2. Shepherd RW, Chin SE, Cleghorn GJ, et al. Malnutrition in children with chronic liver disease accepted for liver transplantation: clinical profile and effect on outcome. J Paediatr Child Health 1991;27(5):295–9.
3. DeRusso PA, Ye W, Shepherd R, et al. Growth failure and outcomes in infants with biliary atresia: a report from the Biliary Atresia Research Consortium. Hepatology 2007;46(5):1632–8.
4. Wayman KI, Cox KL, Esquivel CO. Neurodevelopmental outcome of young children with extrahepatic biliary atresia 1 year after liver transplantation. J Pediatr 1997;131(6):894–8.
5. Stewart SM, Uauy R, Waller DA, et al. Mental and motor development, social competence, and growth one year after successful pediatric liver transplantation. J Pediatr 1989;114(4 Pt 1):574–81.
6. Moukarzel AA, Najm I, Vargas J, et al. Effect of nutritional status on outcome of orthotopic liver transplantation in pediatric patients. Transplant Proc 1990;22(4): 1560–3.
7. Chin SE, Shepherd RW, Thomas BJ, et al. The nature of malnutrition in children with end-stage liver disease awaiting orthotopic liver transplantation. Am J Clin Nutr 1992;56(1):164–8.
8. Laviano A, Cangiano C, Preziosa I, et al. Plasma tryptophan levels and anorexia in liver cirrhosis. Int J Eat Disord 1997;21(2):181–6.
9. Aqel BA, Scolapio JS, Dickson RC, et al. Contribution of ascites to impaired gastric function and nutritional intake in patients with cirrhosis and ascites. Clin Gastroenterol Hepatol 2005;3(11):1095–100.

10. Aranda-Michel J. Nutrition in hepatic failure and liver transplantation. Curr Gastroenterol Rep 2001;3(4):362–70.

11. Dietschy JM. The biology of bile acids. Arch Intern Med 1972;130(4):473–4.

12. Norman K, Pirlich M. Gastrointestinal tract in liver disease: which organ is sick? Curr Opin Clin Nutr Metab Care 2008;11(5):613–9.

13. Yamamoto T, Hamanaka Y, Suzuki T. [Intestinal microflora and bile acids following biliary tract reconstruction]. Nippon Geka Gakkai Zasshi 1991;92(9): 1288–91 [Japanese].

14. Matos C, Porayko MK, Francisco-Ziller N, et al. Nutrition and chronic liver disease. J Clin Gastroenterol 2002;35(5):391–7.

15. Pierro A, Koletzko B, Carnielli V, et al. Resting energy expenditure is increased in infants and children with extrahepatic biliary atresia. J Pediatr Surg 1989;24(6): 534–8.

16. Greer R, Lehnert M, Lewindon P, et al. Body composition and components of energy expenditure in children with end-stage liver disease. J Pediatr Gastroenterol Nutr 2003;36(3):358–63.

17. Dolz C, Raurich JM, Ibanez J, et al. Ascites increases the resting energy expenditure in liver cirrhosis. Gastroenterology 1991;100(3):738–44.

18. Changani KK, Jalan R, Cox IJ, et al. Evidence for altered hepatic gluconeogenesis in patients with cirrhosis using in vivo 31-phosphorus magnetic resonance spectroscopy. Gut 2001;49(4):557–64.

19. Nielsen MF, Caumo A, Aagaard NK, et al. Contribution of defects in glucose uptake to carbohydrate intolerance in liver cirrhosis: assessment during physiological glucose and insulin concentrations. Am J Physiol Gastrointest Liver Physiol 2005; 288(6):G1135–43.

20. Petrides AS, DeFronzo RA. Glucose and insulin metabolism in cirrhosis. J Hepatol 1989;8(1):107–14.

21. Swart GR, van den Berg JW, Wattimena JL, et al. Elevated protein requirements in cirrhosis of the liver investigated by whole body protein turnover studies. Clin Sci (Lond) 1988;75(1):101–7.

22. Bucuvalas JC, Horn JA, Slusher J, et al. Growth hormone insensitivity in children with biliary atresia. J Pediatr Gastroenterol Nutr 1996;23(2):135–40.

23. Holt RI, Miell JP, Jones JS, et al. Nasogastric feeding enhances nutritional status in paediatric liver disease but does not alter circulating levels of IGF-I and IGF binding proteins. Clin Endocrinol (Oxf) 2000;52(2):217–24.

24. Charlton CP, Buchanan E, Holden CE, et al. Intensive enteral feeding in advanced cirrhosis: reversal of malnutrition without precipitation of hepatic encephalopathy. Arch Dis Child 1992;67(5):603–7.

25. Rosen HM, Yoshimura N, Hodgman JM, et al. Plasma amino acid patterns in hepatic encephalopathy of differing etiology. Gastroenterology 1977;72(3): 483–7.

26. Kawahara H, Kamata S, Okada A, et al. The importance of the plasma amino acid molar ratio in patients with biliary atresia. Surgery 1999;125(5):487–97.

27. Munro HN, Fernstrom JD, Wurtman RJ. Insulin, plasma aminoacid imbalance, and hepatic coma. Lancet 1975;1(7909):722–4.

28. Fabbri A, Magrini N, Bianchi G, et al. Overview of randomized clinical trials of oral branched-chain amino acid treatment in chronic hepatic encephalopathy. JPEN J Parenter Enteral Nutr 1996;20(2):159–64.

29. Base W, Barsigian C, Schaeffer A, et al. Influence of branched-chain amino acids and branched-chain keto acids on protein synthesis in isolated hepatocytes. Hepatology 1987;7(2):324–9.

30. Marchesini G, Bianchi G, Merli M, et al. Nutritional supplementation with branched-chain amino acids in advanced cirrhosis: a double-blind, randomized trial. Gastroenterology 2003;124(7):1792–801.
31. Als-Nielsen B, Koretz RL, Kjaergard LL, et al. Branched-chain amino acids for hepatic encephalopathy. Cochrane Database Syst Rev 2003;(2):CD001939.
32. Chin SE, Shepherd RW, Thomas BJ, et al. Nutritional support in children with end-stage liver disease: a randomized crossover trial of a branched-chain amino acid supplement. Am J Clin Nutr 1992;56(1):158–63.
33. Knisely A, Boyle J, Naylor E, et al. Pancreatic dysfunction in Byler disease [abstract]. J Pediatr Gastroenterol Nutr 1995;21:328.
34. Emerick KM, Rand EB, Goldmuntz E, et al. Features of Alagille syndrome in 92 patients: frequency and relation to prognosis. Hepatology 1999;29(3):822–9.
35. Cohen MI, Gartner LM. The use of medium-chain triglycerides in the management of biliary atresia. J Pediatr 1971;79(3):379–84.
36. Makrides M, Neumann M, Simmer K, et al. Are long-chain polyunsaturated fatty acids essential nutrients in infancy? Lancet 1995;345(8963):1463–8.
37. Koletzko B, Agostoni C, Carlson SE, et al. Long chain polyunsaturated fatty acids (LC-PUFA) and perinatal development. Acta Paediatr 2001;90(4):460–4.
38. Hoffman DR, Birch EE, Birch DG, et al. Effects of supplementation with omega 3 long-chain polyunsaturated fatty acids on retinal and cortical development in premature infants. Am J Clin Nutr 1993;57(Suppl 5):807S–12S.
39. Villamor E, Fawzi WW. Effects of vitamin a supplementation on immune responses and correlation with clinical outcomes. Clin Microbiol Rev 2005; 18(3):446–64.
40. Zeng NX, Wang JL, Guo JY. [Clinical investigation of vitamin A deficiency and endotoxemia in patients with liver cirrhosis]. Chinese Journal of Internal Medicine 1992;31(2):77–9 125 [Chinese].
41. Holda ME, Ryan JR. Hepatobiliary rickets. J Pediatr Orthop 1982;2(3):285–7.
42. Okajima H, Shigeno C, Inomata Y, et al. Long-term effects of liver transplantation on bone mineral density in children with end-stage liver disease: a 2-year prospective study. Liver Transpl 2003;9(4):360–4.
43. Argao EA, Specker BL, Heubi JE. Bone mineral content in infants and children with chronic cholestatic liver disease. Pediatrics 1993;91(6):1151–4.
44. Leerbeck E, Sondergaard H. The total content of vitamin D in human milk and cow's milk. Br J Nutr 1980;44(1):7–12.
45. Sokol RJ, Heubi JE, Iannaccone S, et al. Mechanism causing vitamin E deficiency during chronic childhood cholestasis. Gastroenterology 1983;85(5):1172–82.
46. Guggenheim MA, Jackson V, Lilly J, et al. Vitamin E deficiency and neurologic disease in children with cholestasis: a prospective study. J Pediatr 1983; 102(4):577–9.
47. Sokoll LJ, Booth SL, O'Brien ME, et al. Changes in serum osteocalcin, plasma phylloquinone, and urinary gamma-carboxyglutamic acid in response to altered intakes of dietary phylloquinone in human subjects. Am J Clin Nutr 1997;65(3): 779–84.
48. Usui Y, Tanimura H, Nishimura N, et al. Vitamin K concentrations in the plasma and liver of surgical patients. Am J Clin Nutr 1990;51(5):846–52.
49. Yanofsky RA, Jackson VG, Lilly JR, et al. The multiple coagulopathies of biliary atresia. Am J Hematol 1984;16(2):171–80.
50. Tsiaousi ET, Hatzitolios AI, Trygonis SK, et al. Malnutrition in end stage liver disease: recommendations and nutritional support. J Gastroenterol Hepatol 2008;23(4):527–33.

51. Halsted CH. Nutrition and alcoholic liver disease. Semin Liver Dis 2004;24(3): 289–304.
52. Grantham-McGregor S, Ani C. A review of studies on the effect of iron deficiency on cognitive development in children. J Nutr 2001;131(2S-2):649S–66S [discussion: 666S–8S].
53. Stamoulis I, Kouraklis G, Theocharis S. Zinc and the liver: an active interaction. Dig Dis Sci 2007;52(7):1595–612.
54. Thuluvath PJ, Triger DR. Selenium in primary biliary cirrhosis. Lancet 1987; 2(8552):219.
55. Goksu N, Ozsoylu S. Hepatic and serum levels of zinc, copper, and magnesium in childhood cirrhosis. J Pediatr Gastroenterol Nutr 1986;5(3):459–62.
56. Bayliss EA, Hambridge KM, Sokol RJ, et al. Hepatic concentrations of zinc, copper and manganese in infants with extrahepatic biliary atresia. J Trace Elem Med Biol 1995;9(1):40–3.
57. Fitzgerald K, Mikalunas V, Rubin H, et al. Hypermanganesemia in patients receiving total parenteral nutrition. JPEN J Parenter Enteral Nutr 1999;23(6): 333–6.
58. Ikeda S, Yamaguchi Y, Sera Y, et al. Manganese deposition in the globus pallidus in patients with biliary atresia. Transplantation 2000;69(11):2339–43.
59. Guggenheim MA, Ringel SP, Silverman A, et al. Progressive neuromuscular disease in children with chronic cholestasis and vitamin E deficiency: diagnosis and treatment with alpha tocopherol. J Pediatr 1982;100(1):51–8.
60. Beath S, Pearmain G, Kelly D, et al. Liver transplantation in babies and children with extrahepatic biliary atresia. J Pediatr Surg 1993;28(8):1044–7.
61. Sokol RJ, Stall C. Anthropometric evaluation of children with chronic liver disease. Am J Clin Nutr 1990;52(2):203–8.
62. Sann L, Durand M, Picard J, et al. Arm fat and muscle areas in infancy. Arch Dis Child 1988;63(3):256–60.
63. Roggero P, Cataliott E, Ulla L, et al. Factors influencing malnutrition in children waiting for liver transplants. Am J Clin Nutr 1997;65(6):1852–7.
64. Klein S. The myth of serum albumin as a measure of nutritional status. Gastroenterology 1990;99(6):1845–6.
65. Myron Johnson A, Merlini G, Sheldon J, et al. Clinical indications for plasma protein assays: transthyretin (prealbumin) in inflammation and malnutrition. Clin Chem Lab Med 2007;45(3):419–26.
66. Seres DS. Surrogate nutrition markers, malnutrition, and adequacy of nutrition support. Nutr Clin Pract 2005;20(3):308–13.
67. Burke PA, Ling PR, Forse RA, et al. Sites of conditional essential fatty acid deficiency in end stage liver disease. JPEN J Parenter Enteral Nutr 2001;25(4):188–93.
68. Amedee-Manesme O, Mourey MS, Hanck A, et al. Vitamin A relative dose response test: validation by intravenous injection in children with liver disease. Am J Clin Nutr 1987;46(2):286–9.
69. Feranchak AP, Gralla J, King R, et al. Comparison of indices of vitamin A status in children with chronic liver disease. Hepatology 2005;42(4):782–92.
70. Bianchi ML. Osteoporosis in children and adolescents. Bone 2007;41(4): 486–95.
71. Sokol RJ, Heubi JE, Iannaccone ST, et al. Vitamin E deficiency with normal serum vitamin E concentrations in children with chronic cholestasis. N Engl J Med 1984;310(19):1209–12.
72. Ford L, Farr J, Morris P, et al. The value of measuring serum cholesterol-adjusted vitamin E in routine practice. Ann Clin Biochem 2006;43(Pt 2):130–4.

73. Ferland G, Sadowski JA, O'Brien ME. Dietary induced subclinical vitamin K deficiency in normal human subjects. J Clin Invest 1993;91(4):1761–8.

74. Mager DR, McGee PL, Furuya KN, et al. Prevalence of vitamin K deficiency in children with mild to moderate chronic liver disease. J Pediatr Gastroenterol Nutr 2006;42(1):71–6.

75. Zemel BS, Riley EM, Stallings VA. Evaluation of methodology for nutritional assessment in children: anthropometry, body composition, and energy expenditure. Annu Rev Nutr 1997;17:211–35.

76. Bechard LJ, Wroe E, Ellis K. Body composition and growth. In: C Duggan, JB Watkins, WA Walker, editors. Nutrition in pediatrics: basic science, clinical applications. Hamilton, Ontario; Lewiston (NY): BC Decker; 2008. p. 27–39.

77. Schofield WN. Predicting basal metabolic rate, new standards and review of previous work. Hum Nutr Clin Nutr 1985;39(Suppl 1):5–41.

78. Food and Agriculture Organization of the United Nations. World Health Organization, United Nations University. Energy and protein requirements: report of a joint FAO/WHO/UNU expert consultation. Geneva: World Health Organization; 1985. p. 206.

79. Cabre E, Gonzalez-Huix F, Abad-Lacruz A, et al. Effect of total enteral nutrition on the short-term outcome of severely malnourished cirrhotics. A randomized controlled trial. Gastroenterology 1990;98(3):715–20.

80. Kearns PJ, Young H, Garcia G, et al. Accelerated improvement of alcoholic liver disease with enteral nutrition. Gastroenterology 1992;102(1):200–5.

81. Cabre E, Rodriguez-Iglesias P, Caballeria J, et al. Short- and long-term outcome of severe alcohol-induced hepatitis treated with steroids or enteral nutrition: a multicenter randomized trial. Hepatology 2000;32(1):36–42.

82. de Ledinghen V, Beau P, Mannant PR, et al. Early feeding or enteral nutrition in patients with cirrhosis after bleeding from esophageal varices? A randomized controlled study. Dig Dis Sci 1997;42(3):536–41.

83. Plauth M, Cabre E, Riggio O, et al. ESPEN guidelines on enteral nutrition: liver disease. Clin Nutr 2006;25(2):285–94.

84. Moreno LA, Gottrand F, Hoden S, et al. Improvement of nutritional status in cholestatic children with supplemental nocturnal enteral nutrition. J Pediatr Gastroenterol Nutr 1991;12(2):213–6.

85. Guimber D, Michand L, Ategbo S, et al. Experience of parenteral nutrition for nutritional rescue in children with severe liver disease following failure of enteral nutrition. Pediatr Transplant 1999;3(2):139–45.

86. Chin SE, Shepherd RW, Cleghorn GJ, et al. Pre-operative nutritional support in children with end-stage liver disease accepted for liver transplantation: an approach to management. J Gastroenterol Hepatol 1990;5(5):566–72.

87. Feranchak AP, Sokol RJ. Medical and nutritional management of cholestasis in infants and children. In: FJ Suchy, RJ Sokol, WF Balistreri, editors. Liver disease in children. Cambridge, New York: Cambridge University Press; 2007. p. 190–231.

88. Kelly D. Acute and chronic liver disease. In: Duggan C, Watkins JB, Walker WA, editors. Nutrition in pediatrics: basic science, clinical applications. Hamilton, Ontario; Lewiston (NY): BC Decker; 2008. p. 589–97.

89. Kelly DA, Davenport M. Current management of biliary atresia. Arch Dis Child 2007;92(12):1132–5.

90. Ng VL, Balistreri WF. Treatment options for chronic cholestasis in infancy and childhood. Curr Treat Options Gastroenterol 2005;8(5):419–30.

91. Crawford BA, Labio ED, Strasser SI, et al. Vitamin D replacement for cirrhosis-related bone disease. Nat Clin Pract Gastroenterol Hepatol 2006;3(12):689–99.

92. Guichelaar MM, Kendall R, Malinchoc M, et al. Bone mineral density before and after OLT: long-term follow-up and predictive factors. Liver Transpl 2006;12(9): 1390–402.
93. Argao EA, Heubi JE, Hollis BW, et al. d-Alpha-tocopheryl polyethylene glycol-1000 succinate enhances the absorption of vitamin D in chronic cholestatic liver disease of infancy and childhood. Pediatr Res 1992;31(2):146–50.
94. Heubi JE, Hollis BW, Specker B, et al. Bone disease in chronic childhood cholestasis. I. Vitamin D absorption and metabolism. Hepatology 1989;9(2):258–64.
95. Sokol RJ, Butter-Simon N, Conner C, et al. Multicenter trial of d-alpha-tocopheryl polyethylene glycol 1000 succinate for treatment of vitamin E deficiency in children with chronic cholestasis. Gastroenterology 1993;104(6):1727–35.
96. Perlmutter DH, Gross P, Jones HR, et al. Intramuscular vitamin E repletion in children with chronic cholestasis. Am J Dis Child 1987;141(2):170–4.
97. Bancroft J, Cohen MB. Intracranial hemorrhage due to vitamin K deficiency in breast-fed infants with cholestasis. J Pediatr Gastroenterol Nutr 1993;16(1): 78–80.
98. Pereira SP, Shearer MJ, Williams R, et al. Intestinal absorption of mixed micellar phylloquinone (vitamin K1) is unreliable in infants with conjugated hyperbilirubinaemia: implications for oral prophylaxis of vitamin K deficiency bleeding. Arch Dis Child Fetal Neonatal Ed 2003;88(2):F113–8.
99. Otten JJ, Hellwig JP, Meyers LD. DRI, dietary reference intakes: the essential guide to nutrient requirements. Washington, DC: National Academies Press; 2006. xiii, p. 543.
100. Heubi JE, Higgins JV, Argao EA, et al. The role of magnesium in the pathogenesis of bone disease in childhood cholestatic liver disease: a preliminary report. J Pediatr Gastroenterol Nutr 1997;25(3):301–6.

Nutritional Deficiencies in Intestinal Failure

Charmaine H. Mziray-Andrew, MD[a], Timothy A. Sentongo, MD[b],*

KEYWORDS

- Nutritional deficiency • Intestinal failure
- Short bowel syndrome • Sodium depletion • Malabsorption

Intestinal failure (IF) is a clinical state characterized by impaired ability to maintain normal nutrition, fluid, or electrolyte balance secondary to congenital defects, surgical resection, disease-associated malabsorption, or impaired motility of the gastrointestinal tract, thus necessitating dependence on enteral or intravenous supplements.[1,2] IF may be classified as reversible or permanent, depending on potential for becoming independent of parenteral nutrition (PN) therapy (**Table 1**). The primary goal during management of children with potentially reversible IF is to promote intestinal autonomy while supporting normal growth and nutrient status, and preventing complications from PN therapy. The management goals for irreversible IF are to support normal growth and nutrient status while preventing complications from PN and continually assessing eligibility for intestinal transplant. Surgical resection of necrotizing enterocolitis (NEC) is the most frequent cause of short bowel syndrome (SBS) and IF in children.[3] Before the advent of PN, severe SBS was invariably fatal from dehydration, electrolyte deficiencies, and malnutrition.[4] IF is important for its chronic negative impact on growth,[3,5] disproportionately high costs of medical care,[6] and need for intestinal and or liver transplantation in severely affected children.[7]

In patients with IF the risk of developing nutrient deficiencies depends on the postsurgical anatomy and amount of bowel resected. Loss of more than 75% of the small intestine requires specialized nutrition support to avert severe malnutrition.[2] Patients with jejunostomy or massive resections of the ileum experience more problems with fluid imbalance and electrolyte deficiencies.[8] Some nutrient deficiencies may be iatrogenic from inadequately constituted PN solutions, for example, thiamine deficiency and beri beri syndrome from not providing pediatric intravenous multivitamins,[9–14] and refractory anemia, neutropenia, and neurologic symptoms from not providing

[a] Peds GI, Hepatology and Nutrition, University of Chicago, 5839 South Maryland Avenue, MC 4065, Chicago, IL 60637, USA
[b] Peds GI, Hepatology & Nutrition, University of Chicago, 5839 South Maryland Avenue, MC 4065, WP C-474, Chicago, IL 60637, USA
* Corresponding author.
E-mail address: tsentong@peds.bsd.uchicago.edu (T.A. Sentongo).

Pediatr Clin N Am 56 (2009) 1185–1200
doi:10.1016/j.pcl.2009.07.005
0031-3955/09/$ – see front matter. Published by Elsevier Inc.

pediatric.theclinics.com

Table 1
Causes of intestinal failure in children

Intestinal Failure	
Potentially Reversible	Permanent
Congenital[a]	Congenital
Atresia (unique or multiple)	Extensive Hirchsprung disease
Apple peel syndrome	Neuronal intestinal dysplasia
Gastroschisis	Pseudo-obstruction (visceral myopathies)
Congenital volvulus (with	Mitochondrial myopathies
omphalomesenteric duct or	Diseases of intestinal epithelia
intra-abdominal bands)	Tufting enteropathy
	Microvillus inclusion disease
	Congenital chloridorrhea
	Intestinal lymphangiectasia
Acquired[a]	Acquired
Necrotizing enterocolitis	Lupus-induced pseudo-obstruction
Midgut volvulus (malrotation, bands, tumor)	Extreme short bowel syndrome
Complicated intussusception	
Arterial/venous thrombosis	
Posttrauma resection	
Inflammatory bowel disease	
Postinfection pseudo-obstruction[b]	
(cytomegalovirus, Epstein-Barr virus,	
herpes zoster, rotavirus, etc.)[115]	

[a] Disorders resulting in intestinal resection and short bowel syndrome.
[b] Acquired motility disorders with normal bowel length.

copper.[15–19] The risk of developing nutrient deficiencies is also increased in patients with comorbid disease, for example, cystic fibrosis (pancreatic insufficiency) and Crohn disease.[2] This article presents how an improved understanding of digestive pathophysiology is essential for the diagnosis, successful management, and prevention of nutrient deficiencies in children with IF.

DIGESTIVE PHYSIOLOGY AND ITS RELEVANCE IN SHORT BOWEL SYNDROME

The jejunum is the major site for digestion and absorption of most nutrients.[20] The ileum becomes increasingly important in digestion and absorption when large amounts of nutrients are consumed.[21] Hypertonic meals and the degradation products from pancreatic enzyme hydrolysis of macronutrients increase osmolality in the duodenum and jejunum.[22] This process causes an influx or water and electrolytes into the jejunal lumen to make chyme isosmotic with plasma.[23] Loss of the jejunum alone does not result in severe malabsorption, because the ileum has a large capacity to compensate for increased absorption of ingested and endogenous fluids and electrolytes. Patients with jejunostomy or massive loss of the ileum are more prone to malnutrition, excessive fluid losses, and electrolyte deficiencies because the jejunum is more porous and has limited capacity for enhanced absorption.[20] Having an intact or partial colon is advantageous for salvaging water and electrolytes not reabsorbed by the ileum.[24] Unabsorbed carbohydrates are fermented by colonic flora to short-chain fatty acids (SCFA). Absorption of SCFA in the colon is accompanied by sodium and water.[25]

NUTRITIONAL MANAGEMENT OF SHORT BOWEL SYNDROME

Enteral feeding is the most important stimulus for villous growth, intestinal motility, and bowel adaptation.[20,26] Administering enteral nutrition stimulates bile flow and intestinal peristalsis, thus decreasing the risk of bacterial overgrowth and exerting a protective effect against PN-associated cholestasis.[27] Continuously administered enteral feeds are well tolerated, and result in more nutrient absorption than boluses or oral feeds.[28,29] Endogenous secretions constitute a significant proportion of ostomy and fecal output in patients with severe SBS. Therefore, the amount of enteral feeds in children with SBS should be advanced at a slow but controlled rate, for example, by 1 mL/h/d[30] while monitoring ostomy and fecal output to remain less than or equal to 40–50 mL/kg/d.[31] Excessive outputs risk dehydration, and thus necessitate replacement therapy with intravenous fluids and electrolytes.

ENERGY REQUIREMENTS IN PATIENTS WITH INTESTINAL FAILURE

The energy requirements of patients with IF are similar to healthy individuals. Jaksic and colleagues[32] measured resting metabolic rate in infants with SBS on PN therapy, and found an average energy expenditure of 53 ± 5.1 kcal/kg/d, which was within the predicted range (43–60 kcal/kg/d) for healthy infants.[33] Beghin and colleagues[34] found no differences between energy expenditure of children with IF on home PN (age 4.5–15.0 years) and similarly aged healthy controls. Justino and colleagues[35] also found normal energy expenditure in adult patients with SBS. Uncompensated malabsorption is the main cause of protein energy malnutrition in patients with SBS. Therefore, patients with SBS who are fed enterally must consume excess calories to compensate for malabsorption.[2,36] Wolf and colleagues[37] evaluated a group of patients with severe SBS, and found that those who maintained a positive nitrogen balance off PN therapy consumed 127% to 170% of predicted energy requirements. Absorption kinetic studies suggest that diets composed of 48% carbohydrate, 23% protein, and 29% fat (within the recommended composition for normal health[38]) result in absorption of most nutrients over the shortest length of intestine.[39] Therefore, hyperphagia with a normal diet composition should be encouraged in patients with SBS consuming table foods. The protein and energy requirements of patients on PN therapy can be determined using the World Health Organization weight-, age- and gender-based prediction equations.[40] Adjustments for malabsorption are not necessary for intravenous nutrition (PN). On the contrary, patients with SBS fed via the gastrointestinal tract should have energy and protein intakes increased by more than 30% to support normal growth while compensating for malabsorption. Growth should be regularly monitored using proper tools, the anthropometry technique,[41] and plotted on appropriate age- and gender-based growth charts (www.cdc.gov/growthcharts) (Table 2).

NUTRIENT DIGESTIBILITY AND RISK OF MALABSORPTION
Carbohydrates

Simple sugars are more rapidly digested and absorbed compared with oligosaccharides and starches. Glucose, galactose, and rapidly hydrolyzed disaccharides (eg, sucrose) are absorbed in the duodenum and proximal jejunum. Lactose is hydrolyzed much more slowly and is thus more likely to be delivered into the distal jejunum and ileum,[42] and does not induce increased fluid losses in patients with SBS.[43] Ingesting large amounts of less rapidly absorbed simple sugars, for example, fructose and sorbitol, may cause osmotic diarrhea, and therefore should be avoided in patients with SBS. Ingestion of hemicelluloses, cereal bran, and other indigestible complex

Table 2
Frequency for monitoring growth and nutrient status in children with IF

Measurement	Comment	Initial Period[a]	Long-Term Follow-up
Weight, kg	Preterm infants	Daily	2–4 wk
	Age > 1 y	Twice a wk	1–6 mo
Head circumference, cm	Birth to 3 y	2 wk	1–3 mo
Length, cm	Birth to 3 y	2–4 wk	1–3 mo
Height, cm	Age ≥ 2 y	4 wk	1–6 mo
Electrolytes, Ca, PO_4, Mg	(Patients on PN)	Twice a wk	2–4 wk
Hepatic transaminases, direct bilirubin	(Patients on PN)	1–2 wk	1–3 mo
Total protein, Prealbumin		2–4 wk	1–3 mo
Complete blood count, reticulocyte count		2–4 wk	1–3 mo
PT/PTT/INR		Baseline	As indicated
Iron studies (iron, transferrin, % saturation, TIBC)		Baseline	As indicated
Vitamin A		Baseline	3 mo
Vitamin E	Serum α-tocopherol:cholesterol ratio <2.47 mg/g consistent with deficiency[116]	Baseline	3 mo
Vitamin D (25-hydroxyvitamin)	Also consider seasonal factors influencing risk of deficiency	Baseline	3 mo
Vitamin B12	↓plasma B12 accompanied by ↑methylmalonic acid confirms deficiency[75]	Baseline	3–6 mo
Trace minerals (Cu, Zn, Se, Mn)		Baseline	3–6 mo

Abbreviations: INR, international normalized ratio; PT, prothrombin time; PTT, partial thromboplastin time; TIBC, total iron-binding capacity.
[a] Initial period ranges from time of diagnosis to 3 mo.

carbohydrates is associated with increased fecal losses of nitrogen.[40] Hemicelluloses and indigestible complex carbohydrates (fiber) are fermented to SCFA by colonic bacteria. SCFA play an important role in stimulating absorption of sodium and water, and metabolize into energy used by colonocytes.[25] Therefore, consumption of fiber should be encouraged in patients with an intact or remnant colon, but should be restricted in patients with jejunostomy.

Protein Source and Nutritional Benefit

Approximately 70% of digestible protein is absorbed proximal to the midjejunum and the remainder in the distal ileum.[44] Breast milk, hydrolyzed protein formulas, and crystalline amino acid based formulas are well tolerated, and associated with faster weaning from PN therapy than intact whey or casein-protein based formulas.[45,46] Crystalline amino acid based formulas have a high osmolality at standard concentrations, and thus will induce a large influx of water and electrolytes into the jejunum with the associated risk of increased dumping in patients with jejunostomy or severe SBS. Similar effects may occur with intact-protein formulas because following hydrolysis by pancreatic enzymes an increase in jejunal osmolality occurs, which induces an increased influx of endogenous secretions.[22] This osmotic effect may be minimized by initiating feeds with crystalline amino acid formulas diluted to a concentration of 15 kcal/oz (0.53 kcal/mL).

The protein quality of table foods consumed by patients with IF should be judged based on content of "reference proteins." Hen's egg, milk, cheese, meat, and fish contain all the essential amino acids, are completely digested and absorbed, and therefore designated as "reference proteins."[40] Soy, legumes, grains, and corn proteins have relative digestibility of less than 90% compared with the "reference proteins."[40] The lower nutritional value of plant proteins is secondary to intrinsic factors, for example, cell walls that decrease digestibility, presence of fibers, phenols, and tannins that may inhibit digestion, and antinutritional factors (eg, trypsin inhibitors and lectins) that interfere with digestion.[40,47] Therefore, nutritional benefit from dietary protein in patients with IF can be maximized by encouraging greater consumption of "reference proteins."

Fats

Dietary fat is important for its energy content and effects to slow gastrointestinal motility. Patients with jejunostomy or severe SBS develop steatorrhea following increased consumption of dietary fat.[21,36,37,48] Oversen and colleagues[48] investigated the effects of varying the amounts and composition of dietary fat in patients with severe SBS. These investigators found that high intakes did not negatively impact fecal volumes but resulted in steatorrhea and increased fecal losses of calcium, zinc, and magnesium.[48] Nonproximally absorbed medium- and long-chain fatty acids compete with oxalate in the colon to bind with calcium. The unbound oxalate is rapidly absorbed and may predispose to renal oxalate stones.[49] Therefore, increased consumption of fat should be encouraged for its calorie content and lack of detrimental effect on fecal output. However, patients should have calcium, zinc, and magnesium status closely monitored and replenished.

Calcium

Calcium is the most abundant divalent cation in the human body, and has vital structural and regulatory functions. More than 99% of the body's calcium reserves are in skeletal tissue, where it has a structural role. The regulatory functions of calcium include neuromuscular transmission of chemical and electrical stimuli, cellular secretion, and blood clotting. The risk factors for calcium deficiency in patients with IF are inadequate intake of calcium, vitamin D deficiency, intestinal losses secondary to jejunostomy or massive ileal resection, and calciuria from cycling PN.[50,51] Calcium is actively absorbed in the duodenum and passively absorbed in the jejunum and ileum. Active absorption of calcium is enhanced by vitamin D.[52] When calcium intakes are adequate or high (>800 mg/d) passive mechanisms are the major mode of absorption.[52] Passive absorption is enhanced by glucose and galactose.[53] However, simple sugars ingested orally are rapidly absorbed proximal to the jejunum. Lactose is hydrolyzed slowly and is thus delivered more distally into the jejunum and ileum, where its degradation products (glucose and galactose) can enhance passive absorption of calcium.[53] Steatorrhea is associated with increased fecal losses of calcium[48] as nonabsorbable calcium salts of fatty acids. The manifestations of decreased calcium (hypocalcaemia) include muscle cramps, tetany, and poor bone mineralization. Serum concentrations of calcium are regulated by dietary intake and hormonal mechanisms at the expense of skeletal stores. Parathyroid hormone (PTH) and 1,25-hydroxyvitamin D (calcitriol) are produced in response to hypocalcaemia while calcitonin is secreted in response to hypercalcemia. Therefore, assessment of calcium status should include measurements of serum vitamin D (25-hydroxyvitamin D and 1,25-hydroxyvitamin D) and PTH. Decreased 25-hydroxyvitamin D accompanied by increased PTH is consistent with medical rickets. Benefit from calcium supplements is maximized when combined with vitamin D.

Sodium and Electrolytes

Patients with jejunostomy and severe SBS are more prone to increased sodium and electrolyte losses.[54,55] Sodium depletion results in decreased plasma volume, hypotension, secondary hyperaldosteronisim, and reduced urinary excretion of sodium.[54,56] Because simultaneous losses of water occur matching the sodium deficit, serum osmolality and sodium concentrations may be normal in patients with severe sodium depletion.[57] Therefore, decreased urine sodium (<20 mEq/L) is a more reliable indicator of sodium depletion. The dietary content of sodium also influences nutrient absorption and fluid balance in the jejunum. Isotonic low sodium diets induce a large influx of sodium and water into the jejunum, which is associated with greater fluid and electrolyte losses in patients with jejunostomy and severe SBS. Fluid and nutrient absorption in patients with SBS can be maximized by increasing the sodium content of hydration solutions to 90 to 120 mmol/L.[58] On the contrary, hypertonic diets do not require further sodium supplementation to improve absorption. Ehrlein and colleagues[59] supplemented energy-dense formulas with increasing amounts of sodium (30–150 mmol/L), and examined the effect on nutrient absorption and fluid flux in the jejunum. Supplementing energy-dense formulas with sodium did not enhance nutrient absorption, but increased osmolality and endogenous secretions of water and electrolytes into the jejunum,[59] and thus was associated with risk of greater fluid and electrolyte losses in patients with jejunostomy or severe SBS. Nightingale and colleagues[60] investigated sodium balance in patients with jejunostomy, and reported that consumption of sodium 120 mmol/d was associated with positive balance. Therefore, patients with jejunostomy or massive ileal resection on enteral feeds should be counseled to take a daily sodium supplement of 120 mmol/d[60](about 1 "teaspoon" of regular salt) or drink hydration fluids containing sodium, 90 to 120 mmol/L. Homemade hydration fluids containing equimolar concentrations (about 100 mmol/L) of sodium and glucose can be prepared by mixing 1 teaspoon of regular salt (about 6 g of sodium chloride) and 8 teaspoons of sugar (about 35 g of sucrose) mixed in 1000 mL of water.[61]

Potassium

Potassium (K^+) is essential for repolarization of cell membranes during muscle and nerve activity. Lack of K^+ results in persistent hyperpolarization of cell membranes, leading to delayed conductivity and impaired contraction. Symptoms of hypokalemia range from muscular weakness, myalgia, and constipation to flaccid paralysis, hyporeflexia, tetany, respiratory depression, and cardiac arrhythmias. Absorption of K^+ occurs in the small intestine by passive mechanisms that are not disturbed by diarrhea. Negative K^+ balance and hypokalemia occur in SBS secondary to inadequate dietary intake, decreased absorptive surface area, and obligatory losses from combining with nonabsorbed organic anions.[62] Other causes include secondary hyperaldosteronism due to volume contraction following excessive fecal losses of sodium and water, increased consumption of water leading to water diuresis and increased urinary excretion of K^+, and magnesium depletion.[62] Mild hypokalemia (>3.0 mEq/dL) may be treated with oral supplements; however, severe hypokalemia

(<3.0 mEq/dL) requires intravenous supplements. Oral liquid supplements are preferred to tablets in patients with SBS.

Bicarbonate

Bicarbonate loss and metabolic acidosis is a complication of small bowel diarrhea in patients with severe SBS. The mechanism is increased loss of bicarbonate-rich biliary and pancreatic fluids,[63] and normal intestinal secretion of bicarbonate in exchange for reabsorption of chloride.[23] The resulting metabolic acidosis from increased intestinal losses of bicarbonate (hyperchloremic) has a normal anion gap ($[Na] - ([C1] + [HCO_3])$ = ≤ 12). Normal anion gap metabolic acidosis in patients with SBS can be managed by adequate hydration and replacement therapy with Bicitra or Polycitra supplements. The differential diagnosis of increased anion gap (≥ 12) metabolic acidosis includes D-lactic acidosis secondary to small bowel bacterial overgrowth,[64,65] and L-lactic acidosis secondary to thiamine deficiency and beri beri syndrome[14] or bowel ischemia. The management goal for increased anion gap metabolic acidosis is to treat the underlying cause and not merely replenish bicarbonate.

Vitamin B12

The risk of developing vitamin B12 deficiency is increased in patients with a history of surgical resection of greater than 15 to 45 cm of ileum during infancy,[66–68] chronic suppression of gastric acid,[69] and bacterial overgrowth.[70,71] Digestion and release of vitamin B12 from dietary proteins requires hydrolysis by gastric acid. Specialized absorption of vitamin B12 occurs in the terminal ileum. Vitamin B12 deficiency is associated with megaloblastic anemia and potentially irreversible neurocognitive complications.[72] Lack of B12 also causes functional deficiency of cobalamin-dependent enzymes (eg, methylmalonyl coenzyme A mutase), resulting in accumulation of methylmalonic acid.[72–75] Many assays discriminate poorly between serum B12 concentrations in the range of 100 to 400 pg/mL[72]; therefore, deficiency is confirmed by also detecting increased concentrations of methylmalonic acid.[72–75] Persistently elevated serum concentrations of methylmalonic acid despite correction of B12 status may be secondary to absorption of propionate (and methylmalonate derived from it) produced by intestinal flora.[76] B12 deficiency secondary to ileal resection is unresponsive to therapy with oral supplements. This deficiency should be treated with intramuscular injections of cyanocobalamin, 1000 μg administered in aliquots of 100 μg over 10 days. Larger doses of B12 do not result in greater retention because rapid clearance from plasma into urine occurs.[77] Vitamin B12 status should be monitored indefinitely in patients with SBS because time to onset of deficiency may be delayed several years,[72] and requirements increase during pubertal growth.

Folic Acid

Folate is absorbed throughout the small bowel but primarily in the proximal third.[78] The risk of deficiency is low in patients with SBS and other disorders associated with small bowel bacterial overgrowth, because folate synthesized by enteric flora is absorbed and is detectable in plasma.[79,80] In addition, since 1996 it has been a United States Food and Drug Administration regulation to fortify several foods with folate.[81–83] The importance of high folate status in patients with SBS is that hematological changes of vitamin B12 deficiency may be masked, leading to delayed diagnosis.

NUTRITIONAL DEFICIENCIES ASSOCIATED WITH PARENTERAL NUTRITION THERAPY

Vitamins and minerals are essential nutrients required in only small quantities by the body. Nutritional deficiencies should not occur if PN is appropriately constituted and monitored. The basic constituents of PN solutions are dextrose, crystalline amino acids, water, and electrolytes. Intravenous multivitamins (**Table 3**) and trace minerals (copper, zinc, selenium, chromium, and manganese) are added to PN solutions only before administration to the patient. Deficiencies with serious consequences have been reported during unique circumstances when vitamins or minerals were excluded from PN solutions. The reasons for omission included lack of availability,[12] the practice of empirically withdrawing minerals from PN solutions of patients with cholestasis,[18] and nutrition support in patients with suspected hypersensitivity to PN.[84,85] Lack of intake leads to progressive depletion of body stores before onset of biochemical and physiologic consequences.[86] The recommended dose of pediatric multivitamin formula for intravenous infusion (MVI) is 1.5 mL for infants weighing less than 1 kg; 3.25 mL for infants of 1 to 3 kg; and 5 mL for those weighing greater than 3 kg. Children older than 12 years should be given MVI-12.[87] Children receiving nonsupplemented PN solutions and on minimal or no enteral feeds should be closely monitored for risk of developing severe deficiency.

Thiamine

Thiamine deficiency is triggered by administering a large load of carbohydrate without thiamine supplements in patients with malnutrition and poor enteral intake. Time from depletion of thiamine to onset of beri beri symptoms can range from 4 to 40 days of PN therapy without multivitamin supplements.[13] Thiamine (thiamine pyrophosphate) is a coenzyme for transketolase enzyme, which is important for connecting the pentose phosphate pathway to glycolysis, and pyruvate dehydrogenase and α-ketoglutarate dehydrogenase enzymes responsible for oxidative decarboxylation of pyruvate and α-ketoglutarate, respectively. During thiamine deficiency pyruvate is not decarboxylated and thus cannot enter the Krebs cycle. The accumulating pyruvate is converted to lactic acid with the onset of metabolic acidosis. Failure of the Krebs cycle leads to

Table 3		
Composition of standard intravenous multivitamin preparations		
	Pediatric MVI 5 mL	MVI-12 10 mL
Vitamin A (retinol), IU	2300	3300
Vitamin D, IU	400	200
Vitamin E (α-tocopherol), IU	7	10
Vitamin C, mg	80	100
Folate, μg	140	400
Niacin, mg	17	40
Riboflavin, mg	1.4	3.6
Thiamine, mg	1.2	3
Vitamin B6, mg	1	4
Vitamin B12, μg	1	5
Pantothetic acid, mg	5	15
Biotin, μg	20	60
Vitamin K, mg	0.2	[a]

[a] MVI-12 does not contain vitamin K.

an energy deficiency from failed synthesis of adenosine triphosphate.[88] Beri beri clinically manifests as an acute sepsis shocklike state characterized by tachycardia, hypotension, altered mental status, and severe metabolic acidosis (lactic) that is poorly responsive to therapy with bicarbonate. Other symptoms include diplopia (encephalopathy), vomiting, and severe abdominal pain.[10–13,89] The diagnosis is confirmed by rapid improvement of clinical symptoms following intramuscular or intravenous administration of thiamine, 10 to 25 mg. Laboratory diagnosis is based on increased erythrocyte transketolase activity from baseline following addition of thiamine pyrophosphate.[90] Rapid laboratory diagnosis is often unavailable and delayed therapy can be fatal.[90] Therefore, clinical suspicion is adequate for diagnosis and immediate administration of parenteral thiamine.

Copper

Copper deficiency is linked to the practice of empirically withholding trace minerals from PN therapy in patients with cholestasis.[15,18,91] Therefore, removal of copper from PN solutions should be accompanied by regular monitoring of copper status and clinical signs of deficiency.[92] Anemia unresponsive to iron therapy and neutropenia are the most striking abnormalities associated with copper deficiency.[93] Less common manifestations include hair loss, skin depigmentation, neurologic symptoms, and impaired bone mineralization.[93] Deficiency is confirmed by decreased serum copper.[94] Serum concentrations of ceruloplasmin reflect changes only when there is severe copper depletion.[94]

Zinc

Humans do not have a storage form of zinc, therefore status is maintained by continual adequate intake.[95] The risk factors for developing zinc deficiency include increased requirements for normal growth and tissue healing, malabsorption,[37,48] and omission of zinc supplements from PN solutions.[96] Zinc is ubiquitous in human metabolism; therefore, deficiency has widespread consequences including immune dysfunction, dermatitis, impaired wound healing, persistent diarrhea, delayed pubertal development, and stunted growth. Plasma zinc is reliable for assessing zinc status. Plasma alkaline phosphate activity is also decreased during zinc deficiency but responds poorly to changes in intake, and therefore is not reliable for monitoring zinc status.[97]

Selenium

Selenium is among the trace elements routinely added to PN solutions. Therefore, the risk of developing deficiency is also linked to not supplementing PN solutions with trace elements. Clinical signs of deficiency include muscle weakness, pain, wasting, loss of skin and hair pigmentation, whitening of the nail beds, and Keshan cardiomyopathy.[98] Measurement of plasma selenium concentrations is helpful for assessing status and response to supplements.[99]

Choline

Choline is a quaternary amine with several metabolic roles, including source of labile methyl groups, precursor for the neurotransmitter acetylcholine, and structural component of cell membranes, bile, and lipoproteins.[100] The sources of choline are breast milk,[101] infant formulas,[102] regular diets,[103] and endogenous synthesis in the transsulfuration pathway.[100,104] Experimentally induced deficiency is associated with steatosis, with oxidative liver damage in laboratory animals[105,106] and increased hepatic transaminases in humans.[107] Endogenous biosynthesis appears impaired in patients with chronic hepatic dysfunction.[104] Because choline is abundant in diets and is also endogenously synthesized, it is not granted "essential status" mandating routine supplementation in PN solutions. Thus PN therapy in patients on minimal or no enteral feeds is a form of choline-free diet. Infants on chronic PN providing more than 90% of daily calorie intake develop biochemical changes of choline deficiency.[108] More studies are needed to define the efficacy of choline supplements in patients at greatest risk for deficiency (ie, chronic PN therapy with minimal or no enteral feeds).

NUTRIENT DEFICIENCIES RELATED TO MEDICATIONS COMMONLY USED IN INTESTINAL FAILURE

Drugs commonly used during the management of patients with IF may also predispose to nutrient deficiency. For a comprehensive review the reader is referred to the article on drug-induced nutrient deficiencies (Lina Felipez, MD and Timothy Sentongo, MD) in this issue. In summary, the deficiencies pertinent to patients with IF include (1) chronic use of H_2 blockers and proton pump inhibitors to manage SBS associated hyper secretion of gastric acid[109,110] and reflux symptoms, resulting in deficiency of B12 secondary to impaired release from dietary proteins[111]; (2) vitamin K deficiency secondary to eradication of vitamin K synthesizing bacteria by broad-spectrum antibiotics[112] used to control bacterial overgrowth; (3) folate and fat-soluble vitamin malabsorption induced by cholestyramine used to manage bile salt diarrhea[113]; and (4) renal potassium and magnesium wasting induced by therapy with calcineurin inhibitors used for immunosuppression in transplant recipients.[114] Most drug-induced nutrient deficiencies occur randomly; therefore, empirical prescription of supplements based on drug therapy is not justified. The recommended approach is awareness, monitoring, and intervention based on confirmed deficiency.

SUMMARY

IF is the ultimate malabsorption state, with multiple causes, requiring long-term therapy with enteral or intravenous supplements with fluids and nutrients. Any single nutrient can become deficient in patients with IF. The risk of developing some nutrient deficiencies, for example, vitamin B12 and divalent cations, can be anticipated based on the postsurgical anatomy. Improved understanding of digestive pathophysiology and the nutrient composition of foods and supplements should be used to optimize nutrition support in children with IF. The nutritional goals are to achieve independence from PN therapy while sustaining normal growth and nutrient status, and avoidance of metabolic complications. There is no substitute for close monitoring of growth, nutrient status, and continual adjustment of nutritional therapy in children with IF (**Table 2**).

REFERENCES

1. O'Keefe SJD, Buchman AL, Fishbein TM, et al. Short bowel syndrome and intestinal failure: consensus definitions and overview. Clin Gastroenterol Hepatol 2006;4(1):6–10.
2. Jeejeebhoy KN. Management of short bowel syndrome: avoidance of total parenteral nutrition [see comment]. Gastroenterology 2006;130(2 Suppl 1): S60–6.
3. Cole CR, Hansen NI, Higgins RD, et al. Very low birth weight preterm infants with surgical short bowel syndrome: incidence, morbidity and mortality, and growth outcomes at 18 to 22 months. Pediatrics 2008;122(3):e573–82.
4. Goulet O, Ruemmele F. Causes and management of intestinal failure in children [see comment]. Gastroenterology 2006;130(2 Suppl 1):S16–28.

5. Goulet O, Baglin-Gobet S, Talbotec C, et al. Outcome and long-term growth after extensive small bowel resection in the neonatal period: a survey of 87 children. Eur J Pediatr Surg 2005;15(2):95–101.

6. Spencer AU, Kovacevich D, McKinney-Barnett M, et al. Pediatric short-bowel syndrome: the cost of comprehensive care. Am J Clin Nutr 2008;88(6):1552–9.

7. Kaufman SS, Atkinson JB, Bianchi A, et al. Indications for pediatric intestinal transplantation: a position paper of the American Society of Transplantation. Pediatr Transplant 2001;5(2):80–7.

8. Nightingale JM. Management of patients with a short bowel. World J Gastroenterol 2001;7(6):741–51.

9. Naidoo DP, Singh B, Haffejee A, et al. Acute pernicious beriberi in a patient receiving parenteral nutrition. A case report. S Afr Med J 1989;75(11):546–8.

10. Velez RJ, Myers B, Guber MS. Severe acute metabolic acidosis (acute beriberi): an avoidable complication of total parenteral nutrition. JPEN J Parenter Enteral Nutr 1985;9(2):216–9.

11. La Selve P, Demolin P, Holzapfel L, et al. Shoshin beriberi: an unusual complication of prolonged parenteral nutrition. JPEN J Parenter Enteral Nutr 1986;10(1):102–3.

12. Hahn JS, Berquist W, Alcorn DM, et al. Wernicke encephalopathy and beriberi during total parenteral nutrition attributable to multivitamin infusion shortage. Pediatrics 1998;101(1):E10.

13. Kitamura K, Yamaguchi T, Tanaka H, et al. TPN-induced fulminant beriberi: a report on our experience and a review of the literature. Surg Today 1996;26(10):769–76.

14. Cho YP, Kim K, Han MS, et al. Severe lactic acidosis and thiamine deficiency during total parenteral nutrition—case report. Hepatogastroenterology 2004;51(55):253–5.

15. Angotti LB, Post GR, Robinson NS, et al. Pancytopenia with myelodysplasia due to copper deficiency. Pediatr Blood Cancer 2008;51(5):693–5.

16. Bozzetti F, Inglese MG, Terno G, et al. Hypocupremia in patients receiving total parenteral nutrition. JPEN J Parenter Enteral Nutr 1983;7(6):563–6.

17. Fujita M, Itakura T, Takagi Y, et al. Copper deficiency during total parenteral nutrition: clinical analysis of three cases. JPEN J Parenter Enteral Nutr 1989;13(4):421–5.

18. Hurwitz M, Garcia MG, Poole RL, et al. Copper deficiency during parenteral nutrition: a report of four pediatric cases. Nutr Clin Pract 2004;19(3):305–8.

19. Miki H, Kuwayama Y, Hara T, et al. Copper deficiency with pancytopenia, bradycardia and neurologic symptoms. Rinsho Ketsueki 2007;48(3):212–6 [in Japanese].

20. Dowling RH. Compensatory changes in intestinal absorption. Br Med Bull 1967;23(3):275–8.

21. Booth CC, Alldis D, Read AE. Studies on the site of fat absorption: 2 Fat balances after resection of varying amounts of the small intestine in man. Gut 1961;2(2):168–74.

22. Ehrlein H, Haas-Deppe B. Comparison of absorption of nutrients and secretion of water between oligomeric and polymeric enteral diets in pigs. Br J Nutr 1998;80(6):545–53.

23. McDonnell M, Dawson D. Pathophysiology of diarrhea. In: Henderson J, editor. Lippincott's pathophysiology series: gastrointestinal pathophysiology. Philadelphia, New York: Lippincott - Raven; 1996. p. 71–110.

24. Quiros-Tejeira RE, Ament ME, Reyen L, et al. Long-term parenteral nutritional support and intestinal adaptation in children with short bowel syndrome: a 25-year experience [see comment]. J Pediatr 2004;145(2):157–63.

25. Kles KA, Chang EB. Short-chain fatty acids impact on intestinal adaptation, inflammation, carcinoma, and failure [see comment]. Gastroenterology 2006; 130(2 Suppl 1):S100–5.

26. Feldman EJ, Dowling RH, McNaughton J, et al. Effects of oral versus intravenous nutrition on intestinal adaptation after small bowel resection in the dog. Gastroenterology 1976;70(5 PT1):712–9.

27. Kelly DA. Intestinal failure-associated liver disease: what do we know today? [see comment]. Gastroenterology 2006;130(2 Suppl 1):S70–7.

28. Parker P, Stroop S, Greene H. A controlled comparison of continuous versus intermittent feeding in the treatment of infants with intestinal disease. J Pediatr 1981;99(3):360–4.

29. Joly F, Dray X, Corcos O, et al. Tube feeding improves intestinal absorption in short bowel syndrome patients. Gastroenterology 2009;136(3):824–31.

30. Vanderhoof JA, Young RJ. Enteral and parenteral nutrition in the care of patients with short-bowel syndrome. Best Pract Res Clin Gastroenterol 2003;17(6): 997–1015.

31. Wessel JJ, Kocoshis SA. Nutritional management of infants with short bowel syndrome. Semin Perinatol 2007;31(2):104–11.

32. Jaksic T, Shew SB, Keshen TH, et al. Do critically ill surgical neonates have increased energy expenditure? J Pediatr Surg 2001;36(1):63–7.

33. FAO/WHO/UNU. Human Energy Requirements: Report of a Joint FAO/WHO/UNU Expert Committee; 2004.

34. Beghin L, Michaud L, Hankard R, et al. Total energy expenditure and physical activity in children treated with home parenteral nutrition. Pediatr Res 2003; 53(4):684–90.

35. Justino SR, Dias MC, Maculevicius J, et al. Basal energy expenditure and diet-induced modifications to thermogenesis in short bowel syndrome. Clin Nutr 2005;24(1):38–46.

36. Cosnes J, Lamy P, Beaugerie L, et al. Adaptive hyperphagia in patients with postsurgical malabsorption. Gastroenterology 1990;99(6):1814–9.

37. Woolf GM, Miller C, Kurian R, et al. Nutritional absorption in short bowel syndrome. Evaluation of fluid, calorie, and divalent cation requirements. Dig Dis Sci 1987;32(1):8–15.

38. Bier DM, Brosnan JT, Flatt JP, et al. Report of the IDECG Working Group on lower and upper limits of carbohydrate and fat intake. International Dietary Energy Consultative Group. Eur J Clin Nutr 1999;53(Suppl 1):S177–8.

39. Weber E, Ehrlein HJ. Composition of enteral diets and meals providing optimal absorption rates of nutrients in mini pigs. Am J Clin Nutr 1999; 69(3):556–63.

40. FAO/WHO/UNU. Expert consultation. Energy and protein requirements. World Health Organ Tech Rep Ser 1985;724:71–112.

41. Zemel BS, Riley EM, Stallings VA. Evaluation of methodology for nutritional assessment in children: anthropometry, body composition, and energy expenditure. Annu Rev Nutr 1997;17:211–35.

42. Newcomer AD, McGill DB. Distribution of disaccharidase activity in the small bowel of normal and lactase-deficient subjects. Gastroenterology 1966;51(4): 481–8.

43. Marteau P, Messing B, Arrigoni E, et al. Do patients with short-bowel syndrome need a lactose-free diet? Nutrition 1997;13(1):13–6.

44. Gausseres N, Mahe S, Benamouzig R, et al. The gastro-ileal digestion of 15N-labelled pea nitrogen in adult humans. Br J Nutr 1996;76(1):75–85.

45. Andorsky DJ, Lund DP, Lillehei CW, et al. Nutritional and other postoperative management of neonates with short bowel syndrome correlates with clinical outcomes [see comment]. J Pediatr 2001;139(1):27–33.
46. Bines J, Francis D, Hill D. Reducing parenteral requirement in children with short bowel syndrome: impact of an amino acid-based complete infant formula [see comment]. J Pediatr Gastroenterol Nutr 1998;26(2):123–8.
47. Friedman M. Nutritional value of proteins from different food sources. A review. J Agric Food Chem 1996;44:6–29.
48. Ovesen L, Chu R, Howard L. The influence of dietary fat on jejunostomy output in patients with severe short bowel syndrome. Am J Clin Nutr 1983;38(2): 270–7.
49. Nightingale JM. The medical management of intestinal failure: methods to reduce the severity. Proc Nutr Soc 2003;62(3):703–10.
50. Boncompain-Gerard M, Robert D, Fouque D, et al. Renal function and urinary excretion of electrolytes in patients receiving cyclic parenteral nutrition. JPEN J Parenter Enteral Nutr 2000;24(4):234–9.
51. Larchet M, Garabedian M, Bourdeau A, et al. Calcium metabolism in children during long-term total parenteral nutrition: the influence of calcium, phosphorus, and vitamin D intakes. J Pediatr Gastroenterol Nutr 1991;13(4):367–75.
52. Bronner F, Pansu D. Nutritional aspects of calcium absorption. J Nutr 1999; 129(1):9–12.
53. Schuette SA, Knowles JB, Ford HE. Effect of lactose or its component sugars on jejunal calcium absorption in adult man. Am J Clin Nutr 1989;50(5): 1084–7.
54. Ladefoged K, Olgaard K. Sodium homeostasis after small-bowel resection. Scand J Gastroenterol 1985;20(3):361–9.
55. Lennard-Jones JE. Review article: practical management of the short bowel. Aliment Pharmacol Ther 1994;8(6):563–77.
56. Svaninger G, Nordgren S, Palselius IR, et al. Sodium and potassium excretion in patients with ileostomies. Eur J Surg 1991;157(10):601–5.
57. Unwin RJ, Moss S, Peart WS, et al. Renal adaptation and gut hormone release during sodium restriction in ileostomized man. Clin Sci (Lond) 1985;69(3): 299–308.
58. Spiller RC, Jones BJ, Silk DB. Jejunal water and electrolyte absorption from two proprietary enteral feeds in man: importance of sodium content. Gut 1987;28(6): 681–7.
59. Ehrlein H, Haas-Deppe B, Weber E. The sodium concentration of enteral diets does not influence absorption of nutrients but induces intestinal secretion of water in miniature pigs. J Nutr 1999;129(2):410–8.
60. Nightingale JM, Lennard-Jones JE, Walker ER, et al. Oral salt supplements to compensate for jejunostomy losses: comparison of sodium chloride capsules, glucose electrolyte solution, and glucose polymer electrolyte solution. Gut 1992;33(6):759–61.
61. World Health Organization, D.D.C.P. ANNEX 2: Tables for calculating concentrations of sodium and glucose. Available at: http://whqlibdoc.who.int/HQ/1987/WHO_CDD_SER_87.10.pdf. Accessed May 28, 2009.
62. Agarwal R, Afzalpurkar R, Fordtran JS. Pathophysiology of potassium absorption and secretion by the human intestine. Gastroenterology 1994;107(2): 548–71.
63. Perez GO, Oster JR, Rogers A. Acid-base disturbances in gastrointestinal disease. Dig Dis Sci 1987;32(9):1033–43.

64. Dahhak S, Uhlen S, Mention K, et al. D-lactic acidosis in a child with short bowel syndrome. Arch Pediatr 2008;15(2):145–8.
65. Puwanant M, Mo-Suwan L, Patrapinyokul S. Recurrent D-lactic acidosis in a child with short bowel syndrome. Asia Pac J Clin Nutr 2005;14(2):195–8.
66. Valman HB, Roberts PD. Vitamin B12 absorption after resection of ileum in childhood. Arch Dis Child 1974;49(12):932–5.
67. Davies BW, Abel G, Puntis JW, et al. Limited ileal resection in infancy: the long-term consequences. J Pediatr Surg 1999;34(4):583–7.
68. Skidmore MD, Shenker N, Kliegman RM, et al. Biochemical evidence of asymptomatic vitamin B12 deficiency in children after ileal resection for necrotizing enterocolitis. J Pediatr 1989;115(1):102–5.
69. Neale G, Gompertz D, Schonsby H, et al. The metabolic and nutritional consequences of bacterial overgrowth in the small intestine. Am J Clin Nutr 1972; 25(12):1409–17.
70. Giannella RA, Broitman SA, Zamcheck N. Competition between bacteria and intrinsic factor for vitamin B 12: implications for vitamin B 12 malabsorption in intestinal bacterial overgrowth. Gastroenterology 1972;62(2):255–60.
71. Bradford GS, Taylor CT. Omeprazole and vitamin B12 deficiency. Ann Pharmacother 1999;33(5):641–3.
72. Dharmarajan TS, Norkus EP. Approaches to vitamin B12 deficiency. Early treatment may prevent devastating complications. Postgrad Med 2001;110(1):99–105 [quiz: 6].
73. Holleland G, Schneede J, Ueland PM, et al. Cobalamin deficiency in general practice. Assessment of the diagnostic utility and cost-benefit analysis of methylmalonic acid determination in relation to current diagnostic strategies. Clin Chem 1999;45(2):189–98.
74. Stabler SP, Allen RH, Savage DG, et al. Clinical spectrum and diagnosis of cobalamin deficiency [see comment]. Blood 1990;76(5):871–81.
75. Snow CF. Laboratory diagnosis of vitamin B12 and folate deficiency: a guide for the primary care physician [see comment]. Arch Intern Med 1999;159(12):1289–98.
76. Sentongo TA, Azzam R, Charrow J. Vitamin B12 status, methylmalonic acidemia, and bacterial overgrowth in short bowel syndrome. J Pediatr Gastroenterol Nutr 2009;48(4):495–7.
77. Hillman RS. Hematopoietic agents: growth factors, minerals, and vitamins. In: Hardman JG, Limbird LE, Molinoff PB, et al, editors. Goodman & Gilman's the pharmacological basis of therapeutics. 9th edition. New York: McGraw-Hill; 1996. p. 1311–40.
78. Halsted CH. Intestinal absorption and malabsorption of folates. Annu Rev Med 1980;31:79–87.
79. Camilo E, Zimmerman J, Mason JB, et al. Folate synthesized by bacteria in the human upper small intestine is assimilated by the host. Gastroenterology 1996; 110(4):991–8.
80. Russell RM, Krasinski SD, Samloff IM, et al. Folic acid malabsorption in atrophic gastritis. Possible compensation by bacterial folate synthesis. Gastroenterology 1986;91(6):1476–82.
81. Anonymous. Food and Drug Administration. Food standards: amendment of standards of identity for enriched grain products to require addition of folic acid. Fed Regist 1996;61:8781–97.
82. Pfeiffer CM, Caudill SP, Gunter EW, et al. Biochemical indicators of B vitamin status in the US population after folic acid fortification: results from the National Health and Nutrition Examination Survey 1999–2000 [see comment]. Am J Clin Nutr 2005;82(2):442–50.

83. Pfeiffer CM, Johnson CL, Jain RB, et al. Trends in blood folate and vitamin B-12 concentrations in the United States, 1988–2004 [see comment]. Am J Clin Nutr 2007;86(3):718–27.

84. Pomeranz S, Gimmon Z, Ben Zvi A, et al. Parenteral nutrition-induced anaphylaxis. JPEN J Parenter Enteral Nutr 1987;11(3):314–5.

85. Bullock L, Etchason E, Fitzgerald JF, et al. Case report of an allergic reaction to parenteral nutrition in a pediatric patient. JPEN J Parenter Enteral Nutr 1990; 14(1):98–100.

86. Greene HL, Hambidge KM, Schanler R, et al. Guidelines for the use of vitamins, trace elements, calcium, magnesium, and phosphorus in infants and children receiving total parenteral nutrition: report of the subcommittee on pediatric parenteral nutrient requirements from the committee on clinical practice issues of the American Society for Clinical Nutrition. Am J Clin Nutr 1988;48(5): 1324–42.

87. A.S.P.E.N. Parenteral nutrition handbook. In: Canada T, Crill C, Guenter P, editors. How to write parenteral nutrition orders. Silver Spring, (MD): Amercian Society for Parenteral and Enteral Nutrition; 2009.

88. Vitamins. In: Champe P, Harvey P, editors. Lippincott's Illustrated Reviews: Biochemistry. 2nd edition. J.B. Lippincott Company; 1994. p. 319–42.

89. Oriot D, Wood C, Gottesman R, et al. Severe lactic acidosis related to acute thiamine deficiency. JPEN J Parenter Enteral Nutr 1991;15(1):105–9.

90. Doolman R, Dinbar A, Sela BA. Improved measurement of transketolase activity in the assessment of "TPP effect". Eur J Clin Chem Clin Biochem 1995;33(7): 445–6.

91. Fuhrman MP, Herrmann V, Masidonski P, et al. Pancytopenia after removal of copper from total parenteral nutrition. JPEN J Parenter Enteral Nutr 2000; 24(6):361–6.

92. Howard L, Ashley C, Lyon D, et al. Autopsy tissue trace elements in 8 long-term parenteral nutrition patients who received the current U.S. Food and Drug Administration formulation. JPEN J Parenter Enteral Nutr 2007;31(5): 388–96.

93. Uauy R, Olivares M, Gonzalez M. Essentiality of copper in humans. Am J Clin Nutr 1998;67(5 Suppl):952S–9S.

94. Harvey LJ, Ashton K, Hooper L, et al. Methods of assessment of copper status in humans: a systematic review. Am J Clin Nutr 2009;89(6):2009S–24S.

95. King JC, Shames DM, Lowe NM, et al. Effect of acute zinc depletion on zinc homeostasis and plasma zinc kinetics in men. Am J Clin Nutr 2001;74(1):116–24.

96. McGill LC, Boas RN, Zerella JT. Extremity swelling in an infant with copper and zinc deficiency. J Pediatr Surg 1980;15(6):746–7.

97. Lowe NM, Fekete K, Decsi T. Methods of assessment of zinc status in humans: a systematic review. Am J Clin Nutr 2009;89(6):2040S–51S.

98. Ishida T, Himeno K, Torigoe Y, et al. Selenium deficiency in a patient with Crohn's disease receiving long-term total parenteral nutrition. Intern Med 2003;42(2): 154–7.

99. Ashton K, Hooper L, Harvey LJ, et al. Methods of assessment of selenium status in humans: a systematic review. Am J Clin Nutr 2009;89(6):2025S–39S.

100. Zeisel SH. Choline: an essential nutrient for humans. Nutrition 2000;16(7-8): 669–71.

101. Ilcol YO, Ozbek R, Hamurtekin E, et al. Choline status in newborns, infants, children, breast-feeding women, breast-fed infants and human breast milk. J Nutr Biochem 2005;16(8):489–99.

102. Holmes-McNary MQ, Cheng WL, Mar MH, et al. Choline and choline esters in human and rat milk and in infant formulas. Am J Clin Nutr 1996;64(4):572–6.
103. Fischer LM, Scearce JA, Mar M-H, et al. Ad libitum choline intake in healthy individuals meets or exceeds the proposed adequate intake level. J Nutr 2005; 135(4):826–9.
104. Chawla RK, Berry CJ, Kutner MH, et al. Plasma concentrations of transsulfuration pathway products during nasoenteral and intravenous hyperalimentation of malnourished patients. Am J Clin Nutr 1985;42(4):577–84.
105. Koppe SWP, Sahai A, Malladi P, et al. Pentoxifylline attenuates steatohepatitis induced by the methionine choline deficient diet. J Hepatol 2004;41(4):592–8.
106. Sundaram SS, Whitington PF, Green RM. Steatohepatitis develops rapidly in transgenic mice overexpressing Abcb11 and fed a methionine-choline-deficient diet. Am J Physiol Gastrointest Liver Physiol 2005;288(6):G1321–7.
107. Zeisel SH, Blusztajn JK. Choline and human nutrition. Annu Rev Nutr 1994;14: 269–96.
108. Sentongo TA, Kumar P, Karza K, et al. Whole blood free choline and choline metabolites in infants who require chronic parenteral nutrition therapy. J Pediatr Gastroenterol Nutr, in press.
109. Hyman PE, Everett SL, Harada T. Gastric acid hypersecretion in short bowel syndrome in infants: association with extent of resection and enteral feeding. J Pediatr Gastroenterol Nutr 1986;5(2):191–7.
110. Hyman PE, Garvey TQ 3rd, Harada T. Effect of ranitidine on gastric acid hypersecretion in an infant with short bowel syndrome. J Pediatr Gastroenterol Nutr 1985;4(2):316–9.
111. Ruscin JM, Page RL 2nd, Valuck RJ. Vitamin B(12) deficiency associated with histamine(2)-receptor antagonists and a proton-pump inhibitor. Ann Pharmacother 2002;36(5):812–6.
112. Bhat RV, Deshmukh CT. A study of Vitamin K status in children on prolonged antibiotic therapy. Indian Pediatr 2003;40(1):36–40.
113. West RJ, Lloyd JK. The effect of cholestyramine on intestinal absorption. Gut 1975;16(2):93–8.
114. Navaneethan SD, Sankarasubbaiyan S, Gross MD, et al. Tacrolimus-associated hypomagnesemia in renal transplant recipients. Transplant Proc 2006;38(5): 1320–2.
115. Rudolph CD, Hyman PE, Altschuler SM, et al. Diagnosis and treatment of chronic intestinal pseudo-obstruction in children: report of consensus workshop. J Pediatr Gastroenterol Nutr 1997;24(1):102–12.
116. Thurnham DI, Davies JA, Crump BJ, et al. The use of different lipids to express serum tocopherol: lipid ratios for the measurement of vitamin E status. Ann Clin Biochem 1986;23(Pt 5):514–20.

Refeeding Syndrome

Judy Fuentebella, MD*, John A. Kerner, MD

KEYWORDS

- Refeeding syndrome • Pediatric • Hypophosphatemia
- Nutrition support • Malnutrition

Refeeding syndrome (RFS) is a term that describes the metabolic and clinical changes that occur on aggressive nutritional rehabilitation of a malnourished patient. It is a well-described yet often underrecognized entity. Its recognition was heightened in the World War II era when prisoners who had undergone starvation developed cardiac failure and peripheral edema on nutritional replenishment.[1] In Leningrad and The Netherlands, cases of cardiac insufficiency and edema were reported after refeeding survivors of the war who were starved because of scant food supplies.[2] In 1944, Keys and colleagues deliberately starved and refed previously healthy men and observed cardiac decompensation in some patients who were orally fed.[2,3] In the 1960s, the advent of parenteral nutrition (PN) allowed for a more aggressive means of nutritional rehabilitation. Reports of hypophosphatemic hyperalimentation syndrome soon followed in the 1970s. In 1980, Silvis and colleagues[4] noted paresthesias, seizures, or coma in conjunction with hypophosphatemia in patients receiving PN. In the 1980s, Weinsier and Krumdieck[5] wrote a critical paper that described cardiopulmonary complications resulting in the death of two chronically undernourished patients who received PN.

Hypophosphatemia is the hallmark of RFS. Other electrolyte abnormalities are associated with RFS, however, such as hypokalemia and hypomagnesemia. Shifts in glucose, sodium, and fluid balance are also seen in RFS. Consequently, cardiovascular, pulmonary, neuromuscular, hematologic, and gastrointestinal complications occur. This syndrome can emerge with aggressive oral nutrition, enteral nutrition, or PN and can be fatal if not recognized and treated in a timely manner.

PATHOPHYSIOLOGY OF STARVATION

During starvation, the body tries to compensate for the lack of energy by means of changes in metabolism and hormone regulation. The body goes into a state of

This work was supported in part by the Carl and Patricia Dierkes Endowed Fund for Nutrition Support and Home Care.

Division of Pediatric Gastroenterology, Hepatology, and Nutrition, Lucile Packard Children's Hospital, Stanford University Medical Center, 750 Welch Road, Suite 116, Palo Alto, CA 94304, USA

* Corresponding author.

E-mail address: judyf@stanford.edu (J. Fuentebella).

doi:10.1016/j.pcl.2009.06.006
pediatric.theclinics.com

catabolism. A shift from carbohydrate metabolism to fat and protein catabolism occurs, which provides glucose and ketones for energy. This shift to protein catabolism results in a loss of lean body mass, which affects major organs, such as the heart, lungs, intestines, liver, and kidneys. Atrophy of the myocardium results in poor contractility and diminished cardiac output. Liver wasting results in decreased protein synthesis and further alteration in metabolism. Gastrointestinal atrophy causes malabsorption and dysmotility, further exacerbating the malnourished state, and increases the risk for infection. The kidneys also lose their ability to concentrate urine, resulting in diuresis.[6–8]

Cellular mass is also lost, contributing to functional loss of vital organs. Intracellular loss of electrolytes, including potassium, magnesium, and phosphate, occurs as a consequence of this change in metabolism. Insulin secretion decreases and the basal metabolic rate slows down to 20% to 25% to conserve energy.[8] Consequently, the body becomes bradycardic, hypothermic, and hypotensive. Growth and thyroid hormones also decrease.[6] These changes occur in an effort to conserve protein and organ function, which aids in survival. It is important to understand the pathophysiology of starvation and the metabolic shifts that occur, especially when one is about to feed a patient in this state.

PATHOPHYSIOLOGY OF REFEEDING SYNDROME

Once nutrition is reintroduced to a patient who has been starved for an extended period, anabolism begins instantaneously. The body shifts back to carbohydrate metabolism from protein and fat catabolism, and glucose becomes the primary source of energy once again. The increased glucose load, with a corresponding increase in the release of insulin, leads to cellular uptake of glucose, potassium, magnesium, and phosphate. This shift of electrolytes back into the cell causes hypokalemia, hypomagnesemia, and hypophosphatemia. Insulin also exhibits a natriuretic effect on the kidneys. Hence, sodium is retained, causing fluid retention and expansion of the extracellular fluid volume.[6–8]

Anabolism's high requirements may unveil or cause further deficiencies, which may lead to life-threatening circumstances. Rapid correction of undernutrition may cause fluid shifts and intravascular volume overload, which may precipitate congestive heart failure in an undernourished patient with myocardial atrophy.

DETERMINING PATIENTS AT RISK FOR REFEEDING SYNDROME

A critical step in preventing RFS is identifying patients who are at risk before initiating nutrition. These include patients with anorexia nervosa, chronic malnutrition, marasmus, or kwashiorkor; patients underfed or fasting for at least 10 to 14 days; prolonged fasting; prolonged intravenous hydration; and morbid obesity with massive weight loss (**Box 1**). There are several studies and case reports that describe refeeding hypophosphatemia and its consequences in patients with these conditions. Reports continue to emerge in the current literature documenting refeeding complications, notably in patients who have anorexia nervosa. Solomon and Kirby[9] commented that anorexia nervosa serves as a sobering model for the possible calamity inherent in refeeding severely malnourished hospitalized patients. Patients who weigh less than 80% of their ideal body weight or have recent weight loss of 5% to 10% in the past 1 to 2 months are also at risk. A study by Dunn and colleagues[10] showed that one of the most frequent identifiers for a pediatric patient at risk for RFS was a calculated body weight less than 80% of ideal body weight. Additional case reports have documented refeeding hypophosphatemia in children with less than 80% of ideal

---

Box 1
Patients at risk for refeeding syndrome

- Anorexia nervosa

- Less than 80% of ideal body weight

- Patients underfed or not fed for at least 10 to 14 days (including patients receiving prolonged intravenous fluids without adequate calories or protein)

- Acute weight loss of greater than 10% in the past 1 to 2 months (including obese patients with extensive weight loss in a short period)

- Kwashiorkor

- Marasmus

- Chronic conditions causing malnutrition (uncontrolled diabetes mellitus, cancer, congenital heart disease, and chronic liver disease)

- Malabsorptive syndromes (including inflammatory bowel disease, cystic fibrosis, chronic pancreatitis, and short bowel syndrome)

- Cerebral palsy and other conditions causing dysphagia

- Children of neglect

- Postoperative patients, including after bariatric surgery

Data from Refs.[4,6,7,12]

---

body weight. Worley and colleagues[11] describe refeeding hypophosphatemia in children with cerebral palsy and those who are abused and neglected. One recent study had cancer and congenital heart disease as the leading medical diagnoses in those found to have RFS.[10]

In the adult population, patients at risk include those admitted from nursing facilities; those with a history of excessive alcohol intake; and those with chronic diseases causing undernutrition, such as chronic obstructive pulmonary disease and cancer.[8]

INCIDENCE OF REFEEDING SYNDROME

In the past 40 years, the incidence of RFS in adults remains significant. Up to 50% of hospitalized patients are documented to be malnourished.[3] In a study of patients receiving total parenteral nutrition (TPN), the incidence of hypophosphatemia in patients receiving phosphorus ranged from 30% to 38%, and for patients receiving TPN without phosphorus, the incidence was 100%.[8] RFS is seen in up to 25% of adult patients who have cancer.[7,8] The true incidence of RFS in pediatrics in unknown, perhaps as a result of underrecognition or lack of reporting.

CLINICAL MANIFESTATIONS OF REFEEDING SYNDROME

Clinical manifestations of RFS are a direct result of the electrolyte and hormonal changes that occur as the basal metabolic rate rapidly increases. The patient may manifest signs and symptoms of hypophosphatemia, hypokalemia, hypomagnesemia, hyperglycemia, fluid overload, or thiamine deficiency (**Table 1**).

Hypophosphatemia

The one feature that characterizes RFS is hypophosphatemia. During the fasting state, catabolism results in depletion of intracellular phosphate. Rapid introduction of

Table 1
Clinical signs and symptoms of refeeding syndrome

Hypophosphatemia	Hypokalemia	Hypomagnesemia	Vitamin/Thiamine Deficiency	Sodium Retention	Hyperglycemia
Cardiac	Cardiac	Cardiac	Encephalopathy	Fluid overload	Cardiac
Hypotension	Arrhythmias	Arrhythmias	Lactic acidosis	Pulmonary edema	Hypotension
Decreased stroke volume	Respiratory	Neurologic	Death	Cardiac compromise	Respiratory
Respiratory	Failure	Weakness			Hypercapnea
Impaired diaphragm	Neurologic	Tremor			Failure
contractility	Weakness	Tetany			Other
Dyspnea	Paralysis	Seizures			Ketoacidosis
Respiratory failure	Gastrointestinal	Altered mental status			Coma
Neurologic	Nausea	Coma			Dehydration
Paresthesia	Vomiting	Gastrointestinal			Impaired immune
Weakness	Constipation	Nausea			function
Confusion	Muscular	Vomiting			
Disorientation	Rhabdomyolysis	Diarrhea			
Lethargy	Muscle necrosis	Other			
Areflexic paralysis	Other	Refractory hypokalemia			
Seizures	Death	and hypocalcemia			
Coma		Death			
Hematologic					
Leukocyte dysfunction					
Hemolysis					
Thrombocytopenia					
Other					
Death					

Data from Kraft MD, Btaiche IF, Sacks GS. Review of RFS. Nutr Clin Pract 2005;20:625–33.

carbohydrate into the body inhibits fat metabolism and favors glucose metabolism, which causes an insulin surge, promoting cellular uptake and use of glucose and phosphate. The combination of depletion of total body phosphorus stores during catabolic starvation and increased cellular influx of phosphorus during anabolic refeeding leads to severe extracellular (serum) hypophosphatemia.[9] Additionally, when glucose once again becomes the predominant fuel source, a high demand occurs for the production of phosphorylated intermediates of glycolysis (ie, red blood cell ATP, 2-3-diphosphoglycerate [DPG]).[13] Low serum phosphorus levels are directly related to the depletion of ATP and DPG.[9] ATP and DPG are crucial to all processes in the body that depend on energy. Hypophosphatemia can impair neuromuscular function, and the patient may exhibit weakness, impaired muscular contractility, paresthesia, cramps, and seizures. Respiratory muscles can be affected, causing poor ventilatory function and respiratory compromise. Severe hypophosphatemia is also associated with rhabdomyolysis, hemolysis, thrombocytopenia, and leukocyte dysfunction. Psychologic changes include confusion, altered mental status, and coma.[11,13,14] As reported in several cases, even small decreases in serum phosphorus during this delicate state can result in large-scale dysfunction and affect virtually all systems in the body.[15] Refeeding hypophosphatemia can occur within 24 to 72 hours of introducing nutrition.[10] Several papers note the nadir of phosphorus to occur within the first week of refeeding.[12,13]

Hypokalemia

Potassium, which is the major intracellular ion, is also depleted during the catabolic state of starvation. With refeeding, increased insulin secretion leads to cellular uptake of potassium, resulting in hypokalemia. The electrochemical membrane potential is imbalanced, causing arrhythmias and cardiac arrest. Neuromuscular dysfunction, such as weakness, paresthesia, rhabdomyolysis, and respiratory failure, can occur.[10,13]

Hypomagnesemia

The physiology of hypomagnesemia is similar to that of phosphorus and potassium. Magnesium affects membrane potentials, and its imbalance presents in similar ways as hypokalemia. It is also important for the structural integrity of DNA, RNA, and ribosomes and serves as a cofactor for enzymes involved in ATP production and oxidative phosphorylation. Thus, the demand for magnesium increases as the metabolic rate increases. Hypomagnesemia manifests neurologically with weakness, tremors, tetany, seizures, and altered mental status; with cardiac arrhythmias; and with gastrointestinal symptoms, such as nausea, vomiting, and diarrhea. Low magnesium levels may also induce hypokalemia because of impaired Na^+/K^+-ATPase activity. Magnesium is required for parathyroid function, and low levels may induce hypocalcemia.[6,13,15]

Sodium Retention

Sodium retention is also seen in RFS. The infusion of carbohydrates leads to increased insulin secretion. Insulin causes decreased renal excretion of sodium and water. Patients may then develop fluid overload, pulmonary edema, and congestive cardiac failure. Low serum albumin may also contribute to edema during refeeding as a result of low oncotic pressure.[7,10,13,15]

Vitamin Deficiency: Thiamine

Vitamin deficiencies also occur because of inadequate intake. Deficiency in thiamine (vitamin B_1) has important consequences during refeeding. It is an important cofactor for enzymes needed in carbohydrate metabolism, and it is rapidly consumed in glycolysis during refeeding. Deficiency can occur in less than 28 days, because its half-life is 9.5 to 18.5 days.[8] Low levels of thiamine impair glucose metabolism and result in lactic acidosis. Further, thiamine deficiency may result in Wernicke's encephalopathy or Korsakoff's syndrome. Wernicke's encephalopathy is manifested by ataxia, confusion, hypothermia, ocular abnormalities, and coma. Korsakoff's syndrome is associated with amnesia and confabulation.[13-15] Of note, adequate magnesium levels are required for the active form of thiamine.[8]

Hyperglycemia

Administration of glucose in excess amounts leads to hyperglycemia; a high glucose load stops gluconeogenesis and leads to decreased use of amino acids. Thus, the body's ability to metabolize glucose is decreased. Further, a starved patient who is refed is experiencing a stress response that increases circulation of glucocorticoids, exacerbating hyperglycemia.[7] Elevated serum glucose may lead to osmotic diuresis, dehydration, hypotension, metabolic acidosis, and ketoacidosis. Another sequela is lipogenesis, attributable to insulin stimulation, which results in fatty liver, increased carbon dioxide production, hypercapnia, and respiratory failure.[15] Complications of hyperglycemia also include impaired immune function and increased risk for infection. Prolonged hyperglycemia may result in hyperosmolar, hyperglycemic, nonketotic coma.[2,7]

MANAGEMENT OF REFEEDING SYNDROME

There are several recommendations in initiating nutritional support. Regardless of the strategy, a gradual introduction of feeds is recommended. Proposed ranges for starting feeds include 25% to 75% of resting energy expenditure.[2,3,6-8,10,13-15] In adults, reports recommend starting at 20 kcal/kg/d or 1000 kcal/d.[2,8] In pediatric and adult patients, calorie intake is increased 10% to 25% per day or over 4 to 7 days until the calorie goal is met.[10] Advancement of nutrition is based on biochemical stability. The saying "start low, and go slow" serves as a good guideline in approaching a malnourished patient.

Protein is not restricted during nutritional support. Several studies show that high protein intake spares lean muscle mass and helps in its restoration.[3]

Sodium and fluids should be restricted during the initial period of refeeding to prevent fluid overload, especially in a patient at risk for RFS, whose cardiac function may be compromised. Palesty and Dudrick[3] recommend restricting sodium to 20 mEq/d and total fluid to 1000 mL/d or less.

Electrolyte deficiencies should be corrected before starting enteral or parenteral support (Tables 2–4). Of note, the National Institute for Health and Clinical Excellence 2006 guidelines in England and Wales state that correction of fluid and electrolyte abnormalities need not be done before refeeding and can be done while refeeding.[15] Most other investigators advocate correcting electrolyte imbalances before feeding a patient, however. Further, in light of reports of persistent biochemical imbalances despite conservative measures, correcting these abnormalities is prudent before initiating feeds. Miller[2] pointed out that refeeding hypophosphatemia can still occur despite cautious introduction of carbohydrate. Dunn and colleagues[10] also demonstrated similar findings in pediatric patients who showed electrolyte imbalances

Table 2
Guidelines for phosphate replacement

	Intravenous Replacement Dose (Administer Over 6–12 Hours)
Children	0.08–0.24 mmol/kg Maximum single dose: 15 mmol Maximum daily dose: 1.5 mmol/kg
Adults	Initial dose: 0.08 mmol/kg if recent uncomplicated or mild hypophosphatemia[a] 0.16 mmol/kg if prolonged or severe hypophosphatemia[b] Increase dose by 25%–50% if persistent hypophosphatemia Maximum dose: 0.24 mmol/kg per dose

Oral absorption may be unreliable, and the oral form may cause diarrhea.
Serum phosphate should be obtained 2 to 4 hours after completion of infusion.
Patients with impaired renal function should start at 50% or less of the initial dose.[13]
[a] Mild hypophosphatemia: 2.3 to 2.7 mg/dL, moderate hypophosphatemia: 1.5 to 2.2 mg/dL.
[b] Severe hypophosphatemia: less than 1.5 mg/dL. This level of hypophosphatemia can lead to severe neurologic, cardiac, respiratory, and hematologic abnormalities and possibly to death.[13]
Data from Huang T, Wo S, et al. 2007–2009 Housestaff manual Lucile Packard Children's Hospital at Stanford. 8th edition. Hudson (OH): Lexi-Comp, Inc; p. 564–5.

despite using conservative guidelines for nutritional support. Depletion of phosphate in severely malnourished patients is the likely culprit, and higher requirements may be needed. Supplements for potassium and magnesium may be required as well. Sodium and fluid should be limited, however, because there is an inclination to retain these during the initial feeding period. Daily measurement of electrolytes is recommended until stability is met. Weekly prealbumin and albumin levels have also been suggested. Supplementation with multivitamins and thiamine is advisable (**Table 5**).

Close monitoring can help to avoid or minimize the complications of RFS. A patient should be placed on a cardiorespiratory monitor during the initial phase of nutritional support. A patient's neuromuscular and mental status should be assessed on a regular basis. Fluid intake and output should also be carefully measured to avoid fluid overload and its potential sequelae to the cardiorespiratory system. Checking daily weight also ensures proper fluid balance; the goal of weight gain should be no more than 1 kg/wk. Any weight gain greater than this is likely attributable to fluid retention.

Table 3
Guidelines for magnesium replacement

	Intravenous Replacement Dose (Administer Over 4 Hours)
Children	25–50 mg/kg per dose (0.2–0.4 mEq/kg per dose) Maximum single dose: 2000 mg (16 mEq)
Adults	1 g every 6 hours for four doses for mild-moderate hypomagnesemia 8–12 g/d in divided doses for severe hypomagnesemia

Replacement is in the form of magnesium sulfate.
Patients with impaired renal function should start at 50% or less of the initial dose.
Mild hypomagnesemia: 1.5 to 1.8 mg/dL.
Moderate hypomagnesemia: 1 to 1.5 mg/dL.
Severe hypomagnesemia: less than 1 mg/dL.[13]
Data from Huang T, Wo S, et al. 2007–2009 Housestaff manual Lucile Packard Children's Hospital at Stanford. 8th edition. Hudson (OH): Lexi-Comp, Inc; p. 562–4.

Table 4
Guidelines for potassium replacement

	Intravenous Replacement Dose (Administer Over at Least 1 Hour)
Children	0.3–0.5 mEq/kg per dose Maximum dose: 30 mEq per dose
Adults	0.3–0.5 mEq/kg per dose Maximum dose: 30 mEq per dose

Serum potassium should be obtained within 2 hours of completion of infusion.
Ensure that urine output is greater than 0.5 mL/kg/h and that patient is on a cardiac monitor.
Mild to moderate hypokalemia: 2.5 to 3.4 mEq/L.
Severe hypokalemia: less than 2.5 mEq/L or if symptomatic.[13]
Data from Huang T, Wo S, et al. 2007–2009 Housestaff manual Lucile Packard Children's Hospital at Stanford. 8th edition. Hudson (OH): Lexi-Comp, Inc; p. 562–4.

Should the signs and symptoms of RFS emerge, nutritional support should be stopped immediately. Electrolyte abnormalities should be corrected without delay, and supportive measures should be administered, such as the administration of intravenous thiamine for encephalopathy, vasopressors for hypotension, oxygen for respiratory distress, and diuretics for fluid overload. Once these conditions are addressed, nutrition can be restarted. Previous publications recommend restarting nutrition at 50% or less of the previous rate that led to the development of symptoms.[3,13] Health care providers should examine the patient frequently for signs and symptoms of refeeding phenomena. Electrolyte abnormalities usually occur within the first days of initiating feeds, cardiac complications occur within the first week, and altered mental status typically occurs thereafter.[12]

Table 5
Guidelines for thiamine replacement

	Beriberi or Thiamine Deficiency	Deficiency After Bariatric Surgery	Wernicke's Encephalopathy (use Intravenous form)	Dietary Supplement
Children	10–25 mg/d administered IV or IM if extremely ill or 10–50 mg per dose administered PO every day for 2 weeks and then 5–10 mg/d for 1 month	(adolescents) 50 mg/d		0.5–1 mg/d
Adults	5–30 mg per dose 3 times per day, administered IV or IM if extremely ill, and then 5–30 mg/d administered PO for 1 month		Initial:100 mg IV followed by 50–100 mg/d until regular diet resumes	1–2 mg/d

Abbreviations: IM, intramuscular; IV, intravenous; PO, per os.
Data from Huang T, Wo S, et al. 2007–2009 Housestaff manual Lucile Packard Children's Hospital at Stanford. 8th edition. Hudson (OH); Lexi-Comp, Inc; p. 661.

Caring for a malnourished patient requires a well-coordinated multidisciplinary team for optimal results. Nutrition support teams may not be available in some institutions, however. Therefore, raising and maintaining awareness of the dangers of aggressively feeding a starved patient is imperative. Further, it is essential to review the patient's actual nutritional intake (which includes additional glucose, sodium, and fluids in medications) and to compare it with the intended nutritional orders for the patient. Discrepancies between the actual and intended nutritional intake may put the patient at risk, as shown in a study conducted by Dunn and colleagues.[10]

In facing a malnourished patient, there is an instinctive drive for health care providers to re-establish nutrition as rapidly as possible. Starvation develops over time as the body attempts to adapt to the lack of adequate calories and does not occur over a period of hours. Therefore, treatment should not be executed with haste. The pivotal article by Weinsier and Krumdieck[5] opened our eyes to the dangers of aggressive refeeding, and many subsequent papers have continued to echo the same message. Yet, the incidence of refeeding remains significant.[3,7,16] Improved awareness and understanding of RFS, along with a well-coordinated plan of care, are vital in delivering safe and effective nutritional rehabilitation.

SUMMARY

RFS is the result of aggressive enteral or parenteral feeding in a malnourished patient. Hypophosphatemia is the hallmark of RFS. Other metabolic abnormalities, such as hypokalemia and hypomagnesemia, may also occur, along with sodium and fluid retention. Refeeding should be started at a low caloric requirement and advanced slowly only in the setting of metabolic stability. Important in management is close monitoring of signs and symptoms of RFS, in addition to monitoring electrolyte levels while providing electrolyte replacement and vitamin supplementation as needed. Identifying patients at risk for RFS is key to prevention, and awareness of the potential complications involved in reintroducing feeds to an undernourished patient is crucial.

ACKNOWLEDGMENTS

The authors acknowledge Scott Sutherland, MD, for his assistance in the preparation of this article.

REFERENCES

1. Brozek J, Chapman CB, Keys A. Drastic food restriction: effect on cardiovascular dynamics in normotensive and hypertensive conditions. JAMA 1948;137: 1569–74.
2. Miller SJ. Death resulting from overzealous total parenteral nutrition: the refeeding syndrome revisited. Nutr Clin Pract 2008;23(2):166–71.
3. Palesty JA, Dudrick SJ. The Goldilocks paradigm of starvation and refeeding. Nutr Clin Pract 2006;21:147–54.
4. Silvis SE, DiBartolomeo AG, Aaker HM. Hypophosphatemia and neurological changes secondary to oral caloric intake: a variant of hyperalimentation syndrome. Am J Gastroenterol 1980;73:215–22.
5. Weinsier RL, Krumdieck CL. Death resulting from overzealous total parenteral nutrition: the RFS revisited. Am J Clin Nutr 1981;34:393–9.
6. Kerner JA, Hattner JT. Malnutrition and refeeding syndrome in children. In: Hark L, Harrison G, editors. Medical nutrition and disease: a case-based approach. 4th edition. Philadelphia: Wiley-Blackwell; 2009. p. 182–7.

7. Lauts NM. Management of the patient with refeeding syndrome. J Infus Nurs 2005;28(5):337–42.
8. McCray S, Walker S, Parrish CR. Much ado about refeeding. Pract Gastroenterol 2005;29(1):26–44.
9. Solomon SM, Kirby DF. The refeeding syndrome: a review. JPEN J Parenter Enteral Nutr 1990;14:90–7.
10. Dunn RL, Stettler N, Mascarenhas MR. Refeeding syndrome in hospitalized pediatric patients. Nutr Clin Pract 2003;18:327–32.
11. Worley G, Claerhout SJ, Combs SP. Hypophosphatemia in malnourished children during refeeding. Clin Pediatr 1988;37:347–52.
12. Malone AM, Brewer CK. Monitoring for efficacy, complications, and toxicity. Clinical nutrition enteral and tube feeding. 4th edition. Philadelphia: Elsevier Saunders; 1997. p. 286–7.
13. Kraft MD, Btaiche IF, Sacks GS. Review of refeeding syndrome. Nutr Clin Pract 2005;20:625–33.
14. Sobotka L. Refeeding syndrome. Basics in clinical nutrition. 3rd edition. Prague: Galen; 2004. p. 288–90.
15. Mehanna HM, Moledina J, Travis J. Refeeding syndrome: what it is, and how to prevent and treat it. BMJ 2008;336:1495–8.
16. Hernandez-Aranda JC, Gallo-Chico B, Luna-Cruz ML, et al. Malnutrition and total parenteral nutrition: a cohort study to determine the incidence of refeeding syndrome. Rev Gastroenterol Mex 1997;62(4):260–5.

Drug-Induced Nutrient Deficiencies

Lina Felípez, MD, Timothy A. Sentongo, MD*

KEYWORDS

- Pharmacogenomics • Adverse drug reactions
- Nutrient deficiency • Iatrogenic disease • Drug interactions
- Drug therapy • Adverse effects

Drug-induced nutrient deficiencies (DINDs) are an important yet poorly appreciated category of adverse drug reactions (ADRs) in pediatrics. An ADR is an undesirable response associated with use of a drug that compromises therapeutic efficacy, enhances toxicity, or both.[1] It is estimated that approximately 70,000 children hospitalized in the United States experience adverse events every year, of which 19% are secondary to medications.[2] Most reports draw attention to ADRs attributed to errors in dosing frequency, drug interactions, and route of administration or method of dispensing.[2–4] Any drug, no matter how trivial its therapeutic action, has the potential for adverse effects. Therefore, the anticipated benefit from any therapeutic decision should be balanced by potential risks. The etiology of most ADRs can be categorized into "mechanism-based" versus "idiosyncratic".[5] Mechanism-based ADRs are more common and develop as an extension of the principal pharmacologic action of the drug. They can be predicted based on clinical and preclinical trials of the drug,[5] and are therefore potentially preventable. Idiosyncratic ADRs are less frequent but equally important. They usually result from interactions between the drug and unique host factors unrelated to the principal function of the drug. Examples are enhanced folate deficiency during therapy with methotrexate in patients with an inherited methylenetetrahydrofolate reductase deficiency[6] and increased risk for pellagra during therapy with isoniazid in patients with N-acetyltransferase deficiency.[7,8] The burgeoning field of pharmacogenomics may help to predict individuals genetically at risk for altered drug disposition, impaired efficacy, and risk for DINDs and other adverse effects.[9,10]

The magnitude of DINDs is difficult to quantify. Some drugs may cause marginal nutrient deficiencies with serious consequences, such as diuretics contributing to thiamine deficiency and worsening of cardiac failure.[11,12] Disease complexity, drug–drug interactions, and genetic polymorphisms may contribute to previously unrecognized DINDs. The major risk factors for developing DINDs and other ADRs are lack of awareness by the prescribing physician and long duration of drug therapy. Furthermore, susceptibility to DINDs may be greater during periods of increased requirements,

Department of Pediatrics, Section of Pediatric Gastroenterology and Nutrition, University of Chicago, 5839 South Maryland Avenue, MC 4065, WP C-474, Chicago, IL 60637, USA
* Corresponding author.
E-mail address: tsentong@peds.bsd.uchicago.edu (T. A. Sentongo).

Pediatr Clin N Am 56 (2009) 1211–1224
doi:10.1016/j.pcl.2009.06.004
0031-3955/09/$ – see front matter. Published by Elsevier Inc.

pediatric.theclinics.com

such as isoniazid-induced pyridoxine deficiency in neonates,[13] glucocorticoid-induced calcium losses, and malabsorption[14] during pubertal growth. Therefore, physicians should determine and monitor the nutritional risks for children on chronic medications. This article reviews DINDs and their respective mechanisms, risk factors, diagnosis, precautions, and therapy. Awareness of the spectrum of ADRs is an ongoing process that relies on physicians, nurses, and pharmacists voluntarily reporting serious unexpected reactions.[15] Even though it may not be possible to attribute a causal role to a particular drug, it is the professional obligation of every physician to contribute to knowledge by reporting serious suspected ADRs to the US Food and Drug Administration (FDA).[15] An example of the continual need for surveillance and reporting of suspected ADRs was the recent association of complicated hypocupremia with increased use of zinc oxide denture creams,[16] which, in part, may be a sequel of the improvements in preventative dental care and availability of prosthetics.

MECHANISM-BASED DINDs

Drugs may alter nutrient intake, digestion, availability, absorption, storage, metabolism, and excretion. The psychostimulants imipramine, methylphenidate, and dextroamphetamine are the most frequently prescribed chronic drugs in pediatrics with known associations of decreased appetite and slowed growth. The reduced food intake has an equal impact on all nutrients; therefore, no specific deficiency occurs. Growth is mostly affected during the first year of therapy, and the severity is dose

Table 1
Mechanisms of drug-induced nutrient deficiencies

Impaired nutrient digestion	Decreased nutrient availability	Increased intestinal losses
Disaccharidase (α-glucosidase) inhibitors Ascorbase Miglitol Lipase inhibitor Orlistat (tetrahydrolipstatin)	Neomycin (↓enteric vitamin K) Zinc (↑enterocyte retention of copper)	Cholestyramine Mineral oil Sulfasalazine (↓folate) Glucocorticoids (↓calcium absorption) Zinc (↑enteral loss of copper) Oleastra (fat-soluble vitamins)
Decreased storage	Impaired metabolism	Increased urinary losses
Zinc (enterocyte loss with sequestrated copper)	Isoniazid (effect on pyridoxine) Valproate (effect on carnitine) Methotrexate (effect on folate)	Diuretics (effect on electrolytes and minerals) Foscarnet
Idiosyncratic actions		
Isoniazid (effects on niacin) Methotrexate (folate deficiency in patients with MTHFR enzyme def)		

Abbreviation: MTHFR enzyme def, methylenetetrahydrofolate reductase enzyme deficiency.

Table 2
Drugs associated with macronutrient deficiency

Nutrient	Drug	Mechanism of Inducing Nutrient Deficiency	Symptom	Diagnosis	Precautions
Carbohydrate	Ascorbase, miglitol[21,22] (control of postprandial hyperglycemia in diabetes mellitus)	α-Glucosidase inhibitor resulting in carbohydrate malabsorption[21–23]	Diarrhea, flatulence	—	Decrease intake of dietary carbohydrates Gradual increment in ascorbase/miglitol dose
Lipids	Orlistat (tetrahydrolipstatin) Indication: weight management in overweight/obesity, hyperlipidemia	Gastric and pancreas lipase inhibitor; at maximum dose, it may induce malabsorption of up to 30% dietary fat[24]	Diarrhea, steatorrhea, fat-soluble vitamin malabsorption	Steatorrhea Decreased serum concentrations of vitamins A, 25-OHD, and E (α-tocopherol)	Efficacy depends on dose Supplement with fat-soluble vitamins Reduce consumption of dietary fat

Abbreviation: 25-OHD, 25 hydroxy vitamin D.

Table 3
Drugs associated with fat-soluble vitamin deficiency

Nutrient	Drug	Mechanism of Nutrient Deficiency	Risk Factors	Symptoms	Diagnosis	Precautions
Vitamin A	Mineral oil Use: management of constipation[25]		High dose, chronic use, underlying fat malabsorption	N/A	Decreased serum β-carotene[25]	Cautious use in patients with fat malabsorption (eg, cystic fibrosis) Periodically monitor serum β-carotene
Vitamin D	Cholestyramine Use: bile salt malabsorption, bile salt-induced diarrhea, hyperlipidemia[26]	Bile salt deficiency and fat malabsorption Direct binding and impaired absorption[27]	Short gut syndrome	N/A	Decreased serum 25-OHD Increased risk for rickets	Limit dose of cholestyramine Vitamin D supplements Allow 1–4 hours between cholestyramine dose and administering vitamin D[27]
	Phenytoin, phenobarbital, carbamazepine	Cytochrome P450-induced increased degradation of vitamin D[28,29]	Ketogenic diet[30] Immobility, more severe cerebral palsy[30]	N/A	Decreased serum 25-OHD Increased bone alkaline phosphatase	Vitamin D supplements in at-risk patients[29]

Nutrient	Drug	Mechanism	Predisposing condition	Clinical finding	Laboratory findings	Management
Vitamin E	Cholestyramine	See above	SBS	N/A	Serum α-tocopherol/total lipid ratio[a] <0.8 mg/dL[31] Serum α-tocopherol/cholesterol ratio <2.47 mg/g[32]	Limit dose of cholestyramine Vitamin E supplements Allow 1–4 hours between cholestyramine dose and administering vitamin E[27]
Vitamin K	Cholestyramine	See above	SBS Cholestasis	Coagulopathy	Prolonged PT and INR	Vitamin K supplements
	Neomycin, broad-spectrum antibiotics Use: bowel decontamination, bacterial overgrowth	Eradication of vitamin K-synthesizing bacteria[33,34]	SBS Cholestasis Prolonged use	Coagulopathy	Prolonged PT and INR	See above Vitamin K supplements
Vitamins A, D, E, and K	Oleastra (nonabsorbed sucrose polyester substitute for dietary fat)[35]	Solubilizes dietary fats, rendering them unavailable for absorption[36]		Diarrhea Oily stools[37,38]		

Abbreviations: INR, international normalized ratio; 25-OHD, 25 hydroxy vitamin D; N/A, not applicable; PT, prothrombin time; SBS, short bowel syndrome.
[a] Total lipids: cholesterol + triacylglycerols + phospholipids.

Table 4
Drug-inducing water-soluble vitamin deficiency

Nutrient	Drug	Mechanism of Nutrient Deficiency	Risk Factors	Symptoms	Diagnosis	Precautions/Therapy
Vitamin B$_1$ (thiamine)	Loop diuretics (furosemide, bumetanide, ethacrynic acid, torsemide)	Diuretic-induced increased urinary losses[12]	High dose and prolonged use[39] Congestive heart failure Malnutrition	Worsening congestive heart failure	Erythrocyte transketolase activity Red blood cell thiamin concentrations[40,41]	Use alternative diuretic (eg, spironolactone)[42] Thiamine supplements
Vitamin B$_{12}$	PPI and H2 blockers Use: gastric acid suppressants[43]	Lack of gastric acid impairs release of vitamin B$_{12}$ from dietary proteins[43]	Prolonged use		Decreased plasma vitamin B$_{12}$ Increased plasma methylmalonic acid[44]	Monitor B$_{12}$ status Need to justify prolonged gastric acid suppression therapy B$_{12}$ replacement therapy
Folic acid	Methotrexate, pyrimethamine, pentamidine, triamterene	Decreased availability of folate secondary to inhibition of dihydrofolate reductase[45,46]		N/A	Megaloblastic anemia	Supplement with folic acid
	Sulfasalazine	Impaired metabolism and absorption of intestinal folate[47]		N/A	Megaloblastic anemia	
	Phenytoin	Inhibited absorption of pteroylpolyglutamate[47]		N/A	Megaloblastic anemia	
	Cholestyramine	Anionic binding of polyglutamate to cholestyramine resin[48,49]	C677T mutation in the MTHFR gene[10]	N/A	Decreased serum folate	Supplement with folic acid

Niacin	INH	Impaired niacin synthesis secondary to pyridoxine deficiency Competitive inhibition of niacin coenzymes[46,50]	Malnutrition N-acetyl transferase deficiency[7,8] Vegetarian diet Hartnup disease (deficiency of tryptophan)[50]	Pellagra, Photosensitive dermatitis, extensive acne-like rash[7] Manic dementia[8] Diarrhea		Discontinue INH Supplement with nicotinamide[51] Cautious use of INH in populations with high percentage of slow INH acetylators: 60% of Indians, 48% of Europeans[50]
Pyridoxine	Isoniazid	Increased urinary excretion of pyridoxine complexed with INH Competitive inhibition of pyridoxal phosphate[46]	INH dosage >10 mg/kg/d[52] Malnutrition[53]	Peripheral neuropathy Psychosis, convulsions[13,54] Pyridoxine-responsive anemia[46]		Pyridoxine supplements during chronic therapy with INH[53,55]
Carnitine	Valproic acid	Valproic acid-induced carnitine deficiency by formation of valproylcarnitine ester, which is transported out of mitochondria and eliminated in urine[56]	Age <2 years Therapy with multiple AEDs Ketogenic diet Inborn errors of metabolism[57]	Increased fatigue[58]	Plasma total carnitine <25 μmol/L or acylcarnitine/unbound carnitine ratio >0.4[56]	Carnitine supplements in patients with risk factors[57,59]

Abbreviations: AED, antiepilepsy drugs; H2 blockers, histamine receptor 2 blocking drugs (eg, ranitidine, famotidine); INH, isoniazid; MTHFR, methylenetetrahydrofolate reductase; PPI, proton pump inhibitor (eg, omeprazole, lansoprazole, pantoprazole).

Table 5
Drugs associated with electrolyte loss

Nutrient	Drug	Mechanism of Nutrient Deficiency	Risk Factors	Symptoms	Diagnosis	Precautions/Therapy
Sodium	Thiazides diuretics (ie, hydrochlorothiazide, chlorothiazide, chlorthalidone, indapamide, metolazone, Zaroxolyn)	Sodium loss and diuresis through inhibition of distal tubular chloride and sodium transport[60]	Hypokalemia Concurrent use of other diuretics (eg, amiloride)		Na^{2+} <134 mEq/dL Uric acid >4 mg/dL	Exclude SIADH Monitor electrolytes Replace sodium
Potassium	Diuretics: thiazides and loop diuretics	K^+ lost secondary to blocked chloride-associated sodium reabsorption, increased delivery of sodium to collecting tubules, wherein its reabsorption results in excretion of K^{+61}	Increased dose Increased intake of sodium Mg^{2+} depletion	K^+ 3–3.5 mEq/dL Generalized weakness, lassitude, constipation K^+ <2.5 mEq/dL Arrhythmia, paralysis, impaired respiratory function	K^+ <3.5 mEq/dL	Monitor electrolytes K^+ replacements
	Amphotericin (antifungal)	Renal losses of K through inhibition of secretion of hydrogen by collecting duct cells and Mg^{2+} depletion	Mg^{2+} depletion			

Magnesium (Mg^{2+})	Diuretics: loop and thiazide diuretics[62]		Refractory hypocalcemia and hypokalemia[62]	Mg^{2+} <1.8 mEq/dL	Monitor and Mg^{2+} Treatment with magnesium supplements
	Calcineurin inhibitors (eg, tacrolimus, cyclosporine) (immunosuppression)	Renal Mg^{2+} wasting independent of calcineurin[63]	Same	Mg^{2+} <1.8 mEq/dL Magnesium loading test[64]	
	Foscarnet (trisodium phosphonoformate)	Nephrotoxic, renal tubular damage[65]	Dehydration	Mg^{2+} <1.8 mEq/dL Magnesium loading test[64]	Hydrate patients before infusion Monitor and replace magnesium and other electrolytes
	CMV antiviral		Same		

Abbreviations: CMV, cytomegalovirus; SIADH, syndrome of inappropriate secretion of antidiuretic hormone.

Table 6
Drugs inducing mineral losses or deficiency

Nutrient	Drug	Mechanism of Nutrient Deficiency	Risk Factors	Symptoms	Diagnosis	Precautions/Therapy
Calcium	Glucocorticoids	Calcium malabsorption and calciuria[14]	Chronic therapy Inadequate dietary calcium and vitamin D Chronic disease (eg, cystic fibrosis, chronic inflammatory disease)[66]	N/A	Decreased bone mineralization	Adequate calcium and vitamin D intake Thiazide diuretics Minimize glucocorticoid dose
	Diuretics (loop diuretics)	Increased urinary calcium excretion[67]	Chronic use	Hypocalcemic tetany	Hypocalcemia	Thiazide diuretic[14,68]
	Foscarnet	Nephrotoxic[65] Complexes with ionized calcium[69] Magnesium deficiency[70]	Dehydration	Hypocalcemic tetany	Hypocalcemia Hypomagnesinemia Hypokalemia	Hydrate patients before foscarnet infusion Monitor and replace magnesium and other electrolytes
Copper	Zinc supplements[71,72] Zinc oxide denture cream[16]	Zinc induces intestinal metallothionein, which has a greater affinity for copper; this leads to sequestration of copper in the enterocytes, thus blocking further absorption[73]	Chronic use	Sideroblastic anemia Neutropenia[71,74]	Decreased serum copper Decreased ceruloplasmin Increased zinc[75]	Discontinue zinc supplements[71]
Zinc	Thiazide diuretics[76]	Increased urinary excretion of zinc[76]	Chronic use[77] Chronic liver disease[78]	Hypogeusia	Decreased serum zinc[76-78]	Zinc supplements[77]

related. Interventions include dose adjustments and drug holidays.[17] The decision to continue therapy is made based on behavioral response, the individual child's growth, and availability of effective alternative drugs.[17-19] Another medication associated with anorexia and weight loss is sibutramine. Sibutramine is approved for weight management in adolescents and adults. It inhibits norepinephrine and serotonin reuptake, resulting in thermogenesis, increased satiety, and, ultimately, weight loss.[20] This intended therapeutic effect is not categorized as a DINDs. The other drug-induced mechanisms of nutrient deficiency are presented in **Table 1**. The subsequent tables provide more detailed information about mechanisms of DINDs, risk factors, diagnosis, and treatment by nutrient category (ie, macronutrients [**Table 2**], fat-soluble vitamins [**Table 3**], water-soluble vitamins [**Table 4**], electrolytes [**Table 5**], and minerals [**Table 6**]).

SUMMARY

Good clinical care extends beyond mere diagnosis and treatment of disease to appreciation that nutrient deficiencies can be the price of effective drug therapy. Empiric treatment with nutrient supplements on the basis of drug therapy is not justified, and thus does not replace careful monitoring of children who are taking chronic medications for nutrient deficiencies. The exciting field of pharmacogenomics has potential to improve clinical care by detecting patients who might benefit and those at risk for complications of drug therapy. Increased awareness and ultimately, improved patient safety rely on physicians voluntarily reporting serious suspected ADRs.

REFERENCES

1. Availabe at: www.jointcommission.org/sentinelevents/se_glossary.htm. Accessed May 20, 2009.
2. Woods D, Thomas E, Holl J, et al. Adverse events and preventable adverse events in children. Pediatrics 2005;115(1):155–60.
3. Leape LL, Bates DW, Cullen DJ, et al. Systems analysis of adverse drug events. ADE Prevention Study Group. JAMA 1995;274(1):35–43.
4. Holdsworth MT, Fichtl RE, Behta M, et al. Incidence and impact of adverse drug events in pediatric inpatients. Arch Pediatr Adolesc Med 2003;157(1):60–5.
5. Nies A, Spielberg S. Goodman & Gilman's: the pharmacological basis of therapeutics. In: Hardman J, Limbird L, Molinoff P, Ruddon R, Gilman AG, editors. Principles of therapeutics. 9th edition. New York: McGraw-Hill; 1996. p. 43–62.
6. Evans WE. Differing effects of methylenetetrahydrofolate reductase single nucleotide polymorphisms on methotrexate efficacy and toxicity in rheumatoid arthritis. Pharmacogenetics 2002;12(3):181–2.
7. Cohen LK, George W, Smith R. Isoniazid-induced acne and pellagra. Occurrence in slow inactivators of isoniazid. Arch Dermatol 1974;109(3):377–81.
8. Muratake T, Watanabe H, Hayashi S. Isoniazid-induced pellagra and the N-acetyltransferase gene genotype. Am J Psychiatry 1999;156(4):660.
9. McLeod HL, Evans WE. Pharmacogenomics: unlocking the human genome for better drug therapy. Annu Rev Pharmacol Toxicol 2001;41:101–21.
10. Tonstad S, Refsum H, Ose L, et al. The C677T mutation in the methylenetetrahydrofolate reductase gene predisposes to hyperhomocysteinemia in children with familial hypercholesterolemia treated with cholestyramine. J Pediatr 1998;132(2):365–8.
11. McCabe BJ. Prevention of food-drug interactions with special emphasis on older adults. Curr Opin Clin Nutr Metab Care 2004;7(1):21–6.

12. Hanninen SA, Darling PB, Sole MJ, et al. The prevalence of thiamin deficiency in hospitalized patients with congestive heart failure. J Am Coll Cardiol 2006;47(2): 354–61.
13. McKenzie SA, Macnab AJ, Katz G. Neonatal pyridoxine responsive convulsions due to isoniazid therapy. Arch Dis Child 1976;51(7):567–8.
14. Lukert BP, Raisz LG. Glucocorticoid-induced osteoporosis: pathogenesis and management [see comment]. Ann Intern Med 1990;112(5):352–64.
15. Kessler DA. Introducing MEDWatch. A new approach to reporting medication and device adverse effects and product problems. JAMA 1993;269(21):2765–8.
16. Nations SP, Boyer PJ, Love LA, et al. Denture cream: an unusual source of excess zinc, leading to hypocupremia and neurologic disease [see comment]. Neurology 2008;71(9):639–43.
17. Safer DJ, Allen RP, Barr E. Growth rebound after termination of stimulant drugs. J Pediatr 1975;86(1):113–6.
18. Sund AM, Zeiner P. Does extended medication with amphetamine or methylphenidate reduce growth in hyperactive children? Nord J Psychiatry 2002;56(1): 53–7.
19. Charach A, Figueroa M, Chen S, et al. Stimulant treatment over 5 years: effects on growth. J Am Acad Child Adolesc Psychiatry 2006;45(4):415–21.
20. Dunican KC, Desilets AR, Montalbano JK. Pharmacotherapeutic options for overweight adolescents. Ann Pharmacother 2007;41(9):1445–55.
21. Martin AE, Montgomery PA. Acarbose: an alpha-glucosidase inhibitor. Am J Health Syst Pharm 1996;53(19):2277–90 [quiz: 2336–7].
22. Sels JP, Huijberts MS, Wolffenbuttel BH. Miglitol, a new alpha-glucosidase inhibitor. Expert Opin Pharmacother 1999;1(1):149–56.
23. Van de Laar FA, Lucassen PL, Akkermans RP, et al. Alpha-glucosidase inhibitors for people with impaired glucose tolerance or impaired fasting blood glucose. Cochrane Database Syst Rev 2006;(4):CD005061.
24. Hauptman JB, Jeunet FS, Hartmann D. Initial studies in humans with the novel gastrointestinal lipase inhibitor Ro 18-0647 (tetrahydrolipstatin). Am J Clin Nutr 1992;55(Suppl 1):309S–13S.
25. Clark JH, Russell GJ, Fitzgerald JF, et al. Serum beta-carotene, retinol, and alpha-tocopherol levels during mineral oil therapy for constipation. Am J Dis Child 1987; 141(11):1210–2.
26. Knodel LC, Talbert RL. Adverse effects of hypolipidaemic drugs. Med Toxicol Adverse Drug Exp 1987;2:10–32.
27. Bays HE, Dujovne CA. Drug interactions of lipid-altering drugs. Drug Saf 1998; 19(5):355–71.
28. Sheth RD. Metabolic concerns associated with antiepileptic medications. Neurology 2004;63(10 Suppl 4):S24–9.
29. Mintzer S, Boppana P, Toguri J, et al. Vitamin D levels and bone turnover in epilepsy patients taking carbamazepine or oxcarbazepine. Epilepsia 2006; 47(3):510–5.
30. Gissel T, Poulsen CS, Vestergaard P. Adverse effects of antiepileptic drugs on bone mineral density in children. Expert Opin Drug Saf 2007;6(3):267–78.
31. Horwitt MK, Harvey CC, Dahm CH Jr, et al. Relationship between tocopherol and serum lipid levels for determination of nutritional adequacy. Ann N Y Acad Sci 1972;203:223–36.
32. Thurnham DI, Davies JA, Crump BJ, et al. The use of different lipids to express serum tocopherol: lipid ratios for the measurement of vitamin E status. Ann Clin Biochem 1986;23(Pt 5):514–20.

33. Bhat RV, Deshmukh CT. A study of vitamin K status in children on prolonged anti-biotic therapy. Indian Pediatr 2003;40(1):36–40.
34. Alperin JB. Coagulopathy caused by vitamin K deficiency in critically ill, hospital-ized patients. JAMA 1987;258(14):1916–9.
35. Kelly SM, Shorthouse M, Cotterell JC, et al. A 3-month, double-blind, controlled trial of feeding with sucrose polyester in human volunteers. Br J Nutr 1998; 80(1):41–9.
36. Neuhouser ML, Rock CL, Kristal AR, et al. Olestra is associated with slight reduc-tions in serum carotenoids but does not markedly influence serum fat-soluble vitamin concentrations. Am J Clin Nutr 2006;83(3):624–31.
37. Thomson AB, Hunt RH, Zorich NL. Review article: olestra and its gastrointestinal safety. Aliment Pharmacol Ther 1998;12(12):1185–200.
38. Barlam TF, McCloud E. Severe gastrointestinal illness associated with olestra ingestion. J Pediatr Gastroenterol Nutr 2003;37(1):95–6.
39. Zenuk C, Healey T, Donnelly J, et al. Thiamine deficiency in congestive heart failure patients receiving long term furosemide therapy. Can J Clin Pharmacol 2003;10(4):184–8.
40. Bailey AL, Finglas PM, Wright AJ, et al. Thiamin intake, erythrocyte transketolase (EC 2.2.1.1) activity and total erythrocyte thiamin in adolescents. Br J Nutr 1994; 72(1):111–25.
41. Finglas PM. Thiamin. Int J Vitam Nutr Res 1993;63(4):270–4.
42. Rocha RM, Silva GV, de Albuguergue DC, et al. Influence of spironolactone therapy on thiamine blood levels in patients with heart failure. Arquivos Brasileiros de Cardiologia 2008;90(5):324–8.
43. Ruscin JM, Page RL 2nd, Valuck RJ. Vitamin B(12) deficiency associated with histamine(2)-receptor antagonists and a proton-pump inhibitor. Ann Pharmac-other 2002;36(5):812–6.
44. Snow CF. Laboratory diagnosis of vitamin B12 and folate deficiency: a guide for the primary care physician. [see comment]. Arch Intern Med 1999;159(12): 1289–98.
45. Lambie DG, Johnson RH. Drugs and folate metabolism. Drugs 1985;30(2):145–55.
46. Young RC, Blass JP. Iatrogenic nutritional deficiencies. Annu Rev Nutr 1982;2: 201–27.
47. Halsted CH. The intestinal absorption of folates. Am J Clin Nutr 1979;32(4): 846–55.
48. West RJ, Lloyd JK. The effect of cholestyramine on intestinal absorption. Gut 1975;16(2):93–8.
49. Tonstad S, Sivertsen M, Aksnes L, et al. Low dose colestipol in adolescents with familial hypercholesterolaemia. Arch Dis Child 1996;74(2):157–60.
50. Meyrick Thomas RH, Rowland Payne CM, et al. Isoniazid-induced pellagra. Br Med J (Clin Res Ed) 1981;283(6286):287–8.
51. Darvay A, Basarab T, McGregor JM, et al. Isoniazid induced pellagra despite pyridoxine supplementation. Clin Exp Dermatol 1999;24(3):167–9.
52. Pellock JM, Howell J, Kendig EL Jr, et al. Pyridoxine deficiency in children treated with isoniazid. Chest 1985;87(5):658–61.
53. Steichen O, Martinez-Almoyna L, De Broucker T. [Isoniazid induced neuropathy: consider prevention]. Rev Mal Respir 2006;23(2 Pt 1):157–60.
54. Alao AO, Yolles JC. Isoniazid-induced psychosis. Ann Pharmacother 1998;32(9): 889–91.
55. Snider DE Jr. Pyridoxine supplementation during isoniazid therapy. Tubercle 1980;61(4):191–6.

56. De Vivo DC, Bohan TP, Coulter DL, et al. L-carnitine supplementation in childhood epilepsy: current perspectives. Epilepsia 1998;39(11):1216–25.
57. Raskind JY, El-Chaar GM. The role of carnitine supplementation during valproic acid therapy. Ann Pharmacother 2000;34(5):630–8.
58. Van Wouwe JP. Carnitine deficiency during valproic acid treatment. Int J Vitam Nutr Res 1995;65(3):211–4.
59. Lheureux PER, Hantson P. Carnitine in the treatment of valproic acid-induced toxicity. Clinical Toxicol(Phila) 2009;47(2):101–11.
60. Liamis G, Milionis H, Elisaf M. A review of drug-induced hyponatremia. [see comment]. Am J Kidney Dis 2008;52(1):144–53.
61. Gennari FJ. Hypokalemia [see comment]. N Engl J Med 1998;339(7):451–8.
62. al-Ghamdi SM, Cameron EC, Sutton RA. Magnesium deficiency: pathophysiologic and clinical overview [see comment]. Am J Kidney Dis 1994;24(5):737–52.
63. Navaneethan SD, Sankarasubbaiyan S, Gross MD, et al. Tacrolimus-associated hypomagnesemia in renal transplant recipients. Transplant Proc 2006;38(5):1320–2.
64. Arnaud MJ. Update on the assessment of magnesium status. Br J Nutr 2008;99(Suppl 3):S24–36.
65. Jayaweera DT. Minimising the dosage-limiting toxicities of foscarnet induction therapy. Drug Saf 1997;16(4):258–66.
66. Abrams SA, O'Brien KO. Calcium and bone mineral metabolism in children with chronic illnesses. Annu Rev Nutr 2004;24:13–32.
67. Lee CT, Chen HC, Lai LW, et al. Effects of furosemide on renal calcium handling. Am J Physiol Renal Physiol 2007;293(4):F1231–7.
68. Stier CT Jr, Itskovitz HD. Renal calcium metabolism and diuretics. Annu Rev Pharmacol Toxicol 1986;26:101–16.
69. Jacobson MA, Gambertoglio JG, Aweeka FT, et al. Foscarnet-induced hypocalcemia and effects of foscarnet on calcium metabolism. J Clin Endocrinol Metab 1991;72(5):1130–5.
70. Gearhart MO, Sorg TB. Foscarnet-induced severe hypomagnesemia and other electrolyte disorders. Ann Pharmacother 1993;27(3):285–9.
71. Broun ER, Greist A, Tricot G, et al. Excessive zinc ingestion. A reversible cause of sideroblastic anemia and bone marrow depression. JAMA 1990;264(11):1441–3.
72. Fiske DN, McCoy HE 3rd, Kitchens CS. Zinc-induced sideroblastic anemia: report of a case, review of the literature, and description of the hematologic syndrome. Am J Hematol 1994;46(2):147–50.
73. Cai L, Li XK, Song Y, et al. Essentiality, toxicology and chelation therapy of zinc and copper. Curr Med Chem 2005;12(23):2753–63.
74. Fosmire GJ. Zinc toxicity. Am J Clin Nutr 1990;51(2):225–7.
75. Willis MS, Monaghan SA, Miller ML, et al. Zinc-induced copper deficiency: a report of three cases initially recognized on bone marrow examination. Am J Clin Pathol 2005;123(1):125–31.
76. Reyes AJ, Olhaberry JV, Leary WP, et al. Urinary zinc excretion, diuretics, zinc deficiency and some side-effects of diuretics. S Afr Med J 1983;64(24):936–41.
77. Khedun SM, Naicker T, Maharaj B. Zinc, hydrochlorothiazide and sexual dysfunction. Cent Afr J Med 1995;41(10):312–5.
78. Yoshida Y, Higashi T, Nouso K, et al. Effects of zinc deficiency/zinc supplementation on ammonia metabolism in patients with decompensated liver cirrhosis. Acta Med Okayama 2001;55(6):349–55.

Index

Note: Page numbers of article titles are in **boldface** type.

A

Abdominal distension, in kwashiorkor, 1059–1060
Absorption
   in liver disease, 1163
   physiology of, 1186
Acid-base imbalance
   in critical illness, 1154
   in intestinal failure, 1191
Acrodermatitis enteropathica, after bariatric surgery, 1115–1116
Albumin measurement
   in critical illness, 1151–1152
   in protein energy malnutrition, 1062
Allergy diets, 1090–1091
Alopecia, in biotin deficiency, 1043
Anabolism, after starvation, 1202
Anemia
   in iron deficiency, 1035–1037, 1086–1087
     after bariatric surgery, 1112
     in cystic fibrosis, 1131
     in premature infants, 1073–1074
   in protein energy malnutrition, 1062
   in pyridoxine deficiency, 1041
   megaloblastic, 1041–1042
   pernicious, 1041–1042
Anorexia
   in liver disease, 1163
   refeeding syndrome after, 1202
Anthropometric assessment
   in critical illness, 1149
   in liver disease, 1169
Ascorbic acid deficiency. *See* Vitamin C (ascorbic acid) deficiency.
Autism spectrum disorders, restricted diets in, 1095, 1097

B

Bariatric surgery, **1105–1121**
   macronutrient deficiencies after, 1109
   micronutrient deficiencies after, 1109–1115
   nutritional screening and supplementation after, 1110–1111
   pregnancy after, 1116
   procedures for, 1106–1108
   supplementation after, 1108

Pediatr Clin N Am 56 (2009) 1225–1238
doi:10.1016/S0031-3955(09)00144-8
0031-3955/09/$ – see front matter © 2009 Elsevier Inc. All rights reserved.

pediatric.theclinics.com

United States Postal Service

Statement of Ownership, Management, and Circulation
(All Periodicals Publications Except Requestor Publications)

1. Publication Title	2. Publication Number		3. Filing Date
Pediatric Clinics of North America	4 2 4 - 6 6 0 0		9/15/09

4. Issue Frequency	5. Number of Issues Published Annually	6. Annual Subscription Price
Feb, Apr, Jun, Aug, Oct, Dec	6	$162.00

7. Complete Mailing Address of Known Office of Publication (Not printer) (Street, city, county, state, and ZIP+4®)

Elsevier Inc.
360 Park Avenue South
New York, NY 10010-1710

Contact Person
Stephen Bushing
Telephone (Include area code)
215-239-3688

8. Complete Mailing Address of Headquarters or General Business Office of Publisher (Not printer)

Elsevier Inc., 360 Park Avenue South, New York, NY 10010-1710

9. Full Names and Complete Mailing Addresses of Publisher, Editor, and Managing Editor (Do not leave blank)

Publisher (Name and complete mailing address)

John Schrefer, Elsevier, Inc., 1600 John F. Kennedy Blvd. Suite 1800, Philadelphia, PA 19103-2899

Editor (Name and complete mailing address)

Carla Holloway, Elsevier, Inc., 1600 John F. Kennedy Blvd. Suite 1800, Philadelphia, PA 19103-2899

Managing Editor (Name and complete mailing address)

Catherine Bewick, Elsevier, Inc., 1600 John F. Kennedy Blvd. Suite 1800, Philadelphia, PA 19103-2899

10. Owner (Do not leave blank. If the publication is owned by a corporation, give the name and address of the corporation immediately followed by the names and addresses of all stockholders owning or holding 1 percent or more of the total amount of stock. If not owned by a corporation, give the names and addresses of the individual owners. If owned by a partnership or other unincorporated firm, give its name and address as well as those of each individual owner. If the publication is published by a nonprofit organization, give its name and address.)

Full Name	Complete Mailing Address
Wholly owned subsidiary of	4520 East-West Highway
Reed/Elsevier, US holdings	Bethesda, MD 20814

11. Known Bondholders, Mortgagees, and Other Security Holders Owning or Holding 1 Percent or More of Total Amount of Bonds, Mortgages, or Other Securities. If none, check box. ☑ None

Full Name	Complete Mailing Address
N/A	

12. Tax Status (For completion by nonprofit organizations authorized to mail at nonprofit rates) (Check one)
The purpose, function, and nonprofit status of this organization and the exempt status for federal income tax purposes:
☐ Has Not Changed During Preceding 12 Months
☐ Has Changed During Preceding 12 Months (Publisher must submit explanation of change with this statement)

PS Form 3526, September 2007 (Page 1 of 3 (Instructions Page 3)) PSN 7530-01-000-9931 PRIVACY NOTICE: See our Privacy policy in www.usps.com

---

13. Publication Title			14. Issue Date for Circulation Data Below
Pediatric Clinics of North America			June 2009

15. Extent and Nature of Circulation			Average No. Copies Each Issue During Preceding 12 Months	No. Copies of Single Issue Published Nearest to Filing Date
a. Total Number of Copies (Net press run)			5233	4700
b. Paid Circulation (By Mail and Outside the Mail)	(1)	Mailed Outside-County Paid Subscriptions Stated on PS Form 3541. (Include paid distribution above nominal rate, advertiser's proof copies, and exchange copies)	2445	2185
	(2)	Mailed In-County Paid Subscriptions Stated on PS Form 3541 (Include paid distribution above nominal rate, advertiser's proof copies, and exchange copies)		
	(3)	Paid Distribution Outside the Mails Including Sales Through Dealers and Carriers, Street Vendors, Counter Sales, and Other Paid Distribution Outside USPS®	1746	1556
	(4)	Paid Distribution by Other Classes Mailed Through the USPS (e.g. First-Class Mail®)		
c. Total Paid Distribution (Sum of 15b (1), (2), (3), and (4))			4191	3741
d. Free or Nominal Rate Distribution (By Mail and Outside the Mail)	(1)	Free or Nominal Rate Outside-County Copies Included on PS Form 3541	137	114
	(2)	Free or Nominal Rate In-County Copies Included on PS Form 3541		
	(3)	Free or Nominal Rate Copies Mailed at Other Classes Through the USPS (e.g. First-Class Mail)		
	(4)	Free or Nominal Rate Distribution Outside the Mail (Carriers or other means)		
e. Total Free or Nominal Rate Distribution (Sum of 15d (1), (2), (3) and (4))			137	114
f. Total Distribution (Sum of 15c and 15e)			4328	3855
g. Copies not Distributed (See instructions to publishers #4 (page #3))			905	845
h. Total (Sum of 15f and g)			5233	4700
i. Percent Paid (15c divided by 15f times 100)			96.83%	97.04%

16. Publication of Statement of Ownership
☐ If the publication is a general publication, publication of this statement is required. Will be printed in the October 2009 issue of this publication. ☐ Publication not required.

17. Signature and Title of Editor, Publisher, Business Manager, or Owner

Stephen R. Bushing – Subscription Services Coordinator

Date September 15, 2009

I certify that all information furnished on this form is true and complete. I understand that anyone who furnishes false or misleading information on this form or who omits material or information requested on the form may be subject to criminal sanctions (including fines and imprisonment) and/or civil sanctions (including civil penalties).

PS Form 3526, September 2007 (Page 2 of 3)

Moving?

Make sure your subscription moves with you!

To notify us of your new address, find your **Clinics Account Number** (located on your mailing label above your name), and contact customer service at:

Email: journalscustomerservice-usa@elsevier.com

800-654-2452 (subscribers in the U.S. & Canada)
314-447-8871 (subscribers outside of the U.S. & Canada)

Fax number: 314-447-8029

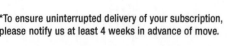

Elsevier Health Sciences Division
Subscription Customer Service
3251 Riverport Lane
Maryland Heights, MO 63043

*To ensure uninterrupted delivery of your subscription, please notify us at least 4 weeks in advance of move.

Printed and bound by CPI Group (UK) Ltd, Croydon, CR0 4YY

03/10/2024

01040462-0001